Cartilage Repair Strategies

CARTILAGE REPAIR STRATEGIES

Edited by

RILEY J. WILLIAMS III, MD

Associate Professor of Orthopaedic Surgery
Weill Medical College of Cornell University
Attending Orthopaedic Surgeon
Director, Institute for Cartilage Repair
Hospital for Special Surgery
New York, NY

With Forewords by

Lars Peterson, MD, PhD

Professor of Orthopaedic Surgery
University of Gothenburg, Gothenburg, Sweden

and

Brian J. Cole, MD, MBA

Departments of Orthopaedics and Anatomy and Cell Biology
and Cartilage Restoration Center at Rush
Rush University Medical Center, Chicago, IL

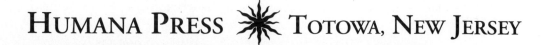

HUMANA PRESS ✳ TOTOWA, NEW JERSEY

Cover design by Karen Schulz

Cover illustrations: Sagittal view magnetic resonance image of the medial compartment of a knee (*left*). There is a full-thickness cartilage lesion on the weightbearing surface of the medial femoral condyle. (*Right*) Sagittal view magnetic resonance image (T2 mapping) of the medial compartment of a knee following implantation of a synthetic biphasic cartilage-bone matrix scaffold. This implant was used to facilitate the repair of a full-thickness cartilage defect of the medial femoral condyle.

For additional copies, pricing for bulk purchases, and/or information about other Humana titles, contact Humana at the above address or at any of the following numbers: Tel.: 973-256-1699; Fax: 973-256-8341; visit our website at www.humanapress.com

This publication is printed on acid-free paper. ∞

ANSI Z39.48-1984 (American National Standards Institute) Permanence of Paper for Printed Library Materials.

E-ISBN 978-1-59745-343-1

Printed in the United States of America. 10 9 8 7 6 5 4 3 2 1

Library of Congress Cataloging-in-Publication Data

Cartilage repair : analysis and strategies / edited by Riley J. Williams III ; with forewords by Lars Peterson and Brian J. Cole.
     p. ; cm.
  Includes bibliographical references and index.
  ISBN 1-58829-629-6 (alk. paper)
  1. Joints--Surgery. 2. Cartilage. 3. Bone marrow--Transplantation. 4. Cartilage cells. I. Williams, Riley J.
  [DNLM: 1. Cartilage, Articular--surgery. 2. Cartilage Diseases--therapy. 3. Cartilage, Articular--physiology. 4. Chondrocytes--transplantation. 5. Chondrogenesis. WE 300 C3275 2007]
  RD686.C37 2007
  617.4'72--dc22
                                                                                          2006019978

FOREWORD

The expansion and development of knee surgery has accelerated during the last three to four decades. Current treatment options for ligament and meniscal injuries have greatly improved the overall quality of life of affected patients. Moreover, more patients are able to return to sports because of their restored knee function.

In dealing with such patients, the typical orthopedic surgeon cannot avoid the problem of articular cartilage injuries in the young and middle-aged. Cartilage injuries in these patients may be catastrophic and career-ending in the young athlete, and disabling in the physically active older patient.

Over the last two decades, the pessimism usually associated with the treatment of cartilage injuries has turned into optimism. Newer treatment techniques are currently available to surgeons worldwide, and have been evaluated in the repair of articular cartilage lesions. Many studies in this area now report good short and long-term results.

The treatment of young patients with articular cartilage injuries, in an attempt to restore joint function and prevent joint deterioration, is the challenge that remains for our specialty.

Among orthopedic scientists and clinicians, it is well known that the spontaneous healing of articular cartilage injuries is poor. In addition, the inability of articular chondrocytes to migrate and repopulate a lesion for the purpose of forming reparative tissue has forced us to investigate the pathophysiology of cartilage degeneration and the healing process.

Current cartilage repair techniques, including bone-marrow stimulating procedures, microfracture, autologous osteochondral grafts transfer, and autologous chondrocyte transplantation/implantation, have given new hope to clinicians in their treatment of symptomatic chondral lesions. The further development of these and future cartilage treatment procedures depends on the collaboration between basic scientists, engineers, and clinicians. This interdisciplinary collaboration has already resulted in the development of new ways of using resorbable scaffolds and membranes in cartilage repair procedures. Such technology may ultimately enable the application of these methods using arthroscopic techniques that would ultimately reduce morbidity and improve clinical results. These new approaches, used in combination with autologous chondrocyte implantation, have created a great interest in the future of cartilage repair.

This is an exciting time. Almost every national or international orthopedic meeting now includes instructional courses, symposiums, and academic papers that focus on the latest methods and research in cartilage repair. I find that these programs generate great interest and fulfill the demand for information in this area from the scientists and physicians.

The area of cartilage repair is rapidly developing. This continuous expansion of the field calls for textbooks that keep the clinician well informed and updated on the research, methodologies, and clinical results of novel treatment techniques.

Cartilage Repair Strategies, edited by Dr. Riley J. Williams, is a welcome contribution to our specialty. This text provides a comprehensive update of the state of cartilage repair and regeneration. *Cartilage Repair Strategies* includes 20 chapters that cover a variety of topics, including discussions of the structure and function of articular cartilage, the evaluation of cartilage repair techniques, and the latest cartilage-sensitive imaging techniques. This book also includes updated information on decision making for both the conservative and surgical treatment of articular cartilage lesions. Front-line updates on current treatment methodologies are given by experts in the field.

In anticipation of the availability of newer cartilage repair techniques, several chapters are included that describe the rationale and application of these procedures. Second generation autologous chondrocyte implantation (ACI), resorbable scaffold-based repair, arthroscopically performed cartilage transplantation, as well as a chapter on the use of allogeneic chondrocytes in cartilage repair are stimulating and report encouraging short-term results by expert authors.

The chapter dealing with the importance of creating an optimal environment for the short and long-term survival of the repair tissue focuses on the indications for concomitant procedures indicated for stabilizing or unloading the affected knee. Osteochondritis dissecans is addressed as a separate issue as well, as is the rationale for meniscal transplantation in the meniscal-deficient knee with cartilage injury. Also, the appropriate application of chondral repair techniques in other joints, including the ankle, hip, and shoulder, is presented.

Last but not least, an update on rehabilitation strategies after cartilage repair is included as this area is of utmost importance in obtaining successful clinical results.

All of the chapters included in *Cartilage Repair Strategies* are of great importance. I recommend reading them for the enhancement of your knowledge and understanding of those issues relevant to the repair of articular cartilage. I believe that the information presented herein will greatly assist you in the challenging treatment of cartilage injuries.

Lars Peterson, MD, PhD

FOREWORD

I remember a particular case during my residency at the Hospital for Special Surgery: a 22-year-old elite female athlete who complained of anterior knee pain with recurrent activity-related effusions underwent "therapeutic" arthroscopy in an effort to relieve her symptoms. The surgery was a simple debridement and chondroplasty for an isolated trochlear cartilage defect. What followed was a sense of frustration for all who were involved in her care. Most importantly, her symptoms remained unchanged, and she never returned to professional basketball. Unlike other areas of orthopedic surgery, where results can be predictable and gratifying, this case was a clear example of the limitations that existed at that time for the treatment of chondral disease.

Over the last 15 years many of us have been fortunate to observe the virtual explosion of information related to the etiology, natural history, and surgical treatment of articular cartilage disease. Although our knowledge base remains limited in this area, we can confidently say that, as surgeons, we are routinely helping patients who not that long ago had no other option other than to live and suffer with the symptoms and dysfunction related to their cartilage injury. The quality of our literature in this area and the innovations derived from the interrelationships between basic scientists, clinicians, industry, and specialty societies allow us to move this field ahead while achieving greater insight into this difficult problem.

The opportunity to perform translational research is perhaps one of the most exciting opportunities in this area. We now routinely move from the preclinical setting to the operating room with increasing efficiency. It is interesting that as orthopedic surgeons, our training has remained technique-focused. Admittedly, knowing how to efficiently and accurately perform a surgical procedure is requisite for a successful clinical outcome. Even more critical is the thought process required to appropriately evaluate and indicate a patient for a specific procedure. This decision-making process is possibly the most difficult aspect of our efforts to treat the cartilage-injured patient. Clinical experience is a critical element to this process, but a foundation is necessary to support this process.

Thus, texts such as *Cartilage Repair Strategies*, edited by Dr. Riley J. Williams, enable the formation of an intellectual forum that permits the clinician to make clinical decisions that are based on peer-reviewed research. The information provided in books such as this addresses what methods are effective, what methods are safe, and what methods will actually lead to an alteration in the generally poor natural history of the articular cartilage injury. In addition, we now understand that we must extend our focus beyond treatment of the defect itself. As this book suggests, we clinicians should be familiar with many issues surrounding articular cartilage disease. *Cartilage Repair Strategies* presents a balanced perspective. An update on the basic science, outcomes analysis, imaging, and patient evaluation provides the initial foundation of knowledge. The inclusion of first and second-generation cell-based repair techniques is important because what we currently use is likely to evolve rapidly over the next 3 to 5 years. The inclusion of many joints is an important advantage of this text, as our biological and technological advances can now be generalized to the treatment of other joints beyond the knee.

As clinicians and scientists we have an implicit obligation to learn from our peers, to critically evaluate our own outcomes, and to convey our experience objectively to the future generations of orthopedic surgeons. Texts such as *Cartilage Repair Strategies* provide fertile ground for the presentation of the existing body of knowledge in an objective fashion. This book is an important contribution in that it consolidates much of the existing information in a uniform format that is easy to read, and includes a thorough representation of future technology. This text will enable the resident, fellow, and experienced orthopedic surgeon to develop or sustain high-level decision-making skills in the face of exciting and evolving technology.

Brian J. Cole, MD, MBA

PREFACE

It is with great pleasure that I present the first edition of *Cartilage Repair Strategies*. Over the past two decades, interest in the area of cartilage reconstruction has grown rapidly. I hoped to harness this great enthusiasm by inviting experts throughout the field to contribute to this comprehensive text.

The need for a book like this is great. My colleagues and I started the Hospital for Special Surgery Cartilage Study Group in 1998. At that time, we felt it important to follow our results critically in an effort to better understand our cartilage repair procedures. And, despite having recorded more than 500 articular cartilage surgeries in our database to date, we still do not understand many of the basic problems that are associated with achieving improved clinical outcomes in patients treated for cartilage lesions. As our group, and many others around the world, continue to analyze their surgical outcomes, the number of publications in the field of articular cartilage repair continues to rise at an amazing rate. The result is that it has become increasingly difficult for the clinician to synthesize this information, and to completely understand the appropriate indications and techniques. I personally have been impressed with the quality of studies in this area, especially over the past 5 years or so. Prospective, outcomes-oriented research is now the norm for clinical studies in this area. Consequently, I have attempted to present useful information that is based on peer-reviewed studies.

Each of the chapters in *Cartilage Repair Strategies* addresses a specific issue that is relevant to the field of articular cartilage surgery. I would strongly urge the reader to focus especially on those chapters that address the basic science of articular cartilage, decision making in cartilage procedures, and rehabilitation. For even as this field continues to evolve, these basic principles will remain unchanged.

As the editor, I would like to thank the clinicians who contributed to this text. Without their expertise and interest, an attempt to compile a book such as this would have been impossible. I also wish to acknowledge the work of Jasmine Zauberer of the Institute for Cartilage Repair at the Hospital for Special Surgery; her dedication is greatly appreciated, and has resulted in the creation of an excellent text. Finally I wish to thank the reader. I sincerely hope that you find this treatise helpful, and I look forward to following the field of articular cartilage surgery as it continues to evolve over the years to come.

Riley J. Williams III, MD

CONTENTS

CONTRIBUTORS

ANSWORTH A. ALLEN, MD • *Associate Professor of Clinical Orthopaedic Surgery, Weill Medical College of Cornell University; Associate Attending Orthopaedic Surgeon, Hospital for Special Surgery, New York, NY*

KARL F. ALMQVIST, MD, PhD • *Professor of Orthopaedic Surgery, Department of Orthopaedic Surgery, Ghent University Hospital, Ghent, Belgium*

BERNARD R. BACH, JR., MD • *Attending Surgeon, Northeast Orthopaedics, LLP, Albany, NY*

KEITH M. BAUMGARTEN, MD • *Sports Medicine and Shoulder Surgery, Orthopedic Institute, Sioux Falls, SD*

ROBERT H. BROPHY, MD • *Resident, Orthopedic Surgery, Hospital for Special Surgery, Weill Medical College of Cornell University, New York, NY*

WILLIAM D. BUGBEE, MD • *Orthopaedic Surgery, Scripps Clinic, La Jolla; Associate Professor of Orthopaedic Surgery, University of California, San Diego, La Jolla, CA*

ROBERT L. BULY, MD • *Assistant Professor of Orthopaedic Surgery, Weill Medical College of Cornell University; Assistant Attending Orthopaedic Surgeon, Hospital for Special Surgery, New York, NY*

MICHAEL D. BUSCHMANN, PhD • *Professor, Chemical and Biomedical Engineering, Canada Research Chair in Cartilage Tissue Engineering, École Polytechnique, Montréal, Qc, Canada*

JOHN T. CAVANAUGH, MEd, PT/ATC • *Senior Physical Therapist, Sports Medicine Performance and Research Center, Department of Rehabilitation, Hospital for Special Surgery; Team Physical Therapist, U.S. Merchant Marine Academy, New York, NY*

TIMOTHY CHARLTON, MD • *Clinical Fellow, Foot and Ankle Surgery, Hospital for Special Surgery, New York, NY*

BRIAN J. COLE, MD, MBA • *Associate Professor, Director, The Rush Cartilage Restoration Center, Rush University Medical Center, Chicago, IL*

JOSEPH J. CZARNECKI, MD • *Harvard Combined Orthopaedic Residency Program, Massachusetts General Hospital, Boston, MA*

JONATHAN T. DELAND, MD • *Assistant Professor of Orthopaedic Surgery, Weill Medical College of Cornell University; Assistant Attending Orthopaedic Surgeon, Chief, Foot and Ankle Surgery, Hospital for Special Surgery, New York, NY*

MARK C. DRAKOS, MD • *Orthopedics Resident, Sports Medicine and Shoulder Service, Hospital for Special Surgery, Weill Medical College of Cornell University, New York, NY*

KYLE R. FLIK, MD • *Attending Surgeon, Northeast Orthopaedics, LLP, Albany, NY*

LI F. FOO, MD • *Research Fellow, Musculoskeletal Magnetic Resonance Imaging, Hospital for Special Surgery, New York, NY*

CAROLINE D. HOEMANN, PhD • *Associate Professor, Chemical and Biomedical Engineering, École Polytechnique, Montréal, Qc, Canada*

Mark B. Hurtig, MVSc, DVM • *Professor, Department of Clinical Studies, Director, Comparative Orthopaedic Research Lab, University of Guelph, Guelph, Ontario, Canada*

Francesco Iacono, MD • *Orthopaedic Surgeon, Rizzoli Orthopaedic Institute, and Biomechanics Laboratory, Bologna, Italy*

Clinton Jambor, MD • *Sports Medicine Fellow, Orthopaedic Surgery, Cleveland Clinic, Cleveland, OH*

Deryk G. Jones, MD • *Section Head, Sports Medicine, Ochsner Clinic Foundation; Assistant Clinical Professor of Orthopaedic Surgery, Tulane University School of Medicine, Professor, Biomedical Engineering, Tulane University, New Orleans, LA*

Bryan T. Kelly, MD • *Associate Professor of Orthopaedic Surgery, Weill Medical College of Cornell University, Assistant Attending Orthopaedic Surgeon, Hospital for Special Surgery, New York, NY*

Mininder S. Kocher, MD, MPH • *Assistant Professor of Orthopaedic Surgery, Harvard Medical School, Harvard School of Public Health; Associate Director, Division of Sports Medicine, Department of Orthopaedic Surgery, Children's Hospital, Boston, MA*

Elizaveta Kon, MD • *Orthopaedic Surgeon, Rizzoli Orthopaedic Institute; Biomechanics Laboratory, Bologna, Italy*

Maurilio Marcacci, MD • *Professor, University of Bologna, Head of IX Orthopaedic Division, and Biomechanics Laboratory, Rizzoli Orthopaedic Institute, Bologna, Italy*

Robert G. Marx, MD, MSc, FRCSC • *Associate Professor of Orthopaedic Surgery and Public Health, Weill Medical College of Cornell University; Associate Attending Orthopaedic Surgeon, Director, Foster Center for Clinical Outcome Research; Orthopaedic Director, The Sports Medicine Institute for Young Athletes, Hospital for Special Surgery, New York, NY*

Anthony Miniaci, MD, FRCSC • *Professor of Orthopaedic Surgery, Lerner College of Medicine, Case Western Reserve University; Executive Director and Section Head, Sports Medicine, Cleveland Clinic, Cleveland, OH*

Maria Pia Neri, MD • *Orthopaedic Surgeon, Rizzoli Orthopaedic Institute, and Biomechanics Laboratory, Bologna, Italy*

Gabriele G. Niederauer, PhD • *Synthetic Resorbable Scaffolds, Director of Research and Development, OsteoBiologics, Inc, San Antonio, TX*

Andrew D. Pearle, MD • *Assistant Attending Orthopedic Surgeon, Sports Medicine and Shoulder Service, Hospital for Special Surgery, New York, NY*

Lars Peterson, MD, PhD • *Professor of Orthopaedic Surgery, University of Gothenburg; Attending Orthopaedic Surgeon, Clinical Director, Department of Orthopaedic Surgery, Gothenburg Medical Center, Gothenburg, Sweden*

Frank A. Petrigliano, MD • *Resident, Department of Orthopedic Surgery, University of California, Los Angeles, Los Angeles, CA*

Hollis G. Potter, MD • *Chief, Division of Magnetic Resonance Imaging, Hospital for Special Surgery; Professor of Radiology, Weill Medical College of Cornell University, New York, NY*

Leonardo Marchesini Reggiano, MD • *Orthopaedic Surgeon, Rizzoli Orthopaedic Institute, and Biomechanics Laboratory, Bologna, Italy*

SCOTT A. RODEO, MD • *Associate Professor of Orthopaedic Surgery, Weill Medical College of Cornell University; Associate Attending Orthopaedic Surgeon and Associate Scientist, Research Division, Hospital for Special Surgery, New York, NY*

MATTHEW S. SHIVE, PhD • *Vice President, Product Development, BioSyntech Canada, Inc., Laval, Qc, Canada*

DANIEL J. SOLOMON, MD • *Sports Medicine and Shoulder Service, Department of Orthopaedic Surgery, Naval Medical Center, San Diego, CA*

PATRICK P. SUSSMANN, MD • *Orthopaedic Department, Balgrist University Hospital, University of Zurich, Zurich, Switzerland*

GUST VERBRUGGEN, MD, PhD • *Professor of Rheumatology, Department of Rheumatology, Ghent University Hospital, Ghent, Belgium*

PETER C. M. VERDONK, MD • *Orthopaedic Surgeon, Department of Orthopaedic Surgery, Ghent University Hospital, Ghent, Belgium*

RENÉ VERDONK, MD, PhD • *Professor of Orthopaedic Surgery, Department of Orthopaedic Surgery, Ghent University Hospital, Ghent, Belgium*

NIKHIL VERMA, MD • *Assistant Professor, Department of Orthopedics, Section of Sports Medicine, Rush University Medical Center, Chicago, IL*

KOENRAAD L. VERSTRAETE, MD, PhD • *Professor of Radiology, Department of Radiology, Ghent University Hospital, Ghent, Belgium*

MONIKA VOLESKY, MD, FRCSC • *Clinical Fellow, Foot and Ankle Surgery, Hospital for Special Surgery, New York, NY*

RUSSELL F. WARREN, MD • *Surgeon-in-Chief Emeritus, Hospital for Special Surgery; Professor of Orthopaedics, Weill Medical College of Cornell University, New York, NY*

THOMAS L. WICKIEWICZ, MD • *Professor of Clinical Orthopaedic Surgery, Weill Medical College of Cornell University; Attending Orthopaedic Surgeon, Hospital for Special Surgery, New York, NY*

RILEY J. WILLIAMS III, MD • *Associate Professor of Orthopaedic Surgery, Weill Medical College of Cornell University, Attending Orthopaedic Surgeon, Director, Institute for Cartilage Repair, Hospital for Special Surgery, New York, NY*

DAVID WOOD, MBBS, MS, FRCS, FRACS • *Head of Unit, Department of Orthopaedic Surgery, Director, Perth Orthopaedic Instiute, Perth Bone and Tissue Bank, University of Western Australia, Nedlands, Western Australia, Australia*

JOSEPH YU, MD • *Fellow, Adult Joint Reconstruction, Department of Orthopaedic Surgery, University of California, San Diego, La Jolla, CA*

STEFANO ZAFFAGNINI, MD • *Orthopaedic Surgeon, Rizzoli Orthopaedic Institute, and Biomechanics Laboratory, Bologna, Italy*

MING HAO ZHENG, PhD, DM, FRCPath • *Director of Research, Orthopaedic Research Laboratories, Department of Orthopaedic Surgery, University of Western Australia, Nedlands, Western Australia, AUSTRALIA*

COLOR PLATES

Color plates follow p. 206.

Articular Cartilage
Structure, Biology, and Function

Kyle R. Flik, MD, Nikhil Verma, MD, Brian J. Cole, MD, MBA, and Bernard R. Bach, Jr., MD

Summary

The dynamic structure and function of articular cartilage is explored in detail in this chapter. Emphasis is placed on the ultrastructure of cartilage and how this provides for its remarkable physical properties.

Key Words: Hyaline cartilage; chondrocyte; proteoglycan; biomechanics; biology.

INTRODUCTION

Articular cartilage has extraordinary mechanical properties and lasting durability even though it is only a few millimeters thick. Its unique structure and composition provides joints with a surface that combines low friction with high lubrication, shock absorption, and wear resistance while bearing large repetitive loads throughout a person's lifetime. These characteristics are clearly unmatched by any synthetic material.

Despite performing with relatively low metabolic activity within a harsh physical environment, healthy articular cartilage has amazing capacity to sustain itself and carry out its functions. Chondrocytes are active in maintaining the tissue's matrix, yet there is limited capability for repair. Damage to cartilage's high level of organization and molecular architecture from trauma or degeneration is a major source of morbidity.

STRUCTURE AND COMPOSITION

A thorough understanding of the complex structure of articular cartilage is essential for understanding its biology and function. Grossly, articular cartilage is a specialized hyaline cartilage found in diarthrodial joints; it has a firm, smooth, slippery surface that resists plastic deformation (Fig. 1). Microscopically, articular cartilage is made up primarily of extracellular matrix (ECM) surrounding a single cell type, the chondrocyte (Fig. 2). There are no blood vessels, lymphatics, or nerves within articular cartilage. In decreasing concentrations, the ECM consists of water, proteoglycan (PG), collagen (primarily type II), and a variety of other proteins and glycoproteins.

The macrostructure of articular cartilage is best described in four distinct zones: superficial, transitional, deep, and calcified. Within each zone, the structure and composition vary. Light microscopy of the different zones reveals variable chondrocyte appearance; unique collagen fibril size, shape, and orientation; as well as different PG and water contents (Fig. 3). The ECM within each zone can also be divided into distinct regions. These regions have been defined as the pericellular region, territorial region, and interterritorial region.

From: *Cartilage Repair Strategies*
Edited by: Riley J. Williams © Humana Press Inc., Totowa, NJ

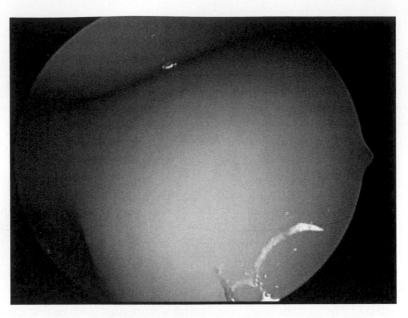

Fig. 1. Gross photograph of human knee articular cartilage.

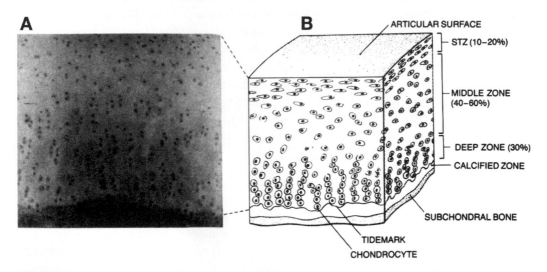

Fig. 2. Healthy articular cartilage structure. Histologic (**A**) and schematic (**B**) views of a section of normal articular cartilage. There are four zones: the superficial tangential zone (STZ), the middle zone, the deep zone, and the calcified zone. The cells in the superficial zone have an ellipsoidal shape and lie parallel to the surface; the cells of the other zones have a more spherical shape. In the deep zone, the chondrocytes align themselves in columns perpendicular to the surface. (Reprinted from ref. *24*. Used with permission.)

Articular Cartilage Zones

The outermost articular gliding surface, or *superficial zone*, is covered by a fine layer called the lamina splendens. Within the superficial zone, the collagen fibrils are oriented parallel to the surface. The chondrocytes are elongated. The PG content is at its lowest; water content is at its highest.

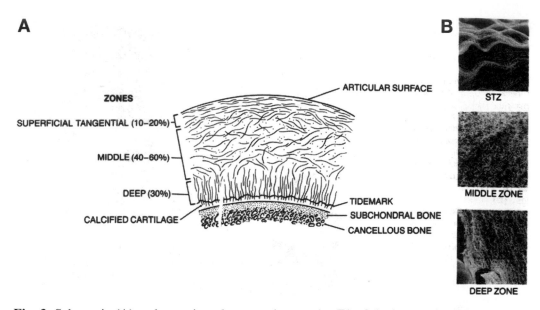

Fig. 3. Schematic (**A**) and scanning electron micrographs (**B**) of the interterritorial matrix collagen fibril orientation and organization in normal articular cartilage. In the superficial tangential zone (STZ), the fibrils lie nearly parallel to the surface. In the middle zone, they assume a more random alignment. In the deep zone, they lie nearly perpendicular to the articular surface. (Reprinted from ref. *24*. Used with permission.)

The *transitional zone* is below the superficial zone and is characterized by larger diameter collagen fibers with less organization. The chondrocytes in this region are rounder and on electron microscopy appear to have intracellular components consistent with a metabolically active cell *(1)*.

Below this zone is the *deep zone;* it contains large-diameter collagen fibers oriented perpendicular to the articular surface. The chondrocytes appear spherical and are arranged in a columnar pattern. PG concentration is the highest in this zone, and the water content is lowest.

The final zone of articular cartilage is called the *calcified zone;* it is separated from the deep zone by the *tidemark*. This deepest layer is a transitional area that anchors the overlying hyaline cartilage to the subchondral bone *(2,3)*. This stiff zone likely blocks the transport of nutrients from the underlying bone, rendering articular cartilage dependent on synovial fluid for nutritional support. The cells in this zone are small and distributed randomly in a matrix filled with apatitic salts.

Articular Cartilage Regions

The ECM of articular cartilage is also divided into regions based on proximity to the chondrocyte. These regions are the pericellular, territorial, or interterritorial and differ in content and in collagen fibril diameter and organization. The *pericellular matrix* completely surrounds the chondrocyte, forming a thin layer around the cell membrane. This matrix region may play a functional biomechanical role for signal transduction within cartilage during loading *(4)*. The pericellular matrix contains PG and noncollagenous matrix components but little or no collagen fibrils.

The *territorial matrix* surrounding the pericellular region contains thin collagen fibrils that form a fibrillar network at its periphery *(5)*. This possibly provides mechanical protection for the chondrocytes during loading *(4)*. The *chondron* is defined as the chondrocyte and its surrounding pericellular and territorial matrix regions.

Finally, the *interterritorial region* is the largest of all regions and contributes most to the material properties of articular cartilage *(6)*. This region encompasses the entire matrix between the territorial matrices of the individual cells. Large collagen fibrils and the majority of the PG reside in this region. The collagen fibrils within the interterritorial region change orientation depending on the zone of articular cartilage. The interterritorial collagen fibrils are arranged parallel to the surface in the superficial zone, obliquely in the middle zone, and perpendicular to the joint surface in the deep zone. Because the tensile stiffness and strength of articular cartilage is provided primarily by collagen, and the interterritorial matrix forms most of the volume, it follows that the biomechanical properties should differ in the various cartilage zones. This has been proven experimentally *(7)*.

Chondrocytes

The chondrocyte is the only cell type within articular cartilage. Despite their presence throughout the tissue, chondrocytes occupy less than 10% of the total volume. Each chondrocyte is surrounded by its ECM, has few cell-to-cell contacts, and relies on diffusion for nutritional support. The chondrocyte shape and size varies depending on its zonal position. The superficial cells are ellipsoidal and are aligned parallel to the surface. The transitional cells are spherical and are randomly distributed. The deep cells form columns aligned perpendicular to the tidemark and the calcified zone.

Chondrocytes are derived from mesenchymal cells. Their primary function is to maintain the ECM, the component of articular cartilage that provides its unique material properties. Chondrocytes rarely divide after skeletal growth is completed. The chondrocyte is metabolically active and able to respond to environmental stimuli and soluble mediators, including growth factors, interleukins, and certain pharmaceuticals. They are responsive to mechanical loads, hydrostatic pressure changes, osmotic pressure changes, and injury and degenerative arthritis.

Extracellular Matrix

In normal articular cartilage, 65–80% of the total weight is water *(8)*. Collagens and PGs are the two major load-bearing macromolecules in articular cartilage. Other classes of molecules make up the remaining ECM; these include lipids, phospholipids, proteins, and glycoproteins.

Water

Water content in articular cartilage varies from approx 80% of the wet weight at the surface to 65% in the deep zone *(8,9)*. A small percentage of water is contained in the intracellular space, approx 30% is found within the collagen in the intrafibrillar space, and the molecular pore space of the matrix holds the balance *(10)*. The extracellular tissue fluid contains inorganic dissolved salts of sodium, calcium, chloride, and potassium. The flow of water through cartilage and across the articular surface aids in the transport of nutrients to chondrocytes.

Tissue water has a crucial biomechanical function in cartilage. Together with its interaction with PGs, water provides articular cartilage with tremendous compressive strength. The small pore size of the ECM causes high frictional resistance to fluid flow. It is this frictional resistance coupled with the pressurization of the water within the ECM that is responsible for the compressive strength and ability of articular cartilage to withstand high joint loads. (Details of this important interaction between tissue fluids and large matrix macromolecules that influences the material properties of articular cartilage are described in the section on biology and function.)

Collagens

A variety of collagen types, synthesized by chondrocytes, compose the major structural macromolecules of the ECM. Collagens contribute approx 60% of the dry weight of cartilage and are distributed throughout the various zones in a relatively uniform concentration but variable orientation as described previously. The unique structure of collagen provides articular cartilage with its tensile strength.

The collagen in articular cartilage is 90–95% type II, with minor contributions by types V, VI, IX, X, and XI. All collagen types are composed of three polypeptide chains (α-chains) wound into a triple helix. The amino acid composition of the polypeptide chains is primarily glycine and proline, with hydroxyproline providing stability via hydrogen bonds along the length of the molecule. In addition, hydroxylysine is involved in creating covalent crosslinks that stabilize the collagen fibrillar structure *(9)*.

The cross-banded fibrils visible on electron microscopy are formed primarily by collagen types II, IX, and XI *(11)*. These extend throughout the tissue to provide tensile stiffness and strength. Importantly, they also act as a meshwork to trap large PGs. Cartilage achieves its compressive strength in part by the swelling of these trapped PGs.

Proteoglycans

Proteoglycans make up approx 10–15% of the wet weight of articular cartilage. Produced by chondrocytes, PGs are secreted into the ECM. The basic structure of a PG is that of a complex macromolecule consisting of a protein core with covalently bound glycosaminoglycan (GAG) side chains. This is called the *PG aggrecan molecule*. The PG aggrecans bind to hyaluronan in the presence of a link protein to form the aggregate. Many aggrecan molecules can bind to a single long hyaluronan chain to form a large PG aggregate (Fig. 4). Aggrecans occupy the interfibrillar space of the cartilage matrix and contribute about 90% to the total cartilage matrix PG *(12)*.

A single GAG is an unbranched chain of repeating disaccharide units, of which there are three major types found in articular cartilage: chondroitin sulfate 4- and 6-isomers, keratin sulfate, and dermatan sulfate. Each disaccharide unit has a negatively charged carboxylate or sulfate group, creating a structure that effectively repels other negatively charged molecules and attracts water and positive counterions such as Ca^{2+} and Na^+ to maintain electroneutrality. These ions are found free floating within the interstitial water. The negative charge of each keratan sulfate and chondroitin sulfate chain repels each other, which tends to maintain the molecules in an expanded form, thus facilitating the trapping of the PGs within the collagen framework.

Hyaluronate, although itself considered a GAG, is not sulfated like those described above, nor is it bound to a protein core. In articular cartilage, hyaluronate is present as large unbranching chains to which the chondroitin and keratin sulfate chains are bound by the link proteins. This provides strong structural stability to this macromolecule, the aggregate. Loss of the link protein to aging or arthritis essentially weakens the ECM of articular cartilage by decreasing the size of the PG aggregate. The length, weight, and composition of an individual aggrecan are variable and are determined primarily by the length of its protein core.

To summarize, the large PG aggregate is composed primarily of chondroitin sulfate and keratin sulfate chains associated with hyaluronic acid filaments and link proteins. In addition,

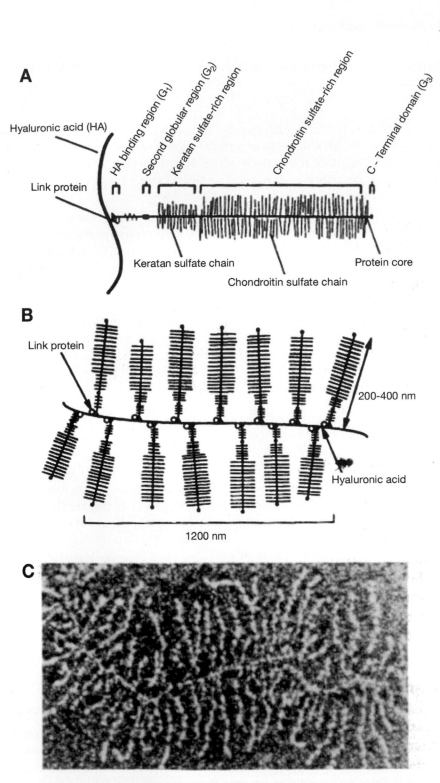

Fig. 4. The structure of proteoglycan. (**A**) Details of proteoglycan monomer structure showing chondroitin sulfate and keratan sulfate chains and the interaction of the monomer with hyaluronate chain and link protein. (**B**) Molecular conformation of a typical proteoglycan aggregate showing size of the molecule. (**C**) An electron micrograph of a proteoglycan aggregate. (Reprinted from ref. *25.* Used with permission.)

biglycan and decorin, two smaller, nonaggregating PGs rich in dermatan sulfate, are found in articular cartilage. Although these are much smaller PGs, they equal the larger aggrecan molecule in total number. Biglycan and decorin are found in association with collagen fibrils.

Noncollagenous Proteins and Glycoproteins

The noncollagenous proteins and glycoproteins are poorly studied proteins with occasional monosaccharides and oligosaccharides attached. They are found within the ECM and are likely involved in maintaining structure. These include anchorin CII, a chondrocyte surface protein; cartilage oligometric protein, an acidic protein found within the territorial matrix; and fibronectin and tenascin.

CARTILAGE BIOLOGY AND FUNCTION

Articular cartilage is a living, active tissue formed and maintained by chondrocytes. These cells are derived from mesenchymal stem cells that differentiate prior to the eighth week of gestation. The chondrocyte survives without blood vessels, lymphatic vessels, or nerves. Standing alone within its matrix, the chondrocyte creates an ordered structure capable of complex interactions that are required to maintain and repair the tissue *(1)*.

It has not been fully elucidated how the chondrocyte obtains nutrition to fuel its metabolism; however, contact between articular cartilage and its vascularized subchondral bone appears to be crucial. In addition, synovial fluid provides chondrocytes with nutrients via diffusion. A double-diffusion barrier requires passage through the synovium first, followed by passage through the ECM to the chondrocyte. Metabolism in articular cartilage is primarily anaerobic in an environment with very low oxygen concentration.

Chondrocytes are metabolically active despite the static appearance of the cells. Basic housekeeping and maintenance of the articular surface requires that chondrocytes turn over the matrix biomacromolecules by replacing degraded matrix components. Chondrocytes must be able to respond to changes in the matrix composition (which occurs with macromolecular degradation) by synthesizing proper types and amounts of these biomacromolecules *(1,5)*.

Biomechanics

Articular cartilage serves the human body by providing for load transmission through joints. The articular cartilage of the knee joint experiences an average load of three times the body weight. With everyday activities, the knee can be exposed to loads ranging up to 10 times body weight during running and 20 times body weight during jumping *(13)*. The structure of articular cartilage enables it to store, transmit, and dissipate this mechanical energy during activity. Articular cartilage must be capable of storing energy; otherwise, it would compress with a permanent loss of thickness, or it would succumb to the forces and tear. In normal conditions, cartilage stores energy as it deforms, and then it dissipates the energy and returns to its form without tearing. Tremendous stresses and strains are developed within the tissue of articular cartilage during normal daily activities.

Articular cartilage has well-defined tensile and compressive properties. The crosslinking among collagen fibrils is primarily responsible for the tensile strength but does little to resist compression. The relationship of PGs and water trapped within the collagen meshwork provides resistance to compression, swelling pressure, and resilience. PGs contain negatively charged GAG chains. These chains attract cations and water and repel each other. By repelling each other, the GAG chains hold the monomers extended, which allows for the filling of the collagen fibril meshwork with water. Compression of the matrix drives the GAG chains together, which increases resistance to further compression as the desire to repel nearby chains remains. Water is forced out of the macromolecules and returns when the compressive load is released.

Articular cartilage is biphasic. It is important to understand this characteristic of articular cartilage as it is essential to its ability to withstand the high repetitive loads to which it is exposed over decades. The solid phase includes the macromolecular framework of collagens, PGs, and noncollagenous proteins; the fluid phase refers to the tissue water composing 65–80% of the total weight. The biomechanical properties of articular cartilage depend on the interaction of these two phases. In general, it is the fluid phase that accounts for deformational behaviors of hydrated soft tissues *(14)*.

The solid matrix is porous and permeable, allowing the water that resides in the microscopic pores to flow through the matrix when loads are applied. Fluid pressure provides a major part of the total load support, thus minimizing the stress appreciated by the solid matrix. This is referred to as stress shielding of the solid matrix. For healthy cartilage, greater than 95% of the applied load in normal activities will be supported by the interstitial fluid *(8,15)*.

Articular cartilage is viscoelastic. Viscoelasticity describes the material property of having stress-strain behavior dependent on strain rate *(14)*. When a constant compressive stress is applied to cartilage, its deformation will increase with time. There are two mechanisms responsible for viscoelasticity in articular cartilage: flow-independent and flow-dependent mechanisms. The flow-independent aspect of its viscoelastic behavior derives from the intermolecular friction of cartilage's PG matrix. The flow-dependent mechanism depends on interstitial fluid flow and its resultant frictional drag. (A fluid's frictional drag is the reciprocal of the permeability, such that a substance with low permeability will have a high frictional drag.) The drag resulting from interstitial fluid flow is the main source for the viscoelastic behavior of healthy articular cartilage. Cartilage in degenerative joint disease has increased permeability and water content and therefore has lower friction drag and less ability to provide a stress-shielding effect to protect the ECM *(8,16)*.

Articular cartilage also demonstrates creep and stress relaxation. These mechanical properties result primarily from fluid flow through the matrix when articular cartilage is compressed *(15)*. *Creep behavior* refers to a viscoelastic material responding with rapid initial deformation when a constant load is applied, followed by further slow deformation up to an equilibrium state. *Stress relaxation behavior* is when a constant deformation leads to high initial stress followed by a slow progressive decrease in the stress required to maintain the deformation.

In sheer, creep and stress relaxation are flow independent and are derived from the intermolecular friction within the collagen-PG matrix and an alteration of the macromolecular framework. The random organization of the collagen architecture through the middle zones contributes most to the sheer properties of articular cartilage.

It is the intact collagen fibril meshwork that restrains the expansion of PGs with tissue fluid. Mechanical failure of the matrix and degenerative arthritis result from a disruption of the collagen fibril framework and the subsequent expansion of PGs with an increased water concentration. This decreases cartilage stiffness and increases matrix permeability, making the tissue less capable to support load *(15)*.

Metabolism

Given the low oxygen content and avascular nature of articular cartilage, a surprisingly high level of metabolism exists. The chondrocyte relies primarily on the anaerobic pathway for energy. Chondrocytes synthesize matrix components, including proteins and GAG chains, and secrete these substances into the ECM. In addition, the chondrocyte is responsible for ECM remodeling via an elaborate group of degradative enzymes. Therefore, it is the chondrocyte that maintains the normal ECM by balancing synthesis of matrix components with their catabolism and release. This metabolic activity of the chondrocyte can be altered by its surrounding chemical and mechanical environment. Cytokines appear to play a role in controlling the balance between matrix macromolecular degradation and synthesis. The ECM plays an important role in transmitting to the chondrocyte chemical, electrical, and mechanical signals created during loading of the articular surface. The chondrocyte responds by altering the matrix structure. Cytokines may be the messenger acting through either autocrine or paracrine means. It is unclear which signals—electrical, mechanical, or physiochemical—are most important in stimulating the activity of the aneural chondrocyte *(4,8,17)*.

PG molecules are synthesized, assembled, sulfated, and secreted into the ECM by the chondrocyte. The control over PG synthesis is responsive to biochemical, mechanical, and physical stimuli. Maintenance of articular cartilage requires continual degradation and release of PGs by articular cartilage. The rate of catabolism is affected by soluble mediators, such as interleukin 1, which accelerates degradation. Joint load can also play a role; for example, immobilization has been found to lead to a loss of PGs from the matrix *(17,18)*. PG fragments such as keratan sulfate can be quantified in body fluids such that synovial fluid concentrations can be used to measure catabolic activity in the cartilage of a particular joint *(19,20)*. Further research on the utility of this information in diagnosis or treatment of early degenerative disease is warranted.

Collagen synthesis and catabolism are both partially under enzymatic control. In addition, growth factors have been found to play an intricate role in cartilage metabolism. The methods by which growth factors influence the chondrocyte are not fully clear; however, cell surface receptor sites are present on the chondrocyte. Platelet-derived growth factor appears to have a mitogenic effect on chondrocytes and may be involved in the healing response in osteoarthritis and lacerative injury *(21)*. Basic fibroblast growth factor, insulinlike growth factors, and insulin are stimulators of deoxyribonucleic acid (DNA) synthesis and matrix production in articular cartilage as well as in the growth plate. Transforming growth factor-β is synthesized by chondrocytes locally and stimulates PG synthesis while suppressing type II collagen synthesis.

Chondrocytes themselves synthesize proteolytic enzymes that are responsible for the breakdown of the cartilage matrix, both in normal turnover and in cartilage degeneration. The primary proteinases involved in cartilage turnover include the metalloproteinases (collagenase, gelatinase, and stromelysin) and the cathepsins (cathepsin B and D), which have the ability to degrade aggrecan. Collagenase is specific in its activity because it cleaves the triple-helical portion of collagen at a single site. Gelatinase then cleaves the denatured α-chains that remain after collagenase activity. Stromelysin acts to break down the protein core of aggrecan. These metalloproteinases all require activation outside the cell by enzymatic modification. For example, collagenase can be activated by plasmin.

Joint motion and loading are required to maintain normal adult articular cartilage structure and function *(1)*. The balance between degradation and synthesis by the chondrocyte is altered when joint loading exceeds or falls below the necessary range *(22)*. Prolonged joint immobilization also leads to cartilage degeneration *(1)*. Normal diffusion of nutrients from the synovial fluid is diminished. In addition, the PG content is decreased, and its structure is altered. Remobilization can reverse the changes in PG *(23)*. Orthopedists today are more

Table 1
Articular Cartilage Composition

Major components	Approximate wet weight (%)
Water	65–80
Type II collagen	10–20
Aggrecan	5

Minor components (<5%)	
Proteoglycans	
Biglycan	
Decorin	
Collagens types V, VI, IX, X, XI	
Link protein	
Hyaluronate	
Fibronectin	
Lipids	

aggressive about maintaining joint motion after injury or surgery because of the increased understanding of the deleterious effects to cartilage of rigid immobilization.

Age-Related Changes

The size of the PG aggregates in the ECM of articular cartilage decreases with age. This occurs as a result of shortening of the hyaluronic acid (HA) chain, such that there are fewer aggrecans attached, or as a result of shortening of the protein core or the GAG chains. In addition, there is a change in the PG at the molecular level such that the concentration of chondroitin sulfate 4 diminishes and chondroitin sulfate 6 increases. However, the overall concentration of chondroitin sulfates decreases and that of keratin sulfate increases. Chondrocytes become larger with aging and acquire increased lysosomal enzymes. The overall protein content increases with aging, and the water content diminishes. As a result of these changes, cartilage stiffness increases, and solubility and elasticity diminish.

Although age-related changes to articular cartilage can be expected eventually in everybody, complex changes to articular cartilage can also result from a variety of intra-articular pathological conditions. It is beyond the scope of this chapter to review the variety of adaptive responses and alterations that take place in articular cartilage in the pathological state.

SUMMARY

Articular cartilage is a dynamic and responsive tissue despite its low metabolic activity and relatively poor ability to heal. The function of articular cartilage is to provide joints with a low-friction and wear-resistant surface that provides shock absorption and high load-bearing capability. The chondrocyte, the only cell type in articular cartilage, is responsible for the production of crucial structural components, including collagen, PGs, and various enzymes, which determine the complex biomechanical properties of the tissue.

The close relationship between articular cartilage's composition and its structural integrity and function enhances our understanding of the effects of aging, degenerative disease, and injury. Although many growth factors have been discovered in the last decade, future investigations are certain to identify an array of articular cartilage growth factors that may lead to important advances in the treatment of articular cartilage pathology.

REFERENCES

1. Buckwalter JA, Mankin HJ. Articular cartilage: tissue design and chondrocyte-matrix interactions. Instr Course Lect 1998;47:477–486.
2. Bullough PG, Jagannath A. The morphology of the calcification front in articular cartilage. Its significance in joint function. J Bone Joint Surg Br 1983;65:72–78.
3. Redler I, Mow VC, Zimny ML, Mansell J. The ultrastructure and biomechanical significance of the tidemark of articular cartilage. Clin Orthop 1975, Oct. (112):357–362.
4. Guilak F, Mow VC. The mechanical environment of the chondrocyte: a biphasic finite element model of cell-matrix interactions in articular cartilage. J Biomech 2000;33:1663–1673.
5. Muir H. The chondrocyte, architect of cartilage. Biomechanics, structure, function and molecular biology of cartilage matrix macromolecules. Bioessays 1995;17:1039–1048.
6. Mow VC, Guo XE. Mechano-electrochemical properties of articular cartilage: their inhomogeneities and anisotropies. Annu Rev Biomed Eng 2002;4:175–209.
7. Roth V, Mow VC. The intrinsic tensile behavior of the matrix of bovine articular cartilage and its variation with age. J Bone Joint Surg Am 1980;62:1102–1117.
8. Mow VC, Ratcliffe A. Structure and Function of Articular Cartilage and Meniscus. 2nd ed. Philadelphia: Lippincott-Raven; 1997.
9. Maroudas A. Physiochemical Properties of Articular Cartilage. Kent, UK: Pitman Medical; 1979.
10. Torzilli PA. Influence of cartilage conformation on its equilibrium water partition. J Orthop Res 1985;3:473–483.
11. Akizuki S, Mow VC, Muller F, Pita JC, Howell DS, Manicourt DH. Tensile properties of human knee joint cartilage: I. Influence of ionic conditions, weight bearing, and fibrillation on the tensile modulus. J Orthop Res 1986;4:379–392.
12. Buckwalter JA, Rosenberg LA, Hunziker EB. Articular Cartilage and Knee Joint Function: Basic Science and Arthroscopy. New York: Raven Press; 1990.
13. Maquet PG, Van de Berg AJ, Simonet JC. Femorotibial weight-bearing areas. Experimental determination. J Bone Joint Surg Am 1975;57:766–771.
14. Buckwalter JA, Einhorn TA, Simon SR. Orthopaedic Basic Science. Chicago: American Academy of Orthopaedic Surgeons; 2000.
15. Mow VC, Holmes MH, Lai WM. Fluid transport and mechanical properties of articular cartilage: a review. J Biomech 1984;17:377–394.
16. Mankin HJ, Thrasher AZ. Water content and binding in normal and osteoarthritic human cartilage. J Bone Joint Surg Am 1975;57:76–80.
17. Kim YJ, Sah RL, Grodzinsky AJ, Plaas AH, Sandy JD. Mechanical regulation of cartilage biosynthetic behavior: physical stimuli. Arch Biochem Biophys 1994;311:1–12.
18. Sah RL, Kim YJ, Doong JY, Grodzinsky AJ, Plaas AH, Sandy JD. Biosynthetic response of cartilage explants to dynamic compression. J Orthop Res 1989;7:619–636.
19. Lohmander LS, Roos H, Dahlberg L, Lark MW. The role of molecular markers to monitor disease, intervention and cartilage breakdown in osteoarthritis. Acta Orthop Scand Suppl 1995; 266:84–87.
20. Lohmander S. Proteoglycans of joint cartilage. Structure, function, turnover and role as markers of joint disease. Baillieres Clin Rheumatol 1988;2:37–62.
21. Mankin HJ, Jennings LC, Treadwell BV, Trippel SB. Growth factors and articular cartilage. J Rheumatol Suppl 1991;27:66–67.
22. Torzilli PA, Grigiene R, Borrelli J Jr, Helfet DL. Effect of impact load on articular cartilage: cell metabolism and viability, and matrix water content. J Biomech Eng 1999;121:433–441.

23. Bachrach NM, Valhmu WB, Stazzone E, Ratcliffe A, Lai WM, Mow VC. Changes in proteogly-can synthesis of chondrocytes in articular cartilage are associated with the time-dependent changes in their mechanical environment. J Biomech 1995;28:1561–1569.
24. Man VC, Proctor CS, Kelly MA, Biomechanics of articular cartilage. Nordin M, Frankel VH. Basic Biomechanics of the Musculoskeletal System. 2nd ed. Philadelphia: Lea and Febiger; 1989:31–57.
25. Buckwalter JA, Mow VC. Basic science and injury of articular cartilage, menisci, and bone. In DeLee J.C. and Drez D.D., eds. Orthopaedic Sports Medicine. Philadelphia: Saunders, 67–119.

2

Evaluating Outcome Following Cartilage Procedures

Robert G. Marx, MD

Summary

Many factors influence the evaluation of outcome following cartilage procedures. The outcome is influenced by the patient, the nature of the lesion, the procedure performed, and the outcome measure utilized. All of these factors must be independently considered in great detail to appropriately evaluate any treatment or procedure for a cartilage lesion. Each of these is reviewed in this chapter.

Key Words: Cartilage; outcome; surgery; evaluation; scale; prognosis.

There are many factors that influence the evaluation of outcome following cartilage procedures. The outcome is influenced by the patient, the nature of the lesion, the procedure performed, and the outcome measure utilized. All of these factors must be independently considered in great detail to appropriately evaluate any treatment or procedure for a cartilage lesion. In this chapter, each of these factors are considered separately to present an organized approach to evaluating the outcome for a patient who has undergone a cartilage regenerative or restorative procedure.

THE PATIENT

Many factors must be considered when evaluating the patient. These factors will have a large effect on the outcome of treatment and must be documented in detail. Patient age as well as the height and weight of the patient have an effect on the outcome. The patient's occupation will also affect outcome because of the inherent relationship with activity level. Patient gender should also be considered.

The duration of symptoms is very important. A patient who has 2 days of pain is very different from an individual who has been in pain chronically for over 2 years. Therefore, an estimation of the duration of symptoms should be determined. In many cases, the patient has sustained trauma in the past; such a history is relevant and should be described in detail regarding the mechanism. When the patient has been injured, the mechanism should be determined.

There are other issues relating to the patient that can also affect outcome. These include prior operations on the knee or other conditions relating to the knee or site of cartilage repair. Other medical problems such as diabetes or heart disease may limit the patient in his or her activity or ability to heal. Medications should also be tracked. If the patient is treated as part of a worker's compensation claim, this has been documented to adversely affect outcome following orthopedic surgery. The surgeon should document whether the patient is in this category.

Perhaps one of the most important prognostic factors following cartilage surgery is the patient's activity level. This is a critical variable because with a decreased level of activity

From: *Cartilage Repair Strategies*
Edited by: Riley J. Williams © Humana Press Inc., Totowa, NJ

many patients can tolerate significant knee pathology. Often, patients with symptomatic cartilage lesions will significantly modify their activities to reduce knee symptoms associated with the lesion. The measurement of patient activity is complex and can be difficult. The Tegner rating scale evaluates patients based on their participation in various sports *(1)*. Although this scale has been used extensively in the past, it has limitations with respect to patients who do not participate in the specific sports measured by the scale. Therefore, individuals who are active but do not participate in one of the sports evaluated in this rating scale may be incorrectly rated as having a lower activity level.

A rating scale that measures patients' activity independent of specific sports is desirable. One such scale has been published that was developed with patient input regarding activities that are important and difficult for them to perform *(2)*. This rating scale asks patients four questions about the frequency with which they perform four activities: running, cutting (changing directions while running), decelerating (coming to a quick stop while running), and pivoting (turning the body with the foot planted, etc.). This scale has been evaluated for reliability and validity in separate groups of patients *(2)*. The use of activity rating scales is recommended in tracking clinical outcomes of cartilage repair procedures.

THE LESION

The characteristics of the cartilage lesion that is repaired have an important impact on the outcome after treatment. These characteristics should be documented in detail prior to surgery to allow an accurate evaluation of the results in light of what was actually treated. Lesion size, location, and character (i.e., whether the lesion involves only cartilage or cartilage plus bone) should also be determined because lesions involving subchondral bone generally require a more involved reconstruction.

The diagnosis will also have an important effect on treatment in many cases. Avascular necrosis leading to a cartilage problem will affect underlying subchondral bone and may be related to systemic health problems. Osteochondritis dissecans also involves the underlying subchondral bone and will often lead to large defects.

The alignment of the lower extremity can also affect outcome depending on the location of the lesion. Alignment is ideally evaluated radiographically using three foot-standing x-rays to determine the anatomical alignment and the mechanical axis. Other intra-articular problems must also be assessed. In general, if the opposing cartilage surface is degenerative, the patient would be diagnosed with arthritis, and cartilage resurfacing may not be appropriate. Therefore, the articular surface opposing the cartilage injury site as well as the articular surfaces elsewhere in the knee must be evaluated.

THE CARTILAGE REPAIR PROCEDURE

When evaluating the results of surgery, there are several factors that should be considered in addition to the actual type of operation performed. The indication for surgery should be documented. In general, the indication for surgery of this type is pain. However, if the indication is not pain and the surgeon is performing the operation to avoid future problems in the knee, this should be explicitly indicated. Prior procedures should also be documented. The postoperative rehabilitation may have an important influence on the outcome. Factors such as use of continuous passive motion, weight bearing and strengthening exercises, as well as the timing of their incorporation can affect the result of the procedure.

Clearly, the operating surgeon is critical in determining the clinical outcome following cartilage repair procedures. When considering cartilage repair procedures, the clinician should honestly assess his or her expertise regarding the specific surgery that is planned. Some methods, autologous chondrocyte implantation, for instance, are technically demanding, and poor technical execution can have a direct bearing on outcome and the need for subsequent procedures.

EVALUATION OF OUTCOME

Objective

There are several objective measures of outcome, such as physical examination, imaging, and tissue biopsy. Although these are generally important to the surgeon, they may not be of any relevance to the patient. Patients are generally more concerned with their symptoms and function. Nevertheless, objective measures are important and often give critical information.

Physical exam is a routine part of follow-up after surgery. For cartilage procedures about the knee, physical exam includes an evaluation of gait, pain on palpation, effusion, range of motion, and stability of the knee. Imaging is also an important part of the evaluation. Radiographs can demonstrate the progression of degenerative disease such as osteophytes, subchondral sclerosis, subchondral cysts, and joint space narrowing. Change in alignment may also be related to degenerative osteoarthritis. However, degenerative changes in the knee often occur over a prolonged period of time, and in the shorter term radiographs may not be relevant.

Magnetic resonance imaging (MRI) has been used as a noninvasive method to evaluate cartilage and cartilage repair *(3,4)*. Because of the direct multiplanar capability and the soft tissue contrast with MRI, the morphology of the cartilage can be assessed accurately. There are cartilage-sensitive sequences that allow the tissue to be distinguished from adjacent joint fluid as well as subchondral bone. The signal characteristics of the cartilage can then be determined to reflect its histopathological state. MRI is currently evolving, and in the present as well as the future, it is an important tool to evaluate cartilage repair in a noninvasive manner.

An evaluation of the repair tissue itself is useful to determine the quality. Routine histology as well as immunohistochemical evaluation have been performed *(5,6)*. Although the information gained by biopsy is valuable, many patients will not consent to this procedure. Despite the potential lack of patient interest in this approach, some authors have been able to evaluate patients with this methodology *(7)*.

Patient-Oriented Outcomes

Issues such as pain and function are of paramount importance to patients who are recovering from cartilage procedures. Symptoms and disabilities are generally evaluated using validated rating scales. There are many that have been published for use in this patient population *(8,9)*. The goal of using rating scales to measure patient outcome is to evaluate concepts that are critical to patients and to do so in a time-efficient manner. Therefore, relatively shorter questionnaires are preferred to limit responder burden.

It is ideal to obtain both a measure of region-specific function as well as an overall measure of health. The latter is usually evaluated using a generic health status instrument such as the Short Form (SF)-36. The SF-36 is a 36-item questionnaire that measures general health *(10–12)*. Its use has been encouraged in conjunction with knee-specific instruments for studies of patients with an injury of the anterior cruciate ligament (ACL) *(13)*. The SF-36 has both a physical component and a mental component summary scale that can be derived from the 36 questions. This instrument is relatively heavily weighted for lower extremity function and is therefore particularly useful for cartilage patients.

Of the available knee rating scales, several are discussed with respect to their usefulness for this patient population. The modified Lysolm scale *(1)* is an eight-item questionnaire that was initially designed to evaluate patients after knee ligament surgery. It has 25 points attributed to knee stability, 25 to pain, 15 to locking, 10 each to swelling and stair climbing, and 5 each to limp, use of support, and squatting. It has been used extensively for clinical research studies mainly for the ACL. However, it has been evaluated and found acceptable for chondral disorders of the knee *(14)*.

The activities of daily living (ADL) scale of the knee outcome survey is a useful instrument for cartilage patients, and we have distributed this questionnaire to evaluate patients at our institution *(15)*. It was developed based on a review of relevant instruments with clinician input. It is designed for patients with disorders of the knee ranging from ACL injury to osteoarthritis. Therefore, it is generally applicable to most cartilage patients. The questions range from relatively simple basic functions to more advanced activity. It has been found to have excellent psychometric properties *(9)*.

The International Knee Documentation Committee developed a rating scale for objective parameters related to knee function. These parameters include effusion, motion, ligament laxity, crepitus, harvest site pathology, radiographic findings, and one-leg-hop tests. Patients were given a grade of normal, nearly normal, abnormal, or severely abnormal for each. The lowest grade for a given group is the patient's final grade. The International Knee Documentation Committee has subsequently developed a questionnaire relating to subjective factors *(16)*. Although this questionnaire has not specifically been validated for patients with articular cartilage disorders, it is likely that it is a useful instrument.

The knee injury and osteoarthritis outcome score (KOOS) was developed using input from patients who underwent meniscal surgery in the past *(17)*. Five separate scores are calculated for pain, symptoms, ADLs, sport and recreational function, and knee-related quality of life. This scale is useful because the Western Ontario and McMaster University's (WOMAC) osteoarthritis index is incorporated into the KOOS *(18)*. The WOMAC involves 24 questions, with 5 relating to pain, 2 to stiffness, and 17 to difficulty with ADLs. The WOMAC is mainly for patients with lower extremity osteoarthritis and therefore can be useful for patients with cartilage disease. The KOOS is a wide-ranging scale because it not only applies to patients with degenerative disease, but also has questions about sport participation. This makes it an attractive alternative for evaluating outcome follow cartilage procedures.

The measurement of activity as a prognostic variable was discussed regarding patient factors. It is worthwhile to mention that this is a critical prognostic variable, and any investigator who chooses to evaluate outcome following cartilage procedures should choose an appropriate measure to evaluate this concept *(2)*.

CONCLUSION

In conclusion, there are a number of factors that affect outcome following cartilage surgery. The evidence available to support cartilage repair surgery is somewhat limited at the present time. However, there have been recent randomized controlled trials specifically comparing different treatment strategies. Surgeons who treat these lesions must be aware of the literature available and how the investigators elected to evaluate the outcome of their patients.

REFERENCES

1. Tegner Y, Lysholm J. Rating systems in the evaluation of knee ligament injuries. Clin Orthop 1985;198:43–49.
2. Marx RG, Stump TJ, Jones EC, Wickiewicz TL, Warren RF. Development and evaluation of an activity rating scale for disorders of the knee. Am J Sports Med 2001;29:213–218.
3. Potter HG, Linklater JM, Allen AA, Hannafin JA, Haas SB. Magnetic resonance imaging of articular cartilage in the knee. An evaluation with use of fast-spin-echo imaging. J Bone Joint Surg Am 1998;80:1276–1284.
4. Brown WE, Potter HG, Marx RG, Wickiewicz TL, Warren RF. Magnetic resonance imaging appearance of cartilage repair in the knee. Clin Orthop 2004;422:214–223.
5. Horas U, Pelinkovic D, Herr G, Aigner T, Schnettler R. Autologous chondrocyte implantation and osteochondral cylinder transplantation in cartilage repair of the knee joint. A prospective, comparative trial. J Bone Joint Surg Am 2003;85:185–192.
6. Knutsen G, Engebretsen L, Ludvigsen TC, et al. Autologous chondrocyte implantation compared with microfracture in the knee. A randomized trial. J Bone Joint Surg Am 2004;86:455–464.
7. Bentley G, Biant LC, Carrington RW, et al. A prospective, randomised comparison of autologous chondrocyte implantation vs mosaicplasty for osteochondral defects in the knee. J Bone Joint Surg Br 2003;85:223–230.
8. Marx RG. Knee rating scales. Arthroscopy 2003;19:1103–1108.
9. Marx RG, Jones EC, Allen AA, et al. Reliability, validity, and responsiveness of four knee outcome scales for athletic patients. J Bone Joint Surg Am 2001;83:1459–1469.
10. McHorney CA, Ware JE, Jr, Rogers W, Raczek AE, Lu JF. The validity and relative precision of MOS short- and long-form health status scales and Dartmouth COOP charts. Results from the Medical Outcomes Study. Med Care 1992;30(5 suppl):MS253–MS265.
11. McHorney CA, Ware JE, Jr, Raczek AE. The MOS 36-Item Short-Form Health Survey (SF-36): II. Psychometric and clinical tests of validity in measuring physical and mental health constructs. Med Care 1993;31:247–263.
12. Ware JE, Jr, Snow KK, Kosinski M, Gandek B. SF-36 Health Survey: Manual and Interpretation Guide. Boston: Health Institute, New England Medical Center; 1993.
13. Shapiro ET, Richmond JC, Rockett SE, McGrath MM, Donaldson WR. The use of a generic, patient-based health assessment (SF-36) for evaluation of patients with anterior cruciate ligament injuries. Am J Sports Med 1996;24:196–200.
14. Kocher MS, Steadman JR, Briggs KK, Sterett WI, Hawkins RJ. Reliability, validity, and responsiveness of the Lysholm knee scale for various chondral disorders of the knee. J Bone Joint Surg Am 2004;86:1139–1145.
15. Irrgang JJ, Snyder-Mackler L, Wainner RS, Fu FH, Harner CD. Development of a patient-reported measure of function of the knee. J Bone Joint Surg Am 1998;80:1132–1145.
16. Irrgang JJ, Anderson AF, Boland AL, et al. Development and validation of the international knee documentation committee subjective knee form. Am J Sports Med 2001;29:600–613.
17. Roos EM, Roos HP, Lohmander LS, Ekdahl C, Beynnon BD. Knee Injury and Osteoarthritis Outcome Score (KOOS)—development of a self-administered outcome measure. J Orthop Sports Phys Ther 1998;28:88–96.
18. Bellamy N, Kaloni S, Pope J, Coulter K, Campbell J. Quantitative rheumatology: a survey of outcome measurement procedures in routine rheumatology outpatient practice in Canada. J Rheumatol 1998;25:852–858.

3

MRI and Articular Cartilage

Evaluating Lesions and Postrepair Tissue

Hollis G. Potter, MD, Li F. Foo, MD, and Andrew D. Pearle, MD

Summary

The ability of noninvasive magnetic resonance imaging (MRI) to obtain reproducible, accurate images of cartilage has enabled early detection of cartilage lesions and provides clinically relevant information when planning cartilage repair. With appropriate pulse sequencing, MRI depicts not only the integrity of the surface cartilage, which would be seen at arthroscopy, but also that of the subchondral bone, which would not be visualized at arthroscopic inspection. This information is vital when planning for complex, sometimes multistage, techniques that require careful size delineation of the cartilage lesion and evaluation of the surrounding subchondral bone. In addition to aiding in preoperative planning, these techniques offer an important objective evaluation of cartilage repair to be correlated with the more subjective clinical outcome instruments and provide insight into the biology of the repair process. Finally, newer matrix assessment techniques will disclose information about the ultrastructure of these individual cartilage repair procedures.

Key Words: Cartilage; cartilage repair; MRI; T_2 mapping.

CARTILAGE IMAGING TECHNIQUES

Arguably one of the greatest contributions that magnetic resonance imaging (MRI) has made in the past decade has been the ability to assess articular cartilage noninvasively and accurately. Despite the increasing availability of sophisticated imaging techniques, conventional radiographs remain the mainstay for assessment of the joint space. It is important to remember that conventional radiographs do not directly depict the articular cartilage but instead provide an indirect measure of cartilage loss. For the knee, a typical initial imaging assessment includes an anteroposterior standing view as well as a posteroanterior semiflexed (30–60°) view, with the latter best suited to assess the posterior margin of the joint space, where cartilage is often initially degraded. Additional lateral and Merchant views are helpful for assessing patellofemoral alignment and joint space. Full hip-to-ankle anteroposterior views are essential when planning for cartilage repair, in order to assess the true mechanical axis of the limb.

Although radiographs remain the standard for this initial assessment, MRI is rapidly supplanting standardized techniques because of its ability to visualize articular cartilage directly and accurately, allowing for accurate, reproducible measurements of cartilage thickness and assessment of morphologic changes over time. MRI is superior to both conventional radiographs and computed tomography because of its direct multiplanar capabilities and superior soft tissue contrast. As such, MRI allows for the detection of isolated full-thickness cartilage

From: *Cartilage Repair Strategies*
Edited by: Riley J. Williams © Humana Press Inc., Totowa, NJ

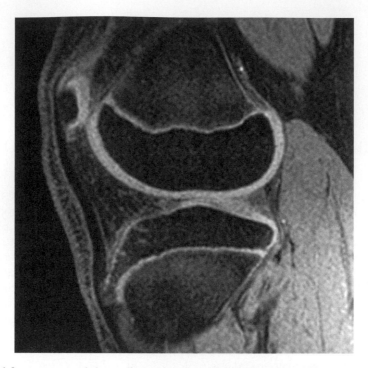

Fig. 1. Sagittal fat-suppressed three-dimensional gradient echo magnetic resonance imaging of the knee in an 11-yr-old boy demonstrates high contrast between the low signal intensity bone and the bright articular and physeal cartilage.

defects; these defects are typically imperceptible on conventional radiographs because of the preservation of joint space and integrity of the subchondral bone.

Many magnetic resonance (MR) pulse sequences are available for assessment of cartilage. It is important to remember that traditional spin echo techniques, including T_1-weighted sequences, are ineffective in assessing cartilage because of the often poor in-plane resolution and tissue contrast *(1,2)*. In particular, on T_1-weighted techniques for which the fatty signal of the cancellous bone is bright, cartilage is poorly differentiated from the surrounding soft tissue as both cartilage and fluid maintain intermediate-to-lower signal intensity. The first validated cartilage pulse sequences (using arthroscopy as a standard) were the three-dimensional (3D) fat-suppressed gradient echo techniques, allowing for very high contrast between the low signal intensity of the suppressed cancellous bone and the high signal intensity of the surrounding cartilage (Fig. 1). Several studies have utilized these techniques with sensitivity ranging between 81 and 93% and specificity ranging between 94 and 97% *(3,4)*.

Volumetric gradient-recalled techniques, particularly when obtained with square voxels, are more amenable to automatic segmentation and volume quantification methods, allowing for 3D assessment of cartilage volume and thickness *(5)*. These techniques have been validated utilizing both clinical and nonclinical models with good degrees of reproducibility *(6)*. These gradient echo techniques, however, are lengthy and subject to susceptibility artifact generated by the metallic debris left by arthroscopy or the presence of instrumentation that may accompany cartilage repair techniques. They are also less sensitive to surface fibrillation.

In an attempt to validate a pulse sequence that was not subject to these limitations, Potter et al. evaluated 88 patients with a fast spin echo (FSE) technique, using arthroscopy as the

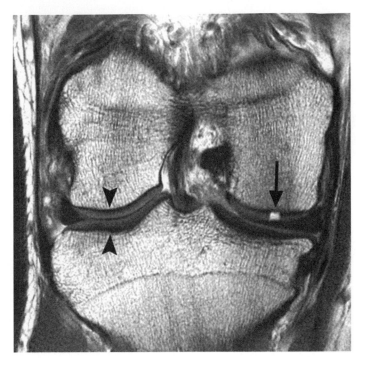

Fig. 2. Coronal fast spin echo magnetic resonance imaging of the knee in a 27-yr-old man demonstrates good gray scale stratification of cartilage (arrowheads) over the lateral compartment with relative low signal intensity in the basilar components. Note the full-thickness cartilage defect over the medial femoral condyle (arrow) without alteration in the signal of the subchondral bone.

standard, and found 87% sensitivity, 94% specificity, and an overall accuracy of 92% (Fig. 2). Interobserver variability was minimal, as indicated by a weighted κ statistic of 0.93 *(7)*. Potter et al.'s study utilized a relatively high in-plane resolution, non-fat-suppressed moderate echo time (TE) pulse sequence utilizing an effective TE of 34 ms, providing differential contrast between synovial fluid, fibrocartilage, and articular cartilage *(7)*.

Soon after, Bredella et al., utilizing fat-suppressed FSE with arthroscopy as the standard, achieved a 94% sensitivity, 99% specificity, and 93% accuracy for detecting cartilage lesions. In this study, the observer variability was not assessed *(8)*. Reproducibility of cartilage evaluation using MRI is important, particularly if imaging of cartilage is intended to serve as a more objective outcome assessment of repair techniques.

Additional pulse sequences have become available in recent years, including 3D driven equilibrium Fourier transfer (DEFT) technique, providing high contrast between cartilage and synovial fluid *(9)*. Yoshioka et al., in a study of 28 patients, noted that the fat-suppressed 3D DEFT images showed the highest fluid-to-cartilage contrast; however, interobserver agreement was highest on the fat-suppressed FSE short TE sequences *(10)*. The choice of imaging parameters and pulse sequence should be made not only based on individual experience, but also reliance on a previously validated cartilage score. Cartilage lesions should ideally be confirmed in two planes of imaging.

Evaluation of cartilage has also been performed at different field strengths. Woertler et al. studied 50 knee specimens at both 0.18 and 1.0 T using a variety of pulse sequences; they found that the high-field system demonstrated significantly better diagnostic performance

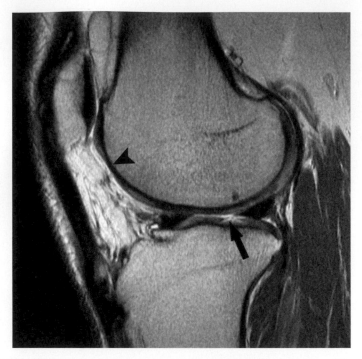

Fig. 3. Sagittal fast spin echo magnetic resonance imaging of the knee in a 50-yr-old man at 0.7 T demonstrates nondisplaced cartilage flap formation (arrow) down to subchondral bone over the central lateral tibial plateau. Also note the high-grade cartilage wear over the trochlea (arrowhead).

using 3D pulse sequences (compared to low-field strength images) when detecting high-grade partial-thickness cartilage lesions *(11)*. The development of higher-field open units, however, has provided the ability to obtain a higher signal-to-noise and superior in-plane resolution compared with standardized low-field strength open constructs (Fig. 3). With increased availability of higher (3T) field strengths, higher in-plane resolution is available, enabling detection of focal cartilage lesions not previously seen at lower field strengths (Fig. 4).

CARTILAGE IMAGING BEYOND MORPHOLOGY: NONINVASIVE INSIGHT INTO STRUCTURE

The signal properties of articular cartilage are dependent on many factors, including the pulse sequence utilized, the cellular composition of collagen, proteoglycans and water, and the orientation of the collagen in the different laminae of cartilage. MRI is purported to be an anatomic study; however, the signal characteristics of the tissue at any point in time reflect their histopathological state. A comparison between MR findings and pathological change as well as a modified Outerbridge classification is provided in Table 1; a non-fat-suppressed FSE sequence was used for the comparison *(12)*.

Although morphological imaging of cartilage and cartilage repair is important, most clinical, standardized cartilage-sensitive pulse sequences do not provide sufficient information to reveal early degenerative changes in the matrix of cartilage *(13)*.

To appreciate the ability of newer MRI techniques, a brief description of cartilage structure is necessary. Hyaline cartilage functions as a low-friction, wear-resistant tissue designed

Table 1
MRI Pathologic/Arthroscopic Correlation

Pathologic change	MRI findings	Modified Outerbridge Classification (12)
Chondral softening	Increased signal in articular cartilage	Grade 1: softening to probe
Fissures/blistering	Linear to ovoid foci of increased signal affecting <50% thickness	Grade 2: fissures/ fibrillation involving <50% thickness
Moderate surface fibrillation	Irregular surface change affecting >50% thickness	Grade 3: fissures/ fibrillation involving >50% thickness
Ulceration to subchondral bone	Surface flap extending to bone Complete loss of articular cartilage	Grade 4: exposed subchondral bone

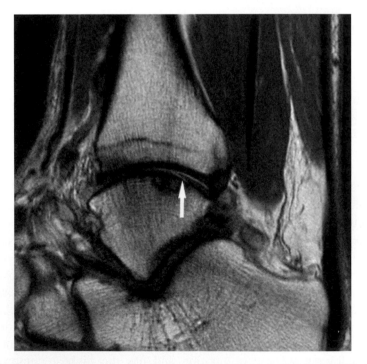

Fig. 4. Sagittal fast spin echo magnetic resonance imaging of the ankle in a 48-yr-old man at 3 T demonstrates osteochondral lesion of the talar dome with cystic change and sclerosis. Flap formation in the adjacent talar articular cartilage is also seen posteriorly (arrow). High-field cartilage imaging is particularly helpful for depicting subtle lesions in areas where cartilage is intrinsically thin.

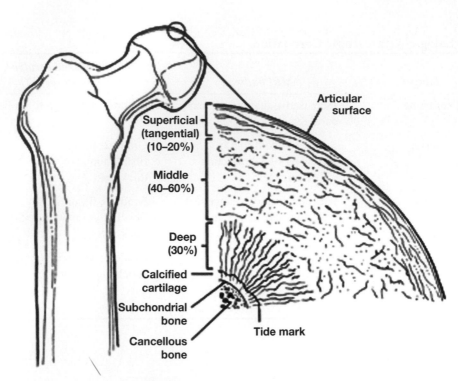

Superficial
(tangential)
(10–20%)

Middle
(40–60%)

Deep
(30%)

Calcified
cartilage

Subchondral
bone

Cancellous
bone

Articular
surface

Tide mark

Fig. 5. Schematic diagram of cartilage zonal histology. (Reproduced with permission from ref. *33*.)

to bear and distribute loads. The major components of the articular cartilage are water, type II collagen, and large aggregating proteoglycans. Water, the most abundant component of articular cartilage *(14)*, is contained within the interstitial space created by a solid matrix consisting of proteoglycan laced in collagen. This abundance of water makes articular cartilage well suited for study with clinical MRI, which tracks the distribution and mobility of water. The mixture of fluid and matrix provides hyaline cartilage with viscoelastic and mechanical properties for efficient load distribution.

Cartilage has an organized layered structure that can be functionally and structurally divided into four zones: the superficial zone, the middle (or transitional) zone, the deep zone, and the zone of calcified cartilage (Fig. 5). The superficial zone is the articulating surface that provides a smooth gliding surface and resists shear. Also known as the tangential zone, this zone makes up approx 10–20% of articular cartilage thickness. Of all the zones, it has the highest collagen content; the collagen fibrils in the superficial zone are densely packed and have a highly ordered alignment parallel to the articular surface *(15)*. The middle zone encompasses 40–60% of the articular cartilage volume. This zone has a higher compressive modulus than the superficial zone and a less-organized arrangement of the collagen fibers. The collagen fibrils of the middle zone are thicker and more loosely packed and have an oblique alignment to the surface. The deep zone makes up 30% of the cartilage and consist of large-diameter collagen fibrils oriented perpendicular to the articular surface. This layer contains the highest proteoglycan and lowest water concentration and has the highest compressive modulus. The tidemark separates the deep zone from the calcified cartilage, which rests directly on the subchondral bone. The calcified cartilage contains small cells in a chondroid matrix speckled with apatitic salts *(15)*.

The signal characteristics of cartilage reflect this highly ordered structure. The majority of the signal emitted from cartilage is accounted for by the free water; however, there is also water that is bound electrostatically to proteoglycan (based on its negative charge) and water associated with the collagen fibers within the macrostructure. More recent MRI techniques can detect alterations in those water pools normally bound by these matrix elements. For assessment of proteoglycan, sodium MRI may be used. The vast majority of clinical MRI uses hydrogen spectroscopy because of its copious concentration in soft tissue. When the excitational radio frequency is peaked on a suitable sodium species (^{23}Na), the relative fixed charge density of cartilage may be evaluated, which is a function of the spatial resolution of charged proteoglycans *(16)*. However, the lower concentration of sodium as well as additional variables make clinical imaging of ^{23}Na difficult, requiring extensive scanning times to achieve adequate signal and requiring specialized coils *(17)*.

Another imaging technique that is able to assess the proteoglycan content of cartilage tissues involves delayed gadolinium-enhanced MRI. This method involves the intravenous injection of a negatively charged salt of a gadolinium MR contrast agent, which in appropriate dosages acts to shorten T_1 relaxation times. Following joint exercise (there is a delay of ~90 min), contrast material diffuses into the cartilage, with distribution based on fixed charged density, indirectly providing a method of tracking areas of depletion of negatively charged glycosaminoglycans *(18)*.

This technique was used in a preliminary study of nine patients who underwent autologous cartilage transplantation (10 grafts). In this study, the authors demonstrated that at more than 12-mo follow-up, transplanted graft articular cartilage had glycosaminoglycan levels that were comparable to adjacent and remote articular cartilage *(19)*. Additional clinical work is necessary to determine the potential of this method in assessing postrepair tissue, specifically the effect of periosteal hypertrophy and hypertrophic synovium (phenomena associated with autologous chondrocyte implantation) on the relative diffusion characteristics of gadolinium salts. Overall, the delayed gadolinium-enhanced MRI technique appears to be promising for assessment of cartilage repair.

A correlation between fixed charged density (reflecting the negatively charged glycosaminoglycans) and $T_{1\rho}$ has been demonstrated in bovine and human explants. These techniques may prove effective in detecting early proteoglycan changes in osteoarthritis and may prove applicable to a clinical cohort of cartilage repair *(20)*.

To assess the collagen component of the extracellular matrix, T_2 mapping has been utilized. T_2 relaxation time is a quantifiable, reproducible MR parameter that reflects the internuclear dephasing that occurs as a result of transverse relaxation of the excited hydrogen dipoles. In the radial zone of articular cartilage, where the collagen is highly organized and perpendicular to the subchondral plate, there is a relative restriction of water; this restriction causes the shorter T_2 relaxation times encountered in this region. In the transitional zone, where the collagen is more randomly oriented, the T_2 values are prolonged, accounting for the higher signal intensity noted, afforded by the relative increased mobility of water (Fig. 6; *see* Color Plate 2, following p. 206). At clinical field strengths of 1.5–3.0 T, the superficial zone cannot be discerned from the transitional zone. Similarly, the low signal intensity line demarcating the cancellous bone from the cartilage reflects both the calcified bone and the subchondral plate, both of which demonstrate very short T_2 values and low signal intensity on all MR pulse sequences.

Studies using high-field microscopy units have disclosed that the spatial variation of T_2 relaxation times reflects collagen architecture. Nieminen et al. studied bovine osteochondral plugs at 9.4 T and demonstrated a linear positive correlation between T_2 relaxation times and

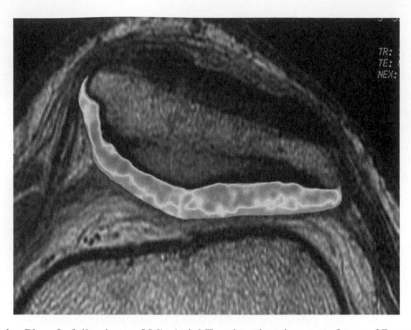

Fig. 6 (Color Plate 2, following p. 206). Axial T_2 relaxation time map from a 27-yr-old man with chronic patellofemoral overload. The color map is coded to capture T_2 values ranging from 5 to 100 ms, with green reflecting longer T_2 values, yellow intermediate, and orange shorter values. Note the stratification of T_2 with shorter values in the radial zone but with foci of prolonged T_2 over the apex and lateral facet because of breakdown in the collagen component in the matrix.

birefringence noted on polarized light microscopy *(21)*. Similarly, Xia et al. studied cartilage samples from the canine shoulder. These authors demonstrated a laminar appearance for all tissue samples, and the T_2 characteristics were statistically equivalent to the histological zones based on collagen fiber orientation for the superficial, transitional, and radial zones *(22)*.

The angular dependence of T_2 relaxation, as seen in articular cartilage, is a reflection of the "magic angle effect." Some components of cartilage are highly ordered, and there is a well-defined relationship between the spinning dipoles within the collagen and the axis of the magnetic field. This relationship reflects the angular anisotropy of the hydrogen dipoles. When the angle between the external field and the dipoles reaches 55°, there is a prolongation of T_2 relaxation time. Recognition of this phenomenon is important as this demonstrates the highly ordered orientation of the collagen in this zone. Further support for this has been demonstrated at high-field microscopy systems *(23)*.

In the clinical setting, some controversy has arisen regarding which zone demonstrates the greatest degree of angular dependence *(24)*. Regional variations in the orientation of the individual components within the cartilage structure over a curved joint surface comprise a complex three-dimensional architectural arrangement that may account for further alterations in the observed clinical T_2 mapping of articular cartilage *(25)*. In addition, care should be utilized in the selection of pulse sequences to acquire the data for T_2 quantification. Although it is more efficient to use a multiecho, multislice sequence to obtain more rapid acquisition of data and joint coverage, caution should be utilized when evaluating the slice profile as added T_1 contrast may result in substantial inaccuracy in T_2 values *(26)*. Despite these issues, the T_2 mapping technique should ultimately allow for the characterization of cartilage repair tissue.

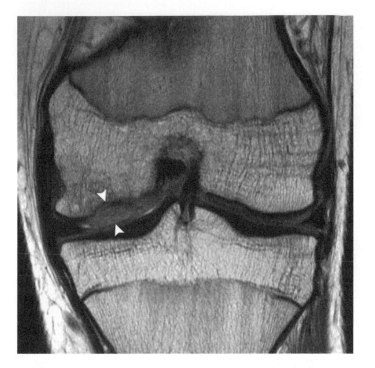

Fig. 7. Coronal fast spin echo magnetic resonance imaging of the knee in a 15-yr-old boy as performed 3 mo following autologous chondrocyte implantation for an osteochondral lesion over the medial femoral condyle; the image demonstrates covering repair cartilage that is slightly proud and hyperintense relative to native cartilage, in keeping with hypertrophy of the periosteal graft (arrowheads).

MRI OF CARTILAGE REPAIR

When evaluating repair cartilage by MRI, multiple variables should be considered. An MRI assessment system for microfracture and autologous cartilage transplantation utilized by Brown et al. studied (1) the relative signal intensity from the repair cartilage compared with the native cartilage (as assessed on a standardized MR workstation using region of interest analysis); (2) morphology (flush, proud, or depressed) with respect to the native cartilage; (3) delamination (in the setting of autologous chondrocyte implantation [ACI]); (4) nature of the interface (presence, absence, or size of fissures) with the adjacent native surface; and (5) percentage fill of the lesion by thirds, using both coronal and sagittal images *(27)*. In addition, the status of the cartilage in the adjacent and opposite articular surfaces should be assessed, particularly in those lesions that may undergo hypertrophy of either the repair cartilage or subchondral bone.

With appropriate in-plane resolution and tissue contrast, MRI may serve as an important objective outcome measure that can be correlated to the subjective (but equally important) clinical assessment of cartilage repair. Brown et al. studied 180 MR examinations obtained in 112 patients who had cartilage-resurfacing techniques, including microfracture and ACI, at a mean of 15 and 13 mo following surgery, respectively. In this observational study, ACI demonstrated consistently better filling at all times compared with microfracture; however, graft hypertrophy was noted in 63% of the lesions *(27)*. The presence of periosteal hypertrophy does account for moderate morbidity and postprocedure debridement, particularly with osteochondritis dissecans (OCD) lesions, likely because of the lack of containment in the intercondylar notch (Fig. 7).

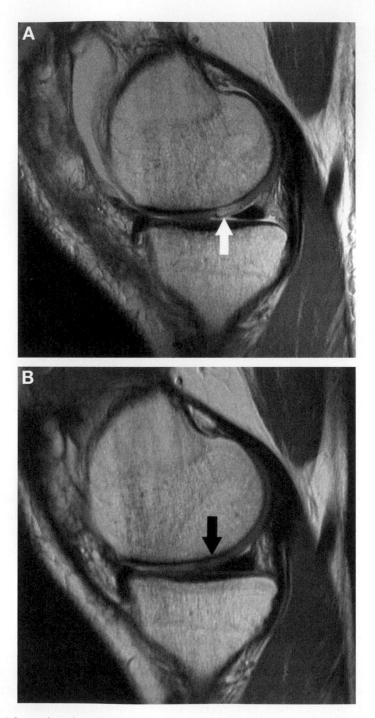

Fig. 8. Sagittal fast spin echo magnetic resonance imaging of the knee in a 31-yr-old man obtained following autologous cartilage implantation. At 6 wk following surgery (**A**), the graft is hyperintense with an intact, hypointense overlying periosteal cover (arrow). At 20 mo following surgery (**B**), there is incorporation of periosteum to now isointense reparative cartilage, such that periosteal cover is no longer distinct (arrow).

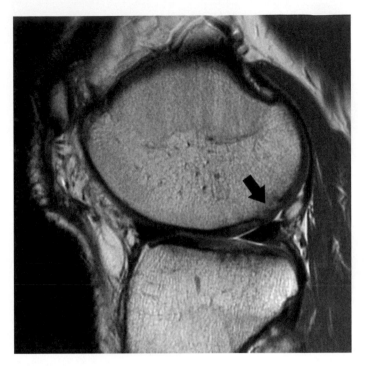

Fig. 9. Sagittal fast spin echo magnetic resonance imaging of the knee in an 18-yr-old man. The image was performed 6 mo following microfracture and demonstrates overgrowth of subchondral bone (arrow) and thin overlying reparative fibrocartilage. Note the hyperintense native cartilage at the anterior interface as well as over the opposite tibial plateau, where there is also deformity of the subchondral plate.

MRIs that are performed early following ACI typically demonstrate hyperintense repair cartilage. This tissue is usually contained by a hypointense periosteum that appears as a separate structure; a more isointense signal is the characteristic appearance over time following the procedure (Fig. 8A,B). The presence of fluid intensity signal between the transplant and the subchondral bone indicates partial or complete repair delamination. In one study, the partial or complete delamination of the periosteal graft was noted in almost half of the transplants, all within the first year following surgery *(27)*. Similarly, Alparslan et al. noted that delamination was most commonly encountered within the first 6 mo following ACI; this was denoted by linear fluid intensity between the repair tissue and subchondral bone *(28)*.

The appearance of the interface between repair and native cartilage is an important feature, and MRI provides an effective way to assess this peripheral integration. Verstraete et al. noted progressive peripheral integration in ACI cartilage with native cartilage. These authors found T_2-weighted images useful for differentiating persistent cartilage defects from maturing cartilage, the latter of which is of lower signal intensity compared to the hyperintense joint fluid *(29)*. They further noted that bone marrow edema progressively disappears, but had been noted to last up to as much as a year following ACI, and that complete edge integration of the transplanted cartilage was noted to take up to 2 yr, denoted as the lack of fluid signal intensity between native and implanted cartilage *(29)*. The ability to assess peripheral integration is largely a function of imaging technique and

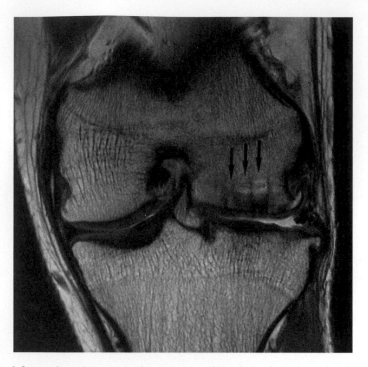

Fig. 10. Coronal fast spin echo magnetic resonance imaging of the knee in a 21-yr-old man. The image was taken 4 mo following mosaicplasty and demonstrates multiple plugs used to restore a large osteochondral defect affecting the lateral femoral condyle (arrows). Although there is good restoration of subchondral bony contour, there is thinning of the overlying cartilage. Note the moderate cartilage wear in the peripheral margin of the lateral tibial plateau.

high in-plane (pixel size), and out-of-plane (slice thickness) resolution is necessary to evaluate the interface comprehensively.

The signal properties of microfracture vary with the time interval between surgery and imaging. The initial signal characteristics of reparative fibrocartilage are largely hyperintense compared to native cartilage; however, variable amounts of isointensity to hypointensity can be observed *(27)*. Alsparslan et al. demonstrated the early appearance of thin, 29 signal intensity repair cartilage in a treated defect with bone marrow edema in the subchondral bone; this early tissue formation was followed by progressive filling of the defect and diminution of the bone marrow edema pattern *(30)*. Brown et al. noted overgrowth of subchondral bone in 42 of 86 microfractures studied; this resulted in thinning of the overlying reparative fibrocartilage *(27)* (Fig. 9).

In a prospective evaluation of 48 patients treated with microfracture and evaluated by both validated outcome instruments, subjective clinical rating and cartilage-sensitive MRI, bony overgrowth was noted on MRI in 25% of patients; however, the presence of bony overgrowth did not have any negative effect on outcome scores *(31)*. In this study, the fill percentage of the repaired defect correlated with knee function scores: All knees with good fill demonstrated improved knee function, and poor fill grade was associated with limited clinical improvement and a decrease in functional scores after 24 mo *(31)*. The signal characteristics of the repair tissue following microfracture were hyperintense compared to normal cartilage; this finding is consistent with less-organized cartilage repair *(27,31)*.

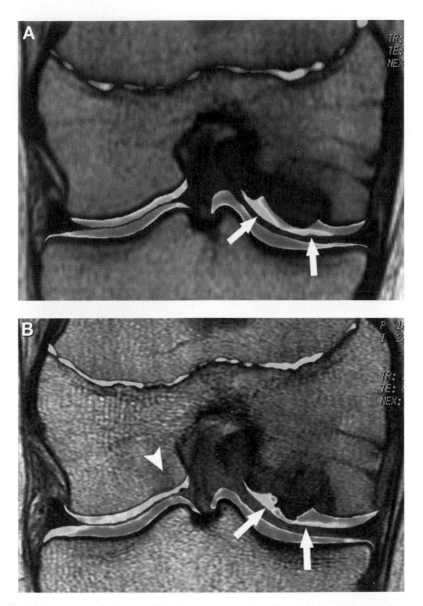

Fig. 11 (Color Plate 1, following p. 206). Coronal T_2 relaxation time maps of the femorotibial articular cartilage of a 13-yr-old girl with osteochondritis dissecans (OCD). The color maps are coded to capture T_2 values ranging from 5 to 100 ms, with green and blue reflecting longer T_2 values, yellow intermediate, and orange shorter values. Preoperative image **(A)** demonstrates a normal lateral compartment with the expected stratification of T_2 values. Note prolongation of T_2 relaxation times at the margins of the osteochondral lesion, affecting the inner margin medial femoral condyle (arrows). At 3 mo following mosaicplasty **(B)**, with harvest of autologous osteochondral plugs from the lateral margin of the intercondylar notch, there is prolongation of T_2 values at the donor site (arrowhead), reflecting the reparative fibrocartilage (and less-organized matrix) that covers this site. Also note persistent prolongation of T_2 values at the margins of the plugs (arrows). There is an intact appearance (albeit with reduced thickness) in the cartilage over the central, slightly proud plug.

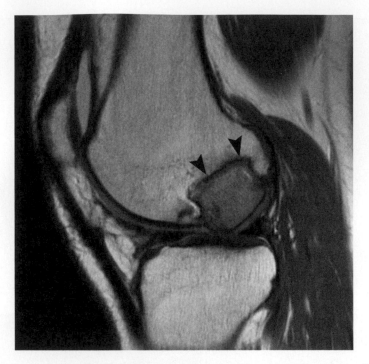

Fig. 12. Sagittal fast spin echo magnetic resonance imaging of the knee in a 33-yr-old woman obtained 20 mo following fresh osteochondral allograft placement for osteonecrosis of the lateral femoral condyle. The fresh osteochondral allograft is proud, with an anterior offset of 7 mm regarding the subchondral plate. There is a low signal intensity line on the recipient side, indicating sclerosis, reactive fibrous interface, and relatively poor allograft incorporation.

Mithoefer et al. noted definable fissures between native and repair cartilage in 96% of microfracture repairs studied *(31)*. Integration is also an issue with osteochondral allografts or autografts (mosaicplasty). In a canine model, Glen et al. noted no statistically significant difference between fresh osteochondral autograft and allografts with respect to bony incorporation, articular cartilage composition, and biomechanical properties up to 6 mo postimplantation, as discerned by histology indentation testing, cartilage-sensitive MRI, and spin echo T_2 mapping *(32)*. Of 36 plugs, 32 were noted to have a cleft between the graft and the host articular surfaces on MRI, and 90% of specimens (both autograft and allograft) demonstrated a cleft on histologic examination *(32)*. Thus, despite good incorporation of the autologous plug into subchondral bone, a persistent cleft existed at the interface, suggesting a lack of peripheral integration and secondary evidence that articular cartilage is unable to regenerate across a physical gap *(32)*.

Peripheral integration is of interest in the clinical arena as well, particularly when multiple plugs are required to restore a defect in bone and cartilage, often created by OCD or avascular necrosis (Fig. 10). MRI detects not only the effective restoration of the radius of curvature of the subchondral bone, but also the degree of congruency that is created on the articular surface. The latter is of significance in that second-look arthroscopy would only visualize the "tip of the iceberg" and will not allow direct visualization of osseous integration of subchondral plate. With the benefit of concomitant T_2 mapping, it is possible to assess not only the morphology of integration but also the signal characteristics and

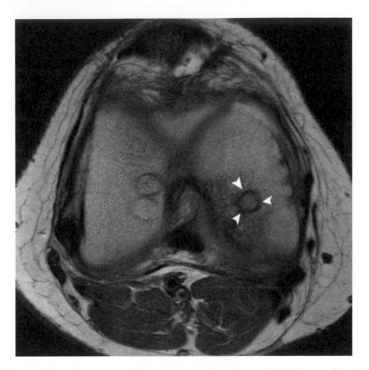

Fig. 13. Axial fast spin echo magnetic resonance imaging of the knee of a 13-yr-old girl. The image was obtained 3 mo following mosaicplasty and demonstrates consolidation of trabeculae around the plug (arrowheads) as a result of the "press fit" fixation.

stratification of expected T_2 relaxation times as they reflect the collagen component of the matrix in both the repair cartilage and the host interface (Fig. 11; *see* Color Plate 1, following p. 206).

When evaluating osteochondral autograft or allografts, additional assessment of the degree of trabecular incorporation should be performed. This requires the use of moderately high in-plane resolution imaging to assess the trabeculae crossing the graft–host interface. The signal characteristics of the osteochondral plug should also be assessed, with the ideal graft demonstrating fatty signal characteristics. The presence of low-signal intensity on all pulse sequences is highly suggestive of a failure of graft incorporation and, in some cases, correlates to bony necrosis (Fig. 12). It is our experience that fresh osteochondral allografts have distinctly different MR signal properties compared to frozen allografts. At our institution, the majority of osteochondral allografts are implanted using a "press fit" fixation; as such, there may be some consolidation of trabeculae adjacent to the plug. This finding should not be mistaken as a failure of osseous integration between the host and donor bone (Fig. 13).

CONCLUSION

Comprehensive imaging of cartilage repair requires standardized plain radiographs for the assessment of axial alignment as well as preoperative MRI to assess the appearance of the lesion and surrounding subchondral bone noninvasively. MRI can prospectively assess the repair for delamination or incorporation, providing an important correlation to more subjective clinical outcome instruments. Finally, newer matrix assessment techniques that target either proteoglycan or collagen in the matrix of cartilage repair will provide important information about structure; in time, this is hoped to obviate the need for second-look biopsy and violation of the repair site.

REFERENCES

1. Hayes CW, Conway WF. Evaluation of articular cartilage: radiographic and cross-sectional imaging techniques. Radiographics 1992;12:409–428.
2. Hayes CW, Sawyer RW, Conway WF. Patellar cartilage lesions: in vitro detection and staging with MR imaging and pathologic correlation. Radiology 1990;176:479–483.
3. Recht MP, Piraino DW, Paletta GA, Schils JP, Belhobek GH. Accuracy of fat-suppressed three-dimensional spoiled gradient-echo FLASH MR imaging in the detection of patellofemoral articular cartilage abnormalities. Radiology 1996;198:209–212.
4. Disler DG, McCauley TR, Wirth CR, Fuchs MD. Detection of knee hyaline cartilage defects using fat-suppressed three-dimensional spoiled gradient-echo MR imaging: Comparison with standard MR imaging and correlation with arthroscopy. Am J Roentgenol 1995;165:377–382.
5. Eckstein F, Westhoff J, Sittek H, et al. In vivo reproducibility of three-dimensional cartilage volume and thickness measurements with MR imaging. Am J Roentgenol 1998;170:593–597.
6. Eckstein F, Schnier M, Haubner M, et al. Accuracy of cartilage volume and thickness measurements with magnetic resonance imaging. Clin Orthop Rel Res 1998;352:137–148.
7. Potter HG, Linklater JM, Allen AA, Hannafin JA, Haas SB. Magnetic resonance imaging of articular cartilage in the knee. An evaluation with use of fast spin echo imaging. J Bone Joint Surg 1998;80A:1276–1284.
8. Bredella MA, Tirman PFJ, Peterfy CG, et al. Accuracy of T_2-weighted fast spin-echo MR imaging with fat saturation in detecting cartilage defects in the knee: comparison with arthroscopy in 130 patients. Am J Roentgenol 1999;172:1073–1080.
9. Hargreaves BA, Gold GE, Lang PK, et al. MR imaging of articular cartilage using driven equilibrium. Magn Reson Med 1999;42:695–703.
10. Yoshioka H, Stevens K, Hargreaves BA, et al. Magnetic resonance imaging of articular cartilage of the knee: comparison between fat-suppressed three-dimensional SPGR imaging, fat-suppressed FSE imaging and fat-suppressed three-dimensional DEFT imaging, and correlation with arthroscopy. J Magn Reson Imaging 2004;20:857–864.
11. Woertler K, Strothmann M, Tombach B, Reimer P. Detection of articular cartilage lesions: Experimental evaluation of low- and high-field-strength MR imaging at 0.18 and 1.0T. J Magn Reson Imaging 2000;11:678–685.
12. Outerbridge RE, Dunlop JAY. The problem of chondromalacia patellae. Clin Orthop Rel Res 1975;110:177–195.
13. Rubenstein JD, Li JG, Majumdar S, Henkelman RM. Image resolution and signal-to-noise ratio requirements for MR imaging of degenerative cartilage. Am J Roentgenol 1997;169:1089–1096.
14. Mankin HJ, Mow VC, Buckwalter JA, Iannotti JB, Ratcliffe A. Articular cartilage structure, composition and function. In: Buckwalter JA, Einhorn TA, Simon SR, eds. Orthopaedic Basic Science: Biology and Biomechanics of the Musculoskeletal System. Rosemont, IL: American Academy of Orthopaedic Surgeons; 1999:440–470.
15. Mow VC, Proctor CS, Kelly MA. Biomechanics of articular cartilage. In: Nordin M, Frankel VH, eds. Basic Biomechanics of the Musculoskeletal System. Philadelphia: Lea and Febiger; 1989:31–57.
16. Shapiro EM, Borthakur A, Gougoutas A. Reddy. ^{23}Na MRI accurately measures fixed charge density in articular cartilage. Magn Reson Med 2002;47:284–291.
17. Gold GE, McCauley TR, Gray ML, Disler DG. What's new in cartilage? Radiographics 2003;23: 1227–1242.
18. Bashir A, Gray ML, Burstein D. Gd-DTPA^{2-} as a measure of cartilage degradation. Magn Reson Med 1996;36:665–673.

19. Gillis A, Bashir A, McKeon B, Scheller A, Gray ML, Burstein D. Magnetic resonance imaging of relative glycosaminoglycan distribution in patients with autologous chondrocyte transplants. Invest Radiol 2001;36:743–748.
20. Wheaton AJ, Casey FL, Gougoutas AJ, et al. Correlation of $T_{1\rho}$ with fixed charge density in cartilage. J Magn Reson Imaging 2004;20:519–525.
21. Nieminen MT, Rieppo J, Töyräs J, et al. T_2 relaxation reveals spatial collagen architecture in articular cartilage: A comparative quantitative MRI and polarized light microscopic study. Magn Reson Med 2001;46:487–493.
22. Xia Y, Moody JB, Burton-Wurster N, Lust G. Quantitative in situ correlation between microscopic MRI and polarized light microscopy studies of articular cartilage. Osteoarthritis Cartilage 2001;9:393–406.
23. Xia Y, Moody JB, Alhadlaq H. Orientational dependence of T_2 relaxation in articular cartilage: microscopic MRI (μMRI) study. Magn Reson Med 2002;48:460–469.
24. Mosher TJ, Smith H, Dardzinski BJ, Schmithorst VJ, Smith MB. MR imaging and T_2 mapping of femoral cartilage: In vivo determination of the magic angle effect. Am J Roentgenol 2001; 177:665–669.
25. Goodwin DW, Wadghiri Z, Zhu H, Vinton CJ, Smith ED, Dunn JF. Macroscopic structure of articular cartilage of the tibial plateau: influence of a characteristic matrix architecture on MRI appearance. Am J Roentgenol 2004;182:311–318.
26. Maier CF, Tan SG, Hariharan H, Potter HG. T_2 quantitation of articular cartilage at 1.5T. J Magn Reson Imaging 2003;17:358–364.
27. Brown WE, Potter HG, Marx RG, Wickiewicz TL, Warren RF. Magnetic resonance imaging appearance of cartilage repair in the knee. Clin Orthop Rel Res 2004;422:214–223.
28. Alparslan L, Minas T, Winalski CS. Magnetic resonance imaging of autologous chondrocyte implantation. Semin Ultrasound CT MRI 2001;22:341–351.
29. Verstraete KL, Almqvist F, Verdonk P, et al. Magnetic resonance imaging of cartilage and cartilage repair. Clin Radiol 2004;59:674–689.
30. Alparslan L, Winalski CS, Boutin RD, Minas T. Postoperative magnetic resonance imaging of articular cartilage repair. Semin Musculoskelet Radiol 2001;5:345–363.
31. Mithoefer K, Williams RJ, Warren RF, et al. Prospective evaluation of the microfracture technique for treatment of articular cartilage defects in the knee. J Bone Joint Surg 2005.
32. Glenn E, McCarty E, Potter HG, Juliao SF, Gordon J, Spindler K. Comparison of fresh osteochondral autografts and allografts: a canine model. Am J sports med 2006, 34(7): 1084–1093. Orthopaedic Society for Sports Medicine; July 20–23, 2003; San Diego, CA.
33. Brinker MR, Miller MD. Fundamentals of Orthopaedics. Philadelphia: Saunders, 1999.

4

Decision Making in Cartilage Repair Procedures

Riley J. Williams III, MD and Robert H. Brophy, MD

Summary

The treatment of isolated articular cartilage lesions remains a difficult clinical problem. Cartilage has a poor intrinsic capacity for repair. Untreated lesions persist indefinitely and can predispose affected joints to pain and dysfunction. Fortunately, the treatment options for these lesions continue to evolve and expand. However, a validated approach to the treatment of such lesions remains elusive. Decision making in these circumstances is highly variable between practitioners. We describe an approach to the patient with a symptomatic articular cartilage lesion. Consideration of certain parameters, including lesion size, lesion location, patient demand, body mass index, limb alignment, and treatment history should be considered when selecting a surgical approach. In addition, surgeons should understand the physiology of the cartilage repair method employed and how this relates to the postoperative rehabilitation program. Cartilage repair strategies are classified into the following: enhancement intrinsic repair response, cell-based, scaffold-based, cell plus scaffold-based, and whole tissue transplantation. A treatment algorithm based on lesion size, patient demand, and treatment (primary vs secondary) is presented.

Key Words: Algorithm; cartilage repair; classification; knee; reconstruction.

INTRODUCTION

Articular cartilage injuries are a serious clinical problem for the orthopedic surgeon. A retrospective review of knee arthroscopies by Curl et al. found that cartilage lesions were present in 63% of knee cases (1). Hijelle et al. prospectively found incidental chondral or osteochondral lesions in 61% of 1000 knee arthroscopies (2). In the Curl study, 19% of the patients were found to have an Outerbridge grade IV lesion, and 4% of all arthroscopies involved a grade IV lesion in patients under 40 yr of age (1). Similarly, the series reported by Hjelle reported grade III or IV lesions at least 1 cm^2 in 5.3% of all arthroscopies in patients younger than 40 yr (2). Thus, it can be inferred that focal symptomatic articular cartilage lesions are common and represent a significant treatment challenge in young patients.

Unfortunately, articular cartilage has a poor intrinsic capacity for healing following injury (3–5). Early in the 18th century, this fact was observed by Hunter, who noted that articular cartilage "once destroyed, is not repaired" (6). Articular cartilage regeneration is poor because of its avascular nature and the extracellular matrix (ECM) structure of collagen and proteoglycan (7,8). This lack of blood flow limits the intrinsic healing process by inhibiting transport of inflammatory mediators to the defect (7). In addition, the ECM does not allow

From: *Cartilage Repair Strategies*
Edited by: Riley J. Williams © Humana Press Inc., Totowa, NJ

cellular migration to the sites of cartilage injury *(8)*. As a result, although chondrocytes do respond initially to tissue injury, they are not capable of repopulating the defect; ultimately, these cells cease their attempts at healing the area of injured cartilage *(9)*. These lesions can become symptomatic and in the long term lead to continued cartilage erosion and osteoarthritis *(10–13)*.

It is clear that isolated articular cartilage lesions are often a cause of debilitating knee pain. Thus, an important question arises: How should the orthopedic surgeon approach this difficult problem? Unfortunately, there is no validated treatment algorithm available for this particular malady. Moreover, this rapidly expanding field is in constant flux. Such consistent change makes the development of a treatment standard even more difficult. The surgeon is reminded that the overall treatment goal of cartilage reconstruction is the durable return of joint function that is achieved with a minimum of morbidity. Currently, there are an increasing number of surgical options for the treatment of articular cartilage lesions. Although there is some confusion regarding which procedures work best in certain patients, there does exist an extensive body of evidence that procedures such as microfracture arthroplasty, mosaicplasty, autologous chondrocyte implantation (ACI), and osteochondral allograft transplantation are effective in restoring knee functions *(14–26)*.

One historic disadvantage was the incidental nature of the articular cartilage defect. Although magnetic resonance imaging (MRI) has for many years been routinely used for the diagnosis of joint injuries, it is only recently that articular cartilage has been sufficiently visualized by MRI *(27)*. Often, surgeons would discover these lesions during procedures that were indicated for other problems, such as meniscal or ligament tears. This scenario created a dilemma for both the patient and treating physician. The discovery of an unanticipated cartilage defect limited the surgeon's ability to plan and address this injury effectively. The ability to detect and treat these lesions accurately has had a positive impact on patient outcomes. We describe our approach to the patient with a symptomatic chondral or osteochondral defect.

CLINICAL APPROACH

When treating lesions of articular cartilage of the knee, the surgeon should focus on the following parameters: cartilage lesion etiology, cartilage lesion quality, knee- and lower extremity-related issues, patient characteristics, surgeon-associated issues, and the literature. Careful consideration of each of these issues will greatly enhance the likelihood of a good clinical outcome following treatment.

Cartilage Lesion Etiology

Articular cartilage lesions typically result from one of three mechanisms: direct trauma, chronic degeneration (mechanical overload), or an abnormality of the underlying subchondral bone (avascular necrosis [AVN], osteochondritits dissecans). Traumatic injury can occur through direct impact or via application shear forces to the joint surface. For example, it is believed that the "bone bruise" that is often noted by MRI following the subluxation of an anterior cruciate ligament (ACL)-deficient knee is caused by the application of shear forces on the knee's lateral femoral condyle by the posterior tibia (Fig. 1). Acute cartilage injury can also be observed in these circumstances (Fig. 2).

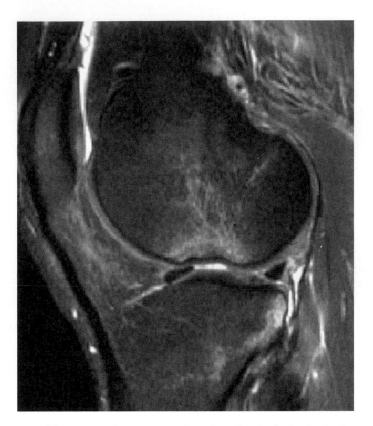

Fig. 1. Cartilage-sensitive magnetic resonance imaging (sagittal view) of a knee that has recently experienced a knee subluxation episode associated with an acute anterior cruciate ligament (ACL) tear. This image demonstrates the typical bone bruise of the posterior lateral tibial plateau and anterior lateral femoral condyle that occurs following a traumatic ACL tear. Note that the image demonstrates an indentation of the chondral surface with an alteration in the signal intensity of the articular cartilage layer. Bone edema (increased bone signal intensity) is also demonstrated.

Degenerative articular cartilage damage can occur after an alteration in joint reactive force. The degenerative cartilage changes that ensue following the removal of meniscal tissue or in cases of severe knee malalignment are believed to occur because of increases in the joint forces that accompany these clinical conditions *(28–30)*. A loss of subchondral bony integrity can result in articular cartilage collapse. Bone forms the structural support for articular cartilage; abnormalities of bone will render the cartilage unable to withstand even normal joint reactive forces. Thus, although the symptoms of an overlying cartilage lesion may be the primary reason that a patient seeks medical attention, it is the bony etiology that must be ultimately addressed along with the chondral surface abnormality.

Consideration of lesion etiology helps the surgeon to focus on how to best correct the underlying cause of the injury. For example, in cases of acute ACL injury in the older patient, MRI performed to assess the ligament injury may also detect chondral lesions, including those on the medial femoral condyle *(1,2)*. A thoughtful analysis of the lesion may suggest that the observed cartilage injury may in fact be a degenerative one that was caused by varus

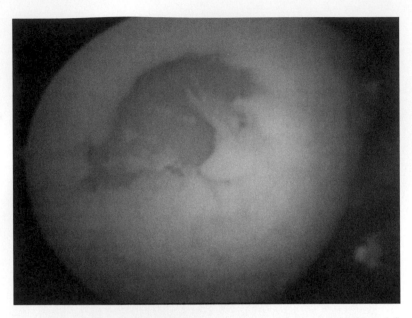

Fig. 2. Intraoperative photograph of a full-thickness chondral lesion of the lateral femoral condyle that was noted at the time of anterior cruciate ligament (ACL) reconstruction.

knee malalignment and not the ACL rupture. Thus, in addition to ACL reconstruction, knee alignment correction (osteotomy) and chondral resurfacing should be considered.

Cartilage Lesion Qualities

In both the preoperative and operative setting, articular cartilage lesions should be described using the following parameters:

    Location
    Grade
    Size
    Morphology/character

Lesion location is typically ascribed to one of the six articular surfaces of the knee: patella, trochlea (above the sulcus terminalis), medial femoral condyle, lateral femoral condyle, medial tibial plateau, and lateral tibial plateau. Lesion location is important as the types of joint reactive forces (compressive, shear) that affect the different areas may have an impact on the surgical decision-making process for a given procedure. Cartilage lesions are graded according to the original classification proposed by Outerbridge or the more recent International Cartilage Repair Society classification *(31–33)* (Table 1). These classifications require careful visualization of the cartilage lesion and can usually be made at arthroscopy. Advances in cartilage-sensitive MRI have facilitated the noninvasive assessment of cartilage lesion grade and a modification of the Outerbridge classification that can also be used *(27)* (Table 1).

When available, cartilage-sensitive MRI should be used to estimate the size and grade of the lesion prior to surgery. At surgery, direct visualization of the lesion should allow accurate verification of preoperative imaging and a determination of size and grade. The size of the lesion is typically reported as the area in square millimeters (mm^2) after measuring the length and width

Table 1
Grading of Cartilage Lesions

Grade	Outerbridge	Modified Outerbridge	International cartilage repair society
0	Normal cartilage	Intact cartilage	Intact cartilage
I	Softening and swelling	Chondral softening or blistering with intact surface	Superficial (soft indentation or superficial fissures and cracks)
II	Fragmentation and fissures in area less than half an inch in diameter	Superficial ulceration, fibrillation, or fissuring less than 50% of depth of cartilage	Lesion less than half the thickness of articular cartilage
III	Fragmentation and fissures in area greater than half an inch in diameter	Deep ulceration, fibrillation, fissuring, or chondral flap more than 50% of cartilage without exposed subchondral bone	Lesion greater than 1/2 thickness of articular cartilage
IV	Exposed subchondral bone	Full-thickness wear with exposed subchondral bone	Lesion extending to subchondral bone

using a marked probe. The morphological distinction between chondral and osteochondral lesions is predicated on the involvement of the underlying subchondral bone as part of the lesion. The depth of any bony involvement is noted. In general, the surgeon must assess the bony involvement and determine the following: Does the degree of bony loss distort the natural architecture of the surface that is affected? If not, then a chondral repair strategy may be employed (i.e., mesenchymal stem cell stimulation, ACI); if the architecture is distorted, then a repair strategy that allows for bony restoration (mosaicplasty, osteochondral allograft) should be chosen.

The Lower Extremity

To treat cartilage lesions of the knee effectively, the surgeon must confirm the structural integrity of the knee joint. In other words, the affected knee should be free from instability, motion loss, or excessive meniscal deficiency. Any history of knee injury and treatment should be deeply explored. The physical exam should carefully assess knee motion, ligament stability, meniscal signs, and lower extremity alignment. If left untreated, then an abnormality of one or more of these anatomic areas could adversely affect the attempted cartilage repair.

Candidates for articular cartilage repair procedures should have normal or correctable ligament stability, a normal or correctable meniscal state, and normal or correctable knee alignment. As such, the cartilage repair surgeon must be facile with other procedures about the knee, including knee osteotomy, ligament reconstruction, and meniscal allograft transplantation. Finally, and perhaps most important, the remaining cartilage surfaces should be free from gross abnormality; an Outerbridge classification of II or less is deemed acceptable in the untreated compartments of the knee.

Although it is possible that an affected knee may have multiple "isolated" defects, this circumstance, more often than not, represents the early stages of a degenerative joint. We urge caution in attempting repairs in such circumstances. Particular attention should be paid to the opposing joint surface in the compartment that is to be treated. Preoperative MRI should be used to assess not only the articular surface but also the subchondral bone. Early degeneration, in the form of subchondral sclerosis or early chondral wear, may be found in the opposing joint surface. And, although this finding may not ultimately preclude an attempted cartilage repair, it may encourage the surgeon to consider a corrective osteotomy to increase the likelihood of clinical success.

The Patient

Certain patient-related characteristics should be considered during the preoperative planning of cartilage repair procedures:

Age
Body habitus or body mass index (BMI)
Hereditary factors
Level of demand
Systemic conditions or disease
Patient functional need
Patient expectation
Ability to comply with rehabilitation

Patient age is relevant to the decision-making process as it has been demonstrated that age may have an adverse effect on certain types of cartilage repair procedures (i.e., microfracture) *(34)*. Some authors haves suggested an upper age limit of 55 yr *(26)*. We suggest that, in most circumstances, a critical assessment of the patient's joint surfaces should be made. If an isolated cartilage lesion is noted and the remaining joint surfaces are in good condition (Outerbridge grade II or less), then a repair strategy may be employed.

Patient weight and BMI should also be considered. Body mass index uses a mathematical formula that takes into account both a person's height and weight. It has been demonstrated that an increased BMI (>30) has an adverse effect on some cartilage repair procedures *(22)*. And, although such an analysis has not been done for all available cartilage repair methods, it remains an important consideration. Having affected patients lose weight prior to moving ahead with cartilage repair may ultimately improve outcome and increase the likelihood of long-term good function.

Patient functional demand should also be considered. For example, the needs of a collegiate or professional athlete differ greatly from that of the 45-yr-old recreational sportsman. The literature does provide some guidance in this area. Success in high-demand athletes following cartilage repair surgery has been reported for both the microfracture technique and ACI procedures *(22,35,36)*. These studies have confirmed the ability of a majority of athletes to return to sport, albeit on the short term (2 years following surgery). Moreover, a short duration of symptoms and short interval between injury and repair have also been shown to correlate positively with a return to sport *(22,37)*. These reports suggest that high-level athletes who are desirous of returning to sport should be treated quickly and aggressively to increase the likelihood of clinical success.

The Surgeon

As the options for resurfacing isolated cartilage defects have grown, so has the interest in treating symptomatic cartilage lesions. However, these techniques have proven to be technically difficult. Certain techniques, in particular mosaicplasty and ACI, require both a deft surgical hand and the ability to think spatially. In determining the procedure that best fits a given clinical scenario, it is also important to assess one's comfort level with the procedure considered *(38)*. As with most orthopedic procedures, there is a learning curve that is overcome with increasing experience. Thus, surgeon expertise should be considered in the indications process.

The Literature

Following the publication of Brittberg and colleagues' landmark 1994 article in the *New England Journal of Medicine* on ACI *(14)*, increasing clinical interest has focused on the problem of treating isolated cartilage lesions. At that time, there was little information available to guide clinicians in the application of ACI and other surgical approaches designed to treat these lesions. Although a validated treatment algorithm for the treatment of these lesions remains elusive, many peer reviewed articles have been published in the field of cartilage repair, and these cover myriad surgical options *(3,14,16,22,25,34,39–43)*.

Careful review of these articles should familiarize the surgeon with the clinical outcomes, technical insights, rehabilitation strategies, and potential pitfalls associated with these cartilage repair strategies. In addition, there are many studies that directly compare cartilage repair methods and address the effectiveness of certain methods in returning athletic individuals to sport *(36,37,43–47)*. As many of these methods are relatively novel, the surgeon seeking to treat articular cartilage defects routinely needs to be current and frequently review the published literature.

CARTILAGE REPAIR INDICATIONS

Our indications for the surgical treatment of chondral or osteochondral lesions of the knee include the following:

Symptoms of knee dysfunction (pain, recurrent effusion, mechanical symptoms)
Isolated chondral or osteochondral lesion of the knee condyles, trochlea, or patella
Normal or correctable knee alignment
Normal or correctable knee ligament stability
Functional meniscus tissue (≥50% native meniscal volume)
Age 15–55 years

Contraindications to cartilage repair surgery include

Degenerative knee osteoarthritis (multiple-compartment disease)
Systemic inflammatory disorders (e.g., rheumatoid arthritis)
Collagen or vascular disorders
Obesity (BMI > 35)
Chronic use of immunosuppressive medication (e.g., corticosteroids)

Potentially treatable lesions should be isolated. The remaining cartilage surfaces should be intact, specifically Outerbridge grade II or less. Patients should have functional meniscal tissue. A gross absence of the posterior horn of either meniscus is worrisome in the setting of articular cartilage repair as such a condition may subject the articular cartilage to excessive joint reactive forces *(48,49)*. Surgeons should consider meniscal allograft transplantation in those patients who have less than 50% of the native meniscus present in the affected knee compartment *(50)*.

PATIENT EVALUATION

The patient evaluation should include a thorough history and physical examination. A specific history of previous diagnoses and treatments is obtained. The initial imaging studies should include the following radiographs of the knee: weight-bearing anteroposterior, weight-bearing 40° posteroanterior, lateral, Merchant's views, and bilateral standing hip-knee-ankle anteroposterior view. If there is clinical suspicion of a cartilage lesion, then a cartilage-sensitive MRI is obtained (27). Imaging studies are critical in understanding lesion quality and should be used extensively in the preoperative planning phase. For patients with a history of previous knee arthroscopy, intraoperative photographs should be obtained and reviewed. Although these lesions can be difficult to diagnose, a growing clinical awareness of this problem combined with improved imaging techniques have made establishing an accurate preoperative diagnosis most achievable (51,52). Assessment of lesion size, location, and grade can accurately be made using the described approach. This information facilitates the creation of a preoperative plan and rehabilitation strategy that can be discussed in detail with surgical candidates.

CURRENT CARTILAGE REPAIR STRATEGIES

A number of repair strategies are currently available for clinical use when treating an articular cartilage lesion. Typically, these strategies fall into one of the following categories:

1. Palliative
2. Intrinsic repair enhancement/marrow stimulation
3. Cell-based repair
4. Scaffold-based repair
5. Cell plus scaffold-based repair
6. Whole tissue transplantation

Each of these strategies has specific objectives, advantages, and disadvantages. The surgeon should consider these points in developing a surgical plan. Palliative options focus on the relief of mechanical symptoms in the cartilage-injured patient and include debridement, lavage, and chondroplasty (53–55). These strategies attempt to remove the mechanical sources of pain but do not result in lesion fill.

The enhancement of intrinsic cartilage repair strategy relies on the local recruitment of marrow-based, pluripotent stem cells to the site of an articular cartilage lesion. Specific treatment options in this group include abrasion arthroplasty, microfracture, and drilling (17–20,34,35,56–60).

Cell-based cartilage repair methods call for the local implantation of chondrogenic cells within a cartilage lesion for the purpose of forming hyalinelike cartilage tissue. ACI or autologous chondrocyte transplantation falls in this category. To date, both periosteum (ACI) and collagen patches (collagen-associated chondrocyte implantation) have been used in cell-based methods (14,15). The cell-based repair strategy has expanded to include the use of chondrocyte-matrix composites (matrix-associated autologous chondrocyte implantation [MACI]; Hyalograft C, Fidia, Abano Terme, Italy) (39,61,62).

Scaffolds alone may also be used as an effective method of treating both chondral and osteochondral defects. A biphasic resorbable synthetic implant is currently available in Europe for primary cartilage repair indication; this implant is also available in the United States with an indication for defect backfill during mosaicplasty (TruFit, Osteobiologics,

Table 2
Cartilage Repair Strategies

Approach	Treatment	Repair tissue	Fill	Known durability
A. Palliative	Arthroscopic debridement	None	None	< 2 yr
B. Intrinsic repair enhancement	1. Microfracture	Fibrocartilage	Partial	
	2. Drilling	Fibrocartilage	Partial	2–6 yr
	3. Abrasion athroplasty	Fibrocartilage	Partial	
C. Whole tissue transplantation	1. Mosaicplasty	Hyaline Cartilage	Near total	2–10 yr
	2. Osteochondral auograft	Hyaline Cartilage	Near total	5–20 yr
D. Cell-based	1. ACI	Hyaline-like	Near total	2–4 yr
	2. MACI	Hyaline-like	Near total	2 yr
	3. Hyalograft C	Hyaline-like	Near total	3 yr
E. Scaffolds	1. TRU-FIT (OBI)	Hyaline-like	Near total	Unknown

San Antonio, TX) (63,64). The whole tissue transplantation strategy relies on the implantation of fully formed osteoarticular constructs into a chondral or osteochondral defect. This tissue can be derived from an autologous source (mosaicplasty) or from an allograft donor *(16,25,42,65,66)*.

These strategies can be sorted further according to the type of repair tissue the approach aims to create, the resulting fill of the lesion, and the durability of the repair tissue (Table 2).

The palliative approach is indicated for grade III or IV lesions covering 0.5–2 cm^2 in older patients with low functional demand. The goal of this technique is to improve the congruency of the articular lesion with the opposing articular surface and to minimize further delamination of the joint surface cartilage. Although this technique is expedient and cost-efficient, it does not result in tissue fill and is a temporizing treatment at best. This approach should be considered as a first-line treatment option only in older, low-demand patients with more generalized cartilage pathology.

Intrinsic repair enhancement is an appropriate first-stage strategy for grade III or IV lesions of the femur covering 0.5–2 cm^2; lesions considered for this method should possess a substantial cartilage rim around the lesion. Higher demand patients with small lesions (less than 2 cm^2) and low-demand patients with larger lesions (greater than 2 cm^2) are appropriate candidates for this treatment approach. Patients with a BMI greater than 30 should not be considered for this approach *(22)*. Both microfracture and drilling of the subchondral bone stimulate the intrinsic repair process by facilitating the formation of a stem cell-rich fibrin clot within the lesion. Such techniques ultimately result in the creation of reparative fibrocartilage.

We recommend the use of the microfracture technique in this category as there are concerns about the thermal effect of drilling on the subchondral bone and local marrow cells. This approach is a single-stage, arthroscopic treatment that is technically easy and cost-effective and results in tissue fill. However, tissue fill can be unpredictable, and bony overgrowth can occur. The durability of the fill created by this repair technique is estimated at to be 2–5 yr in high-demand individuals. Overall, this is a safe, effective first-line treatment with little morbidity and increasingly effective results reported in the literature *(18,21,22,34,35,67,68)*.

Cartilage resurfacing using autologous osteochondral transplantation can be accomplished using multiple small osteochondral cylinders (mosaicplasty) or using a single large plug *(16,66)*. Autologous osteochondral transplantation is indicated for focal, traumatic lesions 1–4 cm^2 in size; such lesions need not be contained. One advantage of this technique is that it can be used for lesions on the patella as well as the femur. This approach uses autogenous tissue to create a hyaline cartilage surface and is cost-effective, with a recovery period similar to microfracture. However, donor graft tissue is limited as this tissue is harvested from alternative sites on the ipsilateral femoral trochlea and notch. Autologous osteochondral transplantation it is a technically demanding procedure that usually requires an arthrotomy for reliable three-dimensional reconstruction of the cartilage surface *(69)*. The technical difficulty of this procedure notwithstanding, autologous osteochondral transplantation is a good option for first-line treatment of focal defects or for treatment of smaller cartilage lesions in high-demand individuals.

Autologous chondrocyte implantation is indicated for large, uncontained lesions (2–10 cm^2) as a first- or second-stage treatment in high-demand patients. Chondral lesions of the femur, trochlea, patella, and tibia can be treated with this technique *(26,70)*. Treatable lesions can be uncontained; multiple lesions can be treated at one sitting. Osteochondral lesions can be treated if there is less than 6 mm bone loss; lesions with greater than 6 mm bone loss should be treated with staged bone grafting prior to ACI. Patients should be between 15 and 55 yr of age with normal or correctable knee alignment and a BMI less than 30. This is a two-stage technique that uses laboratory-expanded autologous chondrocytes. At implantation, these cells are stabilized within the cartilage defect using either a periosteal or a collagen patch. Good clinical results have been reported, even in athletes *(36,37)*. However, the ACI and collagen-associated chondrocyte implantation procedures are technically challenging. Moreover, these procedures have both a high reoperation rate (9–20%) and high cost. Autologous chondrocyte implantation is a reasonable first-line therapy for large cartilage lesions or for patients who have failed other treatment modalities.

Fresh osteochondral allograft transplantation is typically used for large osteochondral lesions (3–12 cm^2 or greater). Large, uncontained chondral lesions; osteochondral lesions; osteochondritis dissecans lesions; AVN lesions; and posttraumatic lesions can all be treated with this approach *(25,42)*. Osteochondral allograft transplantation may also be employed as a salvage procedure for failed first-line treatments. This technique offers the advantage of bony graft fixation. There is no donor site morbidity with this approach. However, allograft specimens are limited in supply and are costly. Moreover, fresh osteochondral allografts can elicit a local host immune response that may compromise healing, and disease transmission remains a remote but real possibility. However, it is important to remember that this method of cartilage resurfacing has the longest history of any method; very good long-term results have been reported *(23,42,71)*. Osteochondral allograft transplantation should be considered a primary option for large osteochondral lesions (osteochondritis dissecans, AVN) and secondary treatment for other failed cartilage repair treatments.

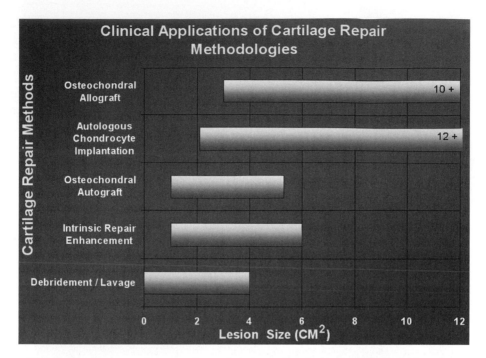

Fig. 3. Cartilage repair strategies and their application according to lesion size.

There is emerging technology in the field of cartilage repair that should further expand the options available to clinicians. Future cartilage repair techniques include those that make use of genetically modified chondrocytes, scaffolds, and growth factors *(3,4,72–75)*. In Europe and Australia, there has been extensive clinical experience with the use of cell-based repair strategies that combine expanded autologous chondrocytes with matrix scaffolds. These so-called third-generation ACI techniques include the Hyalograft C chondrocyte-seeded implant and the MACI method, among others *(39,61,76,77)*.

The Hyalograft C implant uses a hyaluronic acid-based scaffold for the delivery of autologous chondrocytes to the site of a cartilage lesion *(78–80)*. This cartilage repair method has sparked great interest as the implant requires no suture stabilization and may be placed arthroscopically. Studies of this cell-based technique have reported good clinical results with hyaline-like cartilage lesion fill *(39,81)*.

MACI (Verigen AC, Germany) is another third-generation method that is gaining popularity in both Europe and Australia. In this technique, cultured chondrocytes are seeded onto a type I/III porcine collagen membrane. After the membrane is fashioned to the appropriate lesion size, it is ultimately implanted into the articular cartilage defect *(41,62)*. The MACI membrane is easily handled and requires only fibrin glue and a few stabilizing sutures for fixation. Thus, the MACI membrane may be implanted on the femur using a limited arthrotomy. The MACI method results in near-total lesion fill, and good clinical results have been reported at short-term follow-up *(40,62)*.

Both the Hyalograft C and MACI methods are covered in greater detail in this book. These third-generation ACI techniques are quite interesting as they have advanced the application of autologous cells in cartilage repair. Both the MACI and Hyalograft C implants are technically easier to place compared to the original, first-generation ACI technique. And, although

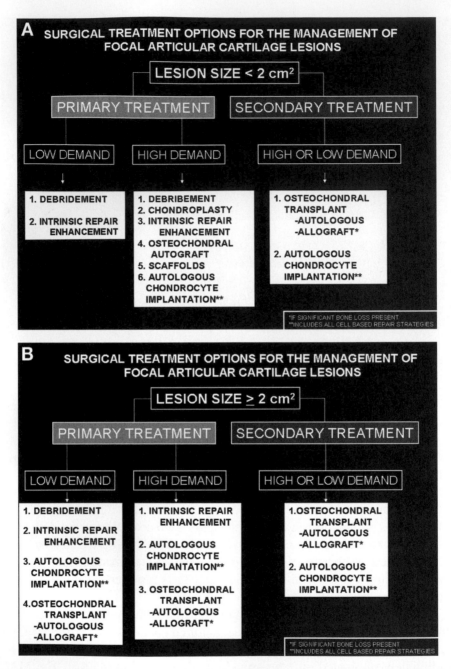

Fig. 4. (A,B) Articular cartilage reconstruction alogorithm. This algorithm considers lesion size, patient demand, and the application of a previous surgical intervention as the primary considerations in determining the appropriate treatment approach. The critical lesion size is 2 cm^2. High-demand patients are defined as those who plan to participate in athletic activities or laborious activities for more than 2 days per week (professional or collegiate athletes, high-demand laborers). Autologous chondrocyte implantation includes the application of all cell-based articular cartilage repair strategies (autologous chondrocyte implantation, matrix-induced autologous chondrocyte implantation, Hyalograft C).

long-term follow-up is still needed to validate the use of the Hyalograft C and MACI matrices for the treatment of symptomatic articular cartilage lesions, these repair methods may enable more surgeons ultimately to treat such lesions successfully.

TREATMENT SELECTION

In light of the ever-increasing number of therapeutic options available for the treatment of articular cartilage lesions, one question remains: How does the clinician go about selecting the appropriate cartilage repair strategy for a specific patient? Although to date no treatment algorithm has been validated in the area of cartilage repair surgery, we put forth in this chapter a systematic method of approaching symptomatic cartilage lesions of the knee. Initially, in developing a treatment plan for such lesions we recommend that lesion size be considered (Fig. 3). Lesion size is estimated from preoperative MRI, prior operative reports, or diagnostic arthroscopy (prior to reconstructive surgery. In addition to lesion size, the history of previous treatment and patient demand are important considerations. Patient demand is a key issue; we define high patient demand as those patients who wish to return to athletic activities or high-demand labor.

A two-part algorithm for the application of cartilage repair procedures that considers lesion size, patient demand, and treatment history is presented (Fig. 4). In the described approach, a lesion area of 2 cm^2 is critical. Once lesion size has been established, patient demand is determined (high vs low). Finally, the surgeon should determine whether the proposed treatment is primary or secondary (revision of failed prior attempt).

CONCLUSION

The treatment of isolated articular cartilage lesions remains a difficult clinical problem. Fortunately, treatment options for these lesions continue to evolve and expand. A thorough evaluation of the patient is important in selecting the optimal treatment modality. Specifically, lesion size, patient demand, and treatment history are considered when selecting a surgical approach. Surgeons should understand the physiology of the cartilage repair method employed and how this relates to the postoperative rehabilitation program. The clarification of other relevant conditions (obesity, limb malalignment) before treating articular cartilage defects will greatly increase the likelihood of a successful clinical outcome. These are difficult patients to treat; often, managing expectations is a major component to a good outcome. Appropriate attention should be paid to surgical technique and rehabilitation protocol to give patients the best chance for an optimal outcome.

REFERENCES

1. Curl W, Krome J, Gordon E, Rushing J, Smith B, Poehling G. Cartilage injuries: a review of 31,516 knee arthroscopies. Arthroscopy 1997;13:456–460.
2. Hijelle K, Solheim E, Strand T, Muri R, Brittberg M. Articular cartilage defects in 1000 knee arthroscopies. Arthroscopy 2002;18:730–734.
3. Hunziker E. Articular cartilage repair: basic science and clinical progress. A review of the current status and prospects. Osteoarthritis Cartilage 2001;10:432–463.
4. Martinek V, Ueblacker P, Imhoff A. Current concepts of gene therapy and cartilage repair. J Bone Joint Surg Br 2003;85B:782–788.
5. Vangsness C, Kurzweil P, Lieberman J. Restoring articular cartilage in the knee. Am J Orthop 2004;33(suppl 2):29–34.

6. Hunter W. On the structure and diseases of articulating cartilages. Philos Trans R Soc Lond 1743;42B:514–521.

7. Mankin H. The response of articular cartilage to mechanical injury. J Bone Joint Surg 1982; 64A:460–466.

8. Newman A. Articular cartilage repair. Am J Sports Med 1998;26:309–324.

9. Buckwalter J. Articular cartilage injuries. Clin Orthop 2002;402:21–37.

10. Buckwalter J, Mankin H. Articular cartilage: degeneration and osteoarthritis, repair, regeneration, transplantation. Instr Course Lect 1998;47:487–504.

11. Buckwalter J, Mankin H. Articular cartilage: tissue design and chondrocyte-matrix interactions. Instr Course Lect 1998;47:477–486.

12. Caplan A, Elyaderani M, Mochizuki Y, Wakitani S, Goldberg V. Principles of cartilage repair and regeneration. Clin Orthop 1997;342:254–269.

13. Lefkoe T, Trafton P, Ehrlich M, et al. An experimental model of femoral condylar defect leading to osteoarthosis. J Orthop Trauma 1993;7:458–467.

14. Brittberg M, Lindhal A, Nilsson A, Ohlsson C, Isaksson O, Peterson L. Treatment of deep cartilage defects in the knee with autologous chondrocyte transplantation of the knee. N Engl J Med 1994;331:889–895.

15. Peterson L, Minas T, Brittberg M, Nilsson A, Sjogren-Jansson E, Lindhal A. Two- to 9-year outcome after autologous chondrocyte transplantation of the knee. Clin Orthop 2000;374:212–234.

16. Hangody L, Kish G, Karpati Z, Udvarhelyi I, Szigeti I, Bely M. Mosaicplasty for the treatment of articular cartilage defects: application in clinical practice. Orthopedics 1998;21:751–756.

17. Johnson L. Clinical methods of cartilage repair. Arthroscopic abrasion arthroplasty. A review. Clin Orthop 2001;391S:306–317.

18. Rodrigo J, Steadman J, Silliman J. Improvement of full-thickness chondral defect healing in the human knee after debridement and microfracture using continuous passive motion. Am J Knee Surg 1994;7:109–116.

19. Rae P, Noble J. Arthroscopic drilling of osteochondral lesions of the knee. J Bone Joint Surg Br 1989;71B:534.

20. Bert J. Role of abrasion arthroplasty and debridement in the management of osteoarthritis of the knee. Rheum Dis Clin North Am 1993;19:725–739.

21. Steadman J, Rodkey W, Rodrigo J. Microfracture: surgical technique and rehabilitation to treat chondral defects. Clin Orthop 2001;391(suppl).

22 Mithoefer K, Williams R, Warren R, et al. The microfracture technique for the treatment of articular cartilage lesions in the knee. A prospective cohort study. J Bone Joint Surg 2005;87A:1911–1920.

23. Meyers M, Akeson W, Convery F. Resurfacing of the knee with fresh osteochondral allograft. J Bone Joint Surg 1989;71A:704–713.

24. Minas T, Chiu R. Autologous chondrocyte implantation. Am J Knee Surg 2000;13:41–50.

25. Bugbee W, Convery F. Osteochondral allograft transplantation. Clin Sports Med 1999;18:67–75.

26. Brittberg M, Tallheden T, Sjogren-Jansson B, Lindhal A, Peterson L. Autologous chondrocytes used for articular cartilage repair: an update. Clin Orthop 2001;391(suppl): S337–S348.

27. Potter H, Linklater J, Allen A, Hannafin J, Haas S. Magnetic resonance imaging of articular cartilage in the knee. An evaluation with use of fast-spin-echo imaging. J Bone Joint Surg 1998;80A:1276–1284.

28. Felson D, Goggins J, Niu J, Zhang Y, Hunter D. The effect of body weight on progression of knee osteoarthritis is dependent on alignment. Arthritis Rheum 2004;50:3904–3909.

29. Tetsworth K, Paley D. Malalignment and degenerative arthropathy. Orthop Clin North Am 1994;25:367–377.

30. Goodman S, Lee J, Smith R, Csongradi J, Fornasier V. Mechanical overload of a single compartment induces early degenerative changes in the rabbit knee: a preliminary study. J Invest Surg 1991;4:161–170.

31. Outerbridge R. The etiology of chondromalacia patellae. J Bone Joint Surg Br 1961;43B: 752–767.

32. Brittberg M, Peterson L. Introduction to an articular cartilage classification. Intl Cartilage Repair Soc Newsl 1998;1–8.
33. Brittberg M. Evaluation of cartilage injuries and cartilage repair. Osteologie 2000;9:17–25.
34. Steadman J, Briggs K, Rodrigo J, Kocher M, Gill T, Rodkey W. Outcomes of microfracture for traumatic chondral defects of the knee: average 11-yr follow-up. Arthroscopy 2003;19:477–484.
35. Blevins F, Steadman J, Rodrigo J, Silliman J. Treatment of articular cartilage defects in athletes: an analysis of functional outcome and lesion appearance. Orthopedics 1998;21:761–767.
36. Mithoefer K, Peterson L, Mandelbaum B, Minas T. Articular cartilage repair in soccer players with autologous chondrocyte transplantation: functional outcome and return to competition. Am J Sports Med 2005;33:1639–1646.
37. Mithoefer K, Minas T, Peterson L, Yeon H, Micheli L. Functional outcome of knee articular cartilage repair in adolescent athletes. Am J Sports Med 2005;33:1147–1153.
38. Peterson L. Autologous Chondrocyte Implantation. Washington, DC: American Academy of Orthopedic Surgeons; 2005.
39. Marcacci M, et al. Articular cartilage engineering with Hyalograft C: 3-yr clinical results. Clin Orthop 2006;435:96–105.
40. Bachmann G, Basad E, Lommel D, Steinmeyer J. MRI in the follow-up of matrix-supported autologous chondrocyte transplantation (MACI) and microfracture [in German]. Radiologe 2004;44:773–782.
41. Behrens P, Ehlers E, Kochermann K, Rohwedel J, Russlies M, Plotz W. New therapy procedure for localized cartilage defects. Encouraging results with autologous chondrocyte implantation [in German]. MMW Fortschr Med 1999;141:49–51.
42. Gross A, Shasha N, Aubin P. Long-term follow-up of the use of fresh osteochondral allografts for posttraumatic knee defects. Clin Orthop 2005;435:79–87.
43. Knutsen G, et al. Autologous chondrocyte implantation compared with microfracture in the knee. A randomized trial. J Bone Joint Surg 2004;86A:455–464.
44. Bentley G, Biant LC, Carrington RW, et al. A prospective, randomised comparison of autologous chondrocyte implantation vs mosaicplasty for osteochondral defects in the knee. J Bone Joint Surg Br 2003;85:223–230.
45. Kish G, Hangody L. A prospective, randomised comparison of autologous chondrocyte implantation vs mosaicplasty for osteochondral defects in the knee. J Bone Joint Surg Br 2004;86:619; author reply 619–620.
46. LaPrade RF. Autologous chondrocyte implantation was superior to mosaicplasty for repair of articular cartilage defects in the knee at 1 yr. J Bone Joint Surg Am 2003;85A:2259.
47. Gudas R, Kalesinskas RJ, Kimtys V, et al. A prospective randomized clinical study of mosaic osteochondral autologous transplantation vs microfracture for the treatment of osteochondral defects in the knee joint in young athletes. Arthroscopy 2005;21:1066–1075.
48. Aagaard H, Verdonk R. Function of the normal meniscus and consequences of meniscal resection. Scand J Med Sci Sports 1999;9:134–140.
49. Wojtys E, Chan D. Meniscus structure and function. Instr Course Lect 2005;54:323–330.
50. Noyes F, Barber-Westin S. Meniscus transplantation: indications, techniques, clinical outcomes. Instr Course Lect 2005;54:341–353.
51. Oberlander M, Shalvoy R, Hughston J. The accuracy of the clinical knee examination documented by arthroscopy. A prospective study. Am J Sports Med 1993;21:773–778.
52. Zamber R, Teitz C, McGuire D, Frost J, Hermanson B. Articular cartilage lesions of the knee. Arthroscopy 1989;5:258–268.
53. Ogilvie-Harris D, Bauer M, Corey P. Prostaglandin inhibition and the rate of recovery after arthroscopic meniscectomy. J Bone Joint Surg Br 1985;67B:567–571.
54. Evans C, Mazzocchi R, Nelson D, Rubash H. Experimental arthritis induced by intraarticular injection of allogeneic cartilaginous particles into rabbit knees. Arthritis Rheum 1984;27:200–207.

55. O'Connor R. The arthroscope in the management of crystal-induced synovitis of the knee. J Bone Joint Surg 1973;55A:1443–1449.
56. Bert J, Maschka K. The arthroscopic treatment of unicompartmental gonarthrosis: a 5-yr follow-up study of abrasion arthroplasty plus arthroscopic debridement and arthroscopic debridement alone. Arthroscopy 1989;5:25–32.
57. Friedman M, Berasi C, Fox J. Preliminary results with abrasion arthroplasty in the osteoarthritic knee. Clin Orthop 1984;182:200–205.
58. Insall J. The Pridie debridement operation for osteoarthritis of the knee. Clin Orthop 1974;101: 61–67.
59. Pridie K. A method of resurfacing osteoarthritic knee joints. J Bone Joint Surg Br 1959; 41B: 618–619.
60. Childers J, Ellwood S. Partial chondrectomy and subchondral bone drilling for chondromalacia. Clin Orthop 1979;144:114–120.
61. Bartlett W, Skinner J, Gooding C, et al. Autologous chondrocyte implantation vs matrix-induced autologous chondrocyte implantation for osteochondral defects of the knee: a prospective, randomized study. J Bone Joint Surg Br 2005;87B:640–645.
62. Marlovits S, Singer P, Zeller P, Mandl I, Haller J, Trattnig S. Magnetic resonance observation of cartilage repair tissue (MOCART) for the evaluation of autologous chondrocyte transplantation: determination of interobserver variability and correlation to clinical outcome after 2 yr. Eur J Radiol 2005.
63. Slivka M, Leatherbury N, Kieswetter K, Niederauer G. Porous, resorbable, fiber-reinforced scaffolds tailored for articular cartilage repair. Tissue Eng 2001;7:767–780.
64. Niederauer G, Slivka M, Leatherbury N, et al. Evaluation of multiphase implants for repair of focal osteochondral defects in goats. Biomaterials 2000;21:2561–2574.
65. Marcacci M, Kon E, Zaffagnini S, et al. Multiple osteochondral arthroscopic grafting (mosaicplasty) for cartilage defects of the knee: prospective study results at 2-yr follow-up. Arthroscopy 2005;21:462–470.
66. Hangody L, Rathonyi G, Duska Z, Vasarhelyi G, Fules P, Modis L. Autologous osteochondral mosaicplasty. Surgical technique. J Bone Joint Surg 2004;86A(suppl 1):65–72.
67. Steadman J, Rodkey W, Briggs K. Microfracture to treat full-thickness chondral defects: surgical technique, rehabilitation, outcomes. J Knee Surg 2002;15:170–176.
68. Steadman J, Miller B, Karas S, Schlegel T, Briggs K, Hawkins R. The microfracture technique in the treatment of full-thickness chondral lesions of the knee in National Football League players. J Knee Surg 2003;16:83–86.
69. Morelli M, Nagamori J, Miniaci A. Management of chondral injuries of the knee by osteochondral autogenous transfer (mosaicplasty). J Knee Surg 2002;15:185–190.
70. Minas T. Autologous chondrocyte implantation for focal chondral defects of the knee. Clin Orthop 2001;391S:S349–S361.
71. Chu C, Convery F, Akeson W, Meyers M, Amiel D. Articular cartilage transplantation. Clinical results in the knee. Clin Orthop 1999;360:159–168.
72. Chen Y. Orthopedic applications of gene therapy. J Orthop Sci 2001;6:199–207.
73. Blunk T, Sieminski A, Gooch K, et al. Differential effects of growth factors on tissue-engineered cartilage. Tissue Eng 2002;8:73–84.
74. Frenkel S, Saadeh P, Mehrara B, et al. Transforming growth factor beta superfamily members: role in cartilage modeling. Plast Reconstr Surg 2000;105:980–990.
75. Trippel S. Growth factors as therapeutic agents. Instr Course Lect 1997;46:473–476.
76. Solchaga L, Dennis J, Goldberg V, Caplan A. Hyaluronic acid-based polymers as cell carriers for tissue-engineered repair of bone and cartilage. J Orthop Res 1999;17:205–213.
77. Solchaga L, Yoo J, Lundberg M, et al. Hyaluronan-based polymers in the treatment of osteochondral defects. J Orthop Res 2000;18:773–780.
78. Campoccia D, Doherty P, Radice M, Brun P, Abatangelo G, Williams D. Semi synthetic resorbable materials from hyaluranon esterification. Biomaterials 1998;19:2101–2127.

79. Grigolo B, Roseti L, Fiorini M, et al. Transplantation of chondrocytes seeded on a hyaluranon derivative (HYAFF 11) into cartilage defects in rabbits. Biomaterials 2001;22/17:2417–2424.
80. Brun P, Abatangelo G, Radice M, et al. Chondrocyte aggregation and reorganization into three-dimensional scaffolds. J Biomed Mater Res 1999;46.
81. Pavesio A, Abatangelo G, Borrione A, et al. Hyaluronan-based scaffolds (Hyalograft C) in the treatment of knee cartilage defects: preliminary clinical findings. Novartis Found Symp 2003; 203–217, 229–233.

5

Nonoperative Treatment Options for Symptomatic Cartilage Lesions

Mark C. Drakos, MD, and Answorth A. Allen, MD

Summary

Chondral injuries represent a spectrum of disorders that include both partial and full-thickness defects. The natural history of full-thickness cartilage lesions remains unclear. Repair or regeneration of normal functioning hyaline cartilage, in the mature adult, has yet to be confirmed following known cartilage restoration procedures and treatments. As such, the initial management of these lesions is largely nonoperative.

Those nonoperative treatment modalities that are available to clinicians include physical therapy, activity modification, bracing, patient education, topical medications, systemic medications, and intra-articular medications. However, it is important to consider that patient responses to these initial treatment modalities are often unpredictable and idiosyncratic. Evidence-based treatment protocols and reliable predictors for identifying efficacious treatment strategies have yet to be established in this group of patients. Given this lack of data, the goals of therapy should be focused on reducing pain and inflammation, increasing flexibility, increasing strength, and optimizing function for a timely return to activities of daily living. This chapter discusses each of these interventions in detail. Current literature and controversies are explored. Ultimately, nonoperative modalities can be effective at relieving pain and improving function in affected patients and as such should be a first-line approach in the management of these lesions.

Key Words: Chondral lesions; NSAIDs; diathermy; chondroitin; glucosamine; viscosupplementation.

INTRODUCTION

Chondral injuries represent a spectrum of disorders that include both partial and full-thickness defects. Approximately 900,000 individuals in the United States suffer an injury that results in a symptomatic chondral lesion each year *(1)* (Fig. 1). In a series by Curl and colleagues, cartilage lesions were found during knee arthroscopy 63% of the time in a review of more than 30,000 cases *(2)* (Fig. 2). Full-thickness lesions of the femur were found in approx 4% of all arthroscopies in patients under 40 yr old *(2)*. Chondral lesions have been reported in 23% of knees with an acute anterior cruciate ligament (ACL) injury and in 54% of patients suffering from chronic ACL insufficiency *(3)*. Thus, symptomatic chondral lesions represent a significant clinical challenge for the practicing orthopedic surgeon.

Unfortunately, the natural history of full-thickness cartilage lesions remains unclear. Repair or regeneration of normal functioning hyaline cartilage in the mature adult has yet to be confirmed following known cartilage restoration procedures and treatments. As such, the initial management of these lesions is largely nonoperative. The focus of this chapter is the development of these lesions and the modalities that represent the currently accepted nonoperative management.

From: *Cartilage Repair Strategies*
Edited by: Riley J. Williams © Humana Press Inc., Totowa, NJ

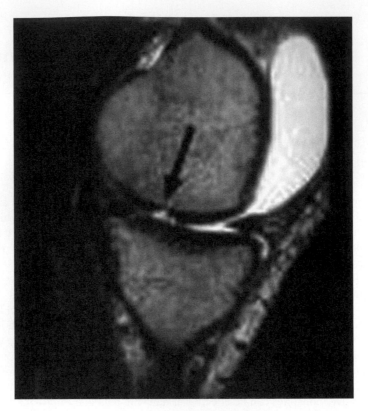

Fig. 1. Magnetic resonance image of a focal chondral defect in the articular cartilage of the femur.

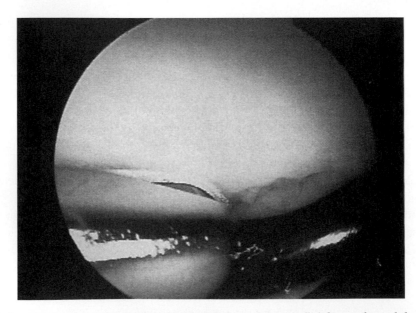

Fig. 2. Arthroscopic view of a partial chondral defect of the medial femoral condyle of the knee.

CLINICAL PRESENTATION AND EVALUATION

Traumatic chondral injuries can occur in any joint but are most common about the knee. Acute injuries are frequently the result of violent shear or twisting motions and often occur in conjunction with other soft tissue injuries (i.e., lateral condylar contusion associated with an ACL tear). Most patients will report a history of knee trauma; however, this is not a uniform finding. Patients will typically report knee pain, recurrent swelling, and mechanic symptoms. Specific complaints include locking, catching, buckling, pain with stairs or after sitting for extended periods, and joint line pain associated with walking or impact activities that improves with rest.

Physical examination of symptomatic patients may reveal the following: joint line tenderness, crepitus, effusion, decreased range of motion, or antalgia. Radiographs should be obtained in these patients as osteochondral defects (i.e., osteochondritis dissecans lesions) can frequently be detected with these studies. However, we suggest the use of cartilage-sensitive magnetic resonance imaging (MRI) for the imaging of articular cartilage lesions. Potter and colleagues showed that MRI had a sensitivity of 87%, a specificity of 94%, an accuracy of 92%, a positive predictive value of 85%, and a negative predictive value of 95% for the detection of a chondral lesions in the knee *(4)*. The authors concluded that it is possible to assess all articular surfaces of the knee accurately with MRI and detect which lesions might be amenable to both operative and nonoperative interventions. The use of cartilage-sensitive MRI is a valuable tool in the workup of patients with symptomatic chondral lesions; this imaging modality is used as part of the standard imaging protocol at our institution.

TREATMENT STRATEGIES

As mentioned, the initial management of patients with symptomatic chondral lesions is typically conservative. The primary focus of the initial treatment regimen is to control symptoms and improve knee function. However, it is important to consider that patient responses to these initial treatment modalities (cryotherapy, anti-inflammatory medications, intra-articular injections) are often unpredictable and idiosyncratic. Evidence-based treatment protocols and reliable predictors for identifying efficacious treatment strategies have yet to be established in this group of patients.

Given this lack of data, the goals of therapy should be focused on reducing pain and inflammation, increasing flexibility, increasing strength, and optimizing function for a timely return to activities of daily living. Those nonoperative treatment modalities that are available to clinicians include physical therapy, activity modification, bracing, patient education, topical medications, systemic medications, and intra-articular medications.

Nonpharmacological, Noninvasive Therapy

There is little information available in the literature on the efficacy of nonpharmacological, noninvasive therapies for the treatment of symptomatic chondral lesions. Deep heat (diathermy) may be useful in ameliorating patient symptoms. When applied prior to physical therapy or exercise, heat causes increased muscle flexibility and joint range of motion. The heat treatment may be delivered by ultrasound or microwave. Diathermy is used commonly by physical therapists and trainers in the treatment of symptomatic knees that are not actively inflamed or effused. However, Falconer and colleagues showed that diathermy provided no benefit with respect to pain reduction or functional gains when added to an exercise program *(5)*.

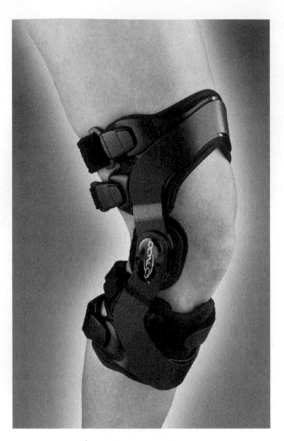

Fig. 3. Don Joy Unloader brace.

The authors suggested that diathermy can be used in those knees in which reestablishing range of motion remains problematic.

Perhaps the most commonly applied modality is cryotherapy; this modality may be applied via ice packs or devices that deliver ice water to the joint via a device that is secured directly to the knee (i.e., Cryocuff, Aircast Inc., Summit, NJ). Cryotherapy is valuable in reducing knee effusion and inflammation that may occur following acute knee injury.

Other modalities include external laser therapy and trancutaneous electric nerve stimulation (TENS). Although the effectiveness of these modalities has yet to be confirmed in the literature, each may be used in the treatment of symptomatic knees.

Bracing

The use of external knee braces has gained favor in the treatment of unicompartmental osteoarthritis (OA) of the knee (Fig. 3). Such braces are designed to decrease the joint reactive forces on either the medial or lateral compartments of the knee for the purposes of decreasing symptoms associated with cartilage damage. These braces include the Bledsoe Thruster (Bledsoe Brace Systems, Grand Prairie, TX), the DonJoy Montana OA (DonJoy Orthopaedic, Vista, CA), and the Generation II Unloader (Generation II Orthotics, Aliso Viejo, CA).

Several studies have demonstrated the effectiveness of putting an externally applied varus moment on valgus knees; the ability of these braces to both decrease the forces applied to arthritic knees and diminish symptoms has been confirmed *(6–9)*. Although not proven to have a similar efficacy for isolated chondral lesions, these braces can be used to aid the clinician in decreasing knee pain in those patients suffering from a symptomatic chondral lesion.

Foot orthoses, including heel wedges, theoretically may also decrease the joint reactive forces of either the medial or lateral compartment of the knee. Such wedges are fitted under the involved extremity to create a varus or valgus moment across the joint and unload the affected compartment. Support of the use of heel wedges and other foot orthoses in the treatment of symptomatic cartilage lesions is largely anecdotal.

Activity Modification/Patient Education

Patient education is of paramount importance for positive outcomes. Perhaps the most effective manner by which symptomatic relief may be obtained by affected patients is activity modification. Patients should make lifestyle adjustments to avoid activities that precipitate pain. In general, patients should decrease stresses on the knee joint. Specifically, impact-loading activities such as running or jogging should be avoided. In addition, heavy weight lifting and activities that require deep knee bends or repetitive knee motion are potential pain-inducing activities in affected patients. Weinberger and colleagues showed that telephone-based counseling with respect to treatment of OA of the knee had statistically significant benefit for patient functional status and the need for subsequent health care *(10)*. The Arthritis Self-Management program is a group patient education community-based intervention based on psychological theory that teaches behavioral modification, reciprocal social interaction, and structure *(11)*. In the program, patients learn the physical and mental skills to help live with their disease.

Physical Therapy and Exercise

Physical therapy has been shown to have the most proven benefit when compared with other nonpharmacological, noninvasive modalities for treatment of chondral lesions. When compared with nonexercising control patients, patients who routinely exercised had a significantly greater improvement in pain symptoms and function over time *(11)*. Activities include education, strengthening, and aerobics. Patients with OA who participated in aerobic activity for 30 min at least three times a week were able to improve their aerobic capacity, reduce their risk of chronic disease, improve psychological health, and enhance their overall quality of life.

With respect to articular cartilage injuries, the physical therapist must try to avoid activities and exercises that might produce excessive shear or compressive forces on the area of cartilage injury. Several studies have advocated the use of continuous passive motion (CPM) devices as a means of decreasing symptoms associated with an articular cartilage lesion *(12)* (Fig. 4). Salter and colleagues demonstrated that CPM was of greater benefit than immobilization or intermittent activity for healing of full-thickness chondral defects *(13)*. Some of the benefits are attributed to the ability of CPM to distribute synovial fluid throughout the joint, thus providing nutrients to damaged intra-articular tissues *(14)*.

In addition to CPM, strengthening the muscles around a joint also helps to protect the articular surfaces. For example, with respect to knee chondral injuries, quadriceps isometric exercises, bicycling, limited arc isotonic quadriceps strengthening, straight leg raises, and closed kinetic chain exercises have all been demonstrated to decrease knee pain in affected knees. In general, we recommend that such exercises be done under the supervision of a licensed physical therapist.

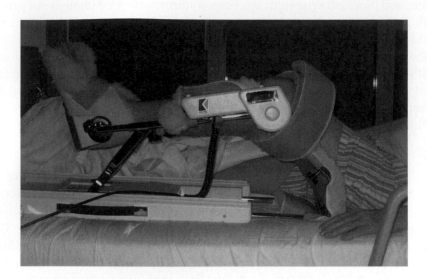

Fig. 4. Continuous passive motion (CPM) machine.

Pharmacotherapies

Analgesics

Acetaminophen has been recommended as a first-line pain control measure in the treatment of OA and chondral lesions. This drug acts on the central nervous system to decrease pain and has been shown to be as efficacious as nonsteroidal anti-inflammatory drugs (NSAIDs) for pain relief *(15)*. Acetaminophen has a safer profile with respect to the incidence of adverse events and is generally thought to be less toxic compared to oral anti-inflammatory medications or narcotics. Caution should be used in the prescription of acetaminophen in those patients with hepatic dysfunction.

Tramadol hydrochloride (Ultram) is a centrally acting opioid analgesic that possesses antidepressant properties as well. This drug prevents the reuptake of norepinephrine and serotonin in the synaptic cleft by acting on central nervous system opioid receptors. It is indicated for the long-term treatment of chronic moderate-to-severe pain as likelihood of the development of chemical dependence is much less with Tramadol compared to other narcotic medication. Potential side effects include lowered seizure threshold, nausea, and dizziness.

Opiod analgesics are usually reserved for those patients with severe pain who otherwise do not respond to the use of acetaminophen, oral NSAIDs, or Tramadol. Narcotic pain-relieving drugs are effective. Unfortunately, prolonged use does typically result in narcotic dependence and decreasing effectiveness. We strongly suggest that patients who present with a chronic articular cartilage injury and a history of prolonged narcotic use be treated adjunctively by a pain management specialist. It is important to remember that these substances are federally controlled with a side-effect profile that includes nausea, constipation, tolerance, dependence, and respiratory depression. Ytterberg et al. showed that opioid analgesics could be used for management of chronic arthritic pain with minimal side effects, although many authors would reserve these drugs for acute flairs *(16)*.

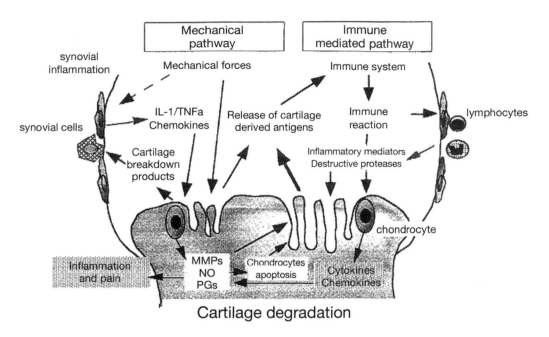

Fig. 5. Chemical mediators of arthritis.

Nonsteroidal Anti-Inflammatory Drugs

The NSAIDs are effective pain relievers and have been used for many years in the management of musculoskeletal pain. Traditionally, OA has been considered an arthritic condition that results from abnormal knee mechanics as opposed to systemically modulated inflammation. However, increased concentrations of inflammatory mediators, such as interleukin 1, tumor necrosis factor-β, and nitric oxide are found in the synovial fluid of cartilage-injured patients and osteoarthritics (Fig. 5). This fact provides the rationale for the use of NSAIDS by affected patients who fail management by other means.

There are more than 15 NSAIDs commercially available, including ibuprofen, naproxen, meloxicam, and indomethacin. These drugs possess both anti-inflammatory and analgesic properties (Fig. 6). The clinical response to these medications is highly idiosyncratic between patients and medications. These drugs act through a nonselective inhibition of cyclo-oxygenase (COX) and lipoxygenase; inhibition of these enzymes results in an overall reduction of prostaglandin synthesis and inhibition of the inflammatory cascade.

Complications associated with the use of NSAIDs include gastrointestinal (GI) bleeding, hepatic dysfunction, renal dysfunction, and platelet inhibition. Some research suggests that these drugs are detrimental to bone and tendon healing *(17)*. Regarding cartilage, there are conflicting reports that the drugs are harmful to cartilage by decreasing prostaglandin synthesis; other data suggest that the drugs are actually chondroprotective.

Selective COX-2 inhibitory drugs were developed in hopes of reducing those side effects typically associated with nonselective anti-inflammatory medications (Fig. 7). These drugs include celecoxib, rofecoxib, and valdecoxib. Although these drugs have demonstrated overall efficacy profiles similar to that of traditional NSAIDs, it is important to note that currently both rofecoxib and valdecoxib are not available because of concerns about the increased incidence of cardiovascular events in some patients taking these drugs (Fig. 8).

Arachidonic acid products

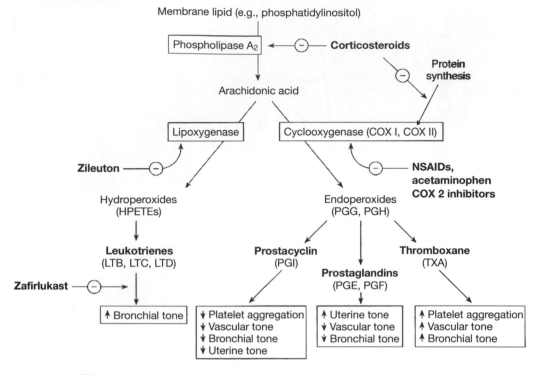

Fig. 6. Mechanism of action of nonsteroidal anti-inflammatory drugs.

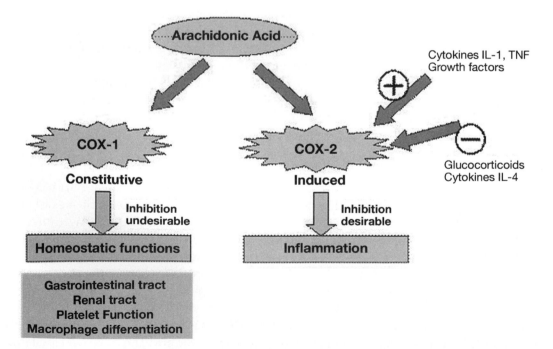

Fig. 7. Selective cyclo-oxygenase enzyme inhibition.

Biochemical Selectivity of COX-2 Inhibitors

Measured in vitro with human whole-blood assays
of COX isozyme activity

Ibuprofen	0.5
Naproxen	0.7
Acetaminophen	1.6
Indomethacin	1.9
Meloxicam	18.0
Nimesulide	19.0
Diclofenac	29.0
Celecoxib	30.0
Rofecoxib	267.0

Fig. 8. Biochemical selectivity of common anti-inflammatory drugs.

Although the COX-2 enzyme is relatively specific for peripheral inflammation, the COX-1 enzyme mediates normal maintenance of the GI mucosa, liver, kidneys, and platelets. Thus, in development the selective inhibition of COX-2 and not COX-1 represented a huge potential benefit as it was thought that the incidence of GI side effects would decrease markedly with the use of drugs in this class compared to traditional NSAIDs. The importance of this drug class is more significant in light of a study that attributed 20–30% of all peptic ulcer deaths to NSAID use *(18)*. COX-2 inhibitors have led to an overall decrease in GI complications. Use of traditional NSAIDs with gastroprotective therapy such as misoprostol has also been advocated by some *(19)*.

Both rofecoxib (Vioxx) and valdecoxib (Bextra) were withdrawn from the market. A recent 3-yr trial involving Vioxx and its role in the prevention of recurrent polyps was stopped by the Data Safety Monitoring Board. It had been observed that those individuals taking Vioxx had a statistically significant increase in the risk of adverse cardiovascular events, specifically stroke and heart attack. The finding was particularly evident in those participants taking Vioxx for more than 18 mo. Vioxx had been associated with hypertension in the past, but in light of these findings, was voluntarily withdrawn from the market.

Glucosamine and Chondroitin Sulfate

The theoretical basis for the use of oral glucosamine and chondroitin in patients with cartilage injury suggests that by increasing the concentration of these ground substance materials into the affected joint, one could facilitate a decrease in knee pain symptoms and promote cartilage repair *(25)*. The substrates are ingested, absorbed in the GI tract, enter the plasma, and are filtered into the synovial fluid. Glucosamine is a simple amino sugar that serves as a building block for glycosaminoglycan (GAG) and hyaluronic acid (HA) synthesis (Fig. 9). Roden et al. demonstrated increased GAG production when glucosamine was added to cartilage-derived fibroblast cell cultures *(19a)*. Veterinary medical trials have shown the efficacy of these drugs *(20)*. Furthermore, numerous human studies have shown improvement in pain scores as well as a decrease in arthritis progression when compared to controls *(20–26)*. In addition, this drug does not have the adverse effects of NSAIDs with respect to the GI or hematopoietic systems.

Chondroitin sulfate is a mucopolysaccharide and a constituent of aggrecan. Chondroitin sulfate and keratin sulfate bond to a protein core to make aggrecan (Fig. 10). This complex interacts with hyaluron to form a macromolecule largely responsible for the biomechanical

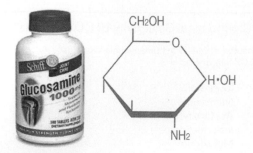

Fig. 9. Molecular composition of glucosamine.

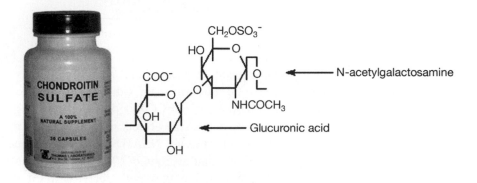

Fig. 10. Molecular composition of chondroitin sulfate.

properties of articular cartilage. As individuals age, the ratio of keratin sulfate to chondroitin sulfate increases, thus reflecting a relative lack of chondroitin sulfate. This is further evidenced by the shorter chondroitin sulfate side chains in diseased cartilage. The pain-relieving effects of this drug are comparable to other oral ground substance supplements. The side-effect profile is also favorable, with few GI complications and good bioavailability (Fig. 11).

Both chondroitin and glucosamine have grown in popularity, partly because of widespread media coverage and their availability for direct purchase that requires no prescription. However, the true efficacy has yet to be established, and many studies have been met with skepticism in the scientific community.

In 2001, Reginster and colleagues reported the results of a double-blind clinical trial involving 212 people with OA who took either glucosamine or a placebo daily (24). Patients were evaluated by both clinical measures and radiographs after 1 and 3 yr. Symptoms were scored by the Western Ontario and McMaster Universities (WOMAC) OA index. WOMAC scores improved by more than 20% in the glucosamine group but worsened slightly in the placebo group. Radiographic evaluation revealed a mean joint space loss after 3 yr of 0.31 mm in the placebo group compared to 0.06 mm in the 106 patients on glucosamine sulfate. These data has been questioned because of their standardization methods. In addition, there was little correlation between the joint space changes and the symptoms.

Other studies have shown similar radiographic data with chondroitin sulfate. Verbruggen and colleagues found that chondroitin sulfate led to a decrease in the radiological progression of the anatomical lesions in pathological finger joints over a 3-yr period. Thus, chondroitin may not improve disease but rather slow the progression of disease (26).

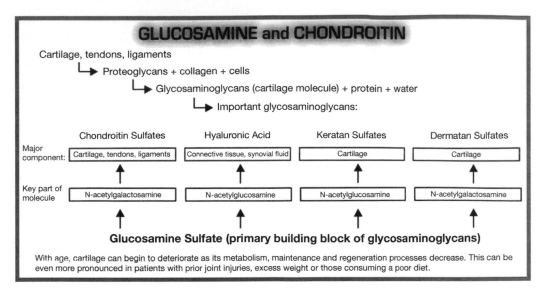

Fig. 11. Proposed mechanism of glucosamine and chondroitin sulfate.

A large meta-analysis of these two drugs published in the *Journal of the American Medical Association* revealed favorable clinical results without commenting on the progression of OA *(22)*. However, most of the individual studies were subsidized by the product's manufacturer and had serious design flaws. The authors concluded:

> Trials of glucosamine and chondroitin preparations for OA symptoms demonstrate moderate to large effects, but quality issues and likely publication bias suggest that these effects are exaggerated. Nevertheless, some degree of efficacy appears probable for these preparations. *(22)*

An accompanying editorial warned

> As with many nutraceuticals that currently are widely touted as beneficial for common but difficult-to-treat disorders, the promotional enthusiasm often far surpasses the scientific evidence supporting clinical use. Until high-quality studies, such as the National Institutes of Health study, are completed, work such as [the meta-analysis] is the best hope for providing physicians with information necessary to advise their patients about the risks and benefits of these therapies. *(25)*

Topical Analgesics

For individuals with mild-to-moderate symptoms associated with cartilage injury, the use of topical agents may be appropriate. Capsaicin cream has an unknown mechanism of action but seems to deplete A, delta, and C neural fibers of substance P, a molecule that is integral in the conduction of pain impulses. This has had the effect of attenuating articular pain pathways and decreasing joint inflammation. Capsaicin has minimal side effects and has been advocated as adjunctive treatment or monotherapy and can be applied up to four times daily *(27)*. Topical NSAIDs have also been proposed as a treatment modality. Skepticism has arisen regarding its overall safety and efficacy as compared to its oral counterpart.

Intra-Articular Medical Therapies

Intra-articular corticosteroid injections were first described by Hollander in the 1950s. Although their benefit, with specific regard to pain relief, is generally accepted, enthusiasm for the use of such injections is tempered by the relative short-term effect, idiosyncratic response, and paucity of clinical studies that support their efficacy. Intra-articular injections are ideally indicated for the management of acute joint pain or inflammation that is associated with known cartilage injury. Such patients usually have failed attempts at the use of oral NSAIDs and physical therapy. Cartilage degradation (chondrolysis) and Charcot arthropathy occur with repeated intra-articular injections so more than three injections are not recommended per year in any one joint *(28)*. Those patients who require repeated injections of corticosteroids should be considered for operative repair as this is not a long-term treatment strategy.

HA is large viscoelastic GAG that is present in both articular cartilage and synovial fluid. The viscosity of HA contributes important biomechanical properties to the synovial fluid. HA aids in the absorption and distribution of forces during high-impact activities such as running and jumping; HA acts as a viscous lubricant during slow movements.

Viscosupplementation is the process by which pathological synovial fluid is removed and replaced with HA-based products (Synvisc, Hyalgan, Supartz). Typically, these injection are administered via weekly intra-articular injections *(3–5)*. It is believed that by increasing the HA concentration to normal levels (levels found in the healthy joint) the viscoelasticity properties might approach those of normal synovial fluid. Several clinical studies have demonstrated a benefit in the majority of patients within a heterogeneous OA population, with improvement in symptoms from months to years. However, there is no evidence to support a persistent increase in HA content after the initial increase from the injection *(29)*. Side effects include local inflammatory reactions (3%) and septic joint-like symptoms (<0.2%), which increase with injections that miss the intra-articular space.

Injection technique is critical to the procedure. Prior to injection, the synovial fluid should be aspirated so the HA injection is not diluted; an intra-articular concentration of HA that is greater than 2 µg/mL at the time of injection is desired. The injection should be administered at the superolateral margin of the knee joint as this approach facilitates avoidance of the anterior fat pad. Injection into the infrapatellar fat pad may compromise diffusion of the HA into the knee space, cause further knee joint inflammation, and decrease the effectiveness of the HA injection series. Ultrasound-guided aspirations and injection can be used but are generally not necessary.

To date, the experience with viscosupplementation has been encouraging. However, the clinician must consider that there is a distinct lack of prospective outcome studies that have analyzed the effective of HA injection, especially as the use of these drugs relates to patients suffering from isolated cartilage defects.

SUMMARY

Chondral lesions are commonly encountered by the practicing orthopedic surgeon. Many patients who present with a symptomatic cartilage lesion will likely undergo repair. However, as the natural history of these lesions remains poorly understood, the clinician should employ a course of nonoperative treatment immediately following the injury to confirm that the lesion is indeed persistently symptomatic. The described nonoperative modalities can be effective at relieving pain and improving function in affected patients.

REFERENCES

1. Minas T, Nehrer S. Current concepts in the treatment of articular cartilage defects. Orthopedics 1997;20:525–538.
2. Curl WW, Krome J, Gordon ES, Rushing J, Smith BP, Poehling GG. Cartilage injuries: a review of 31,516 knee arthroscopies. Arthroscopy 1997;13:456–460.
3. Shelbourne KD, Jari S, Gray T. Outcome of untreated traumatic articular cartilage defects of the knee: a natural history study. J Bone Joint Surg Am 2003;85A(suppl 2):8–16.
4. Potter HG, Linklater JM, Allen AA, Hannafin JA, Haas SB. Magnetic resonance imaging of articular cartilage in the knee. An evaluation with use of fast-spin-echo imaging. J Bone Joint Surg Am 1998;80:1276–1284.
5. Falconer J, Hayes KW, Chang RW. Effect of ultrasound on mobility in osteoarthritis of the knee. A randomized clinical trial. Arthritis Care Res 1992;5:29–35.
6. Keating EM, Faris PM, Ritter MA, Kane J. Use of lateral heel and sole wedges in the treatment of medial osteoarthritis of the knee. Orthop Rev 1993;22:921–924.
7. Lindenfeld TN, Hewett TE, Andriacchi TP. Joint loading with valgus bracing in patients with varus gonarthrosis. Clin Orthop 1997:290–297.
8. Matsuno H, Kadowaki KM, Tsuji H. Generation II knee bracing for severe medial compartment osteoarthritis of the knee. Arch Phys Med Rehabil 1997;78:745–749.
9. Smith EM, Juvinall RC, Corell EB, Nyboer VJ. Bracing the unstable arthritic knee. Arch Phys Med Rehabil 1970;51:22–28 passim.
10. Weinberger M, Tierney WM, Booher P, Katz BP. Can the provision of information to patients with osteoarthritis improve functional status? A randomized, controlled trial. Arthritis Rheum 1989;32:1577–1583.
11. Pate RR, Pratt M, Blair SN, et al. Physical activity and public health. A recommendation from the Centers for Disease Control and Prevention and the American College of Sports Medicine. JAMA 1995;273:402–407.
12. Buckwalter JA. Effects of early motion on healing of musculoskeletal tissues. Hand Clin 1996;12:13–24.
13. Salter RB, Simmonds DF, Malcolm BW, Rumble EJ, MacMichael D, Clements ND. The biological effect of continuous passive motion on the healing of full-thickness defects in articular cartilage. An experimental investigation in the rabbit. J Bone Joint Surg Am 1980;62: 1232–1251.
14. Rubak JM, Poussa M, Ritsila V. Effects of joint motion on the repair of articular cartilage with free periosteal grafts. Acta Orthop Scand 1982;53:187–191.
15. Bradley JD, Brandt KD, Katz BP, Kalasinski LA, Ryan SI. Comparison of an antiinflammatory dose of ibuprofen, an analgesic dose of ibuprofen, and acetaminophen in the treatment of patients with osteoarthritis of the knee. N Engl J Med 1991;325:87–91.
16. Ytterberg SR, Mahowald ML, Woods SR. Codeine and oxycodone use in patients with chronic rheumatic disease pain. Arthritis Rheum 1998;41:1603–1612.
17. Cohen DB, Kawamura S, Ehteshami JR, Rodeo SA. Indomethacin and celecoxib impair rotator cuff tendon-to-bone healing. Am J Sports Med 2006;34:362–369.
18. Griffin MR, Ray WA, Schaffner W. Nonsteroidal anti-inflammatory drug use and death from peptic ulcer in elderly persons. Ann Intern Med 1988;109:359–363.
19. Lanza FL. A guideline for the treatment and prevention of NSAID-induced ulcers. Members of the Ad Hoc Committee on Practice Parameters of the American College of Gastroenterology. Am J Gastroenterol 1998;93:2037–2046.
19a. Roden L, Koerner T, Olson C, Schwartz NB. Mechanisms of chain initiation in the biosynthesis of connective tissue polysaccharides. Fed Proc 1985;44(2):373–380.
20. Lippiello L, Woodward J, Karpman R, Hammad TA. In vivo chondroprotection and metabolic synergy of glucosamine and chondroitin sulfate. Clin Orthop 2000:229–240.

21. Brief AA, Maurer SG, Di Cesare PE. Use of glucosamine and chondroitin sulfate in the management of osteoarthritis. J Am Acad Orthop Surg 2001;9:71–78.
22. McAlindon TE, LaValley MP, Gulin JP, Felson DT. Glucosamine and chondroitin for treatment of osteoarthritis: a systematic quality assessment and meta-analysis. JAMA 2000;283: 1469–1475.
23. Pavelka K, Gatterova J, Olejarova M, Machacek S, Giacovelli G, Rovati LC. Glucosamine sulfate use and delay of progression of knee osteoarthritis: a 3-yr, randomized, placebo-controlled, double-blind study. Arch Intern Med 2002;162:2113–2123.
24. Reginster JY, Deroisy R, Rovati LC, et al. Long-term effects of glucosamine sulphate on osteoarthritis progression: a randomised, placebo-controlled clinical trial. Lancet 2001;357: 251–256.
25. Tanveer E, Anastassiades T. Glucosamine and chondroitin for treating symptoms of osteoarthritis: evidence is widely touted but incomplete. JAMA 2000;283:1483–1484.
26. Verbruggen G, Goemaere S, Veys EM. Chondroitin sulfate: S/DMOAD (structure/disease modifying anti-osteoarthritis drug) in the treatment of finger joint OA. Osteoarthritis Cartilage 1998;6(suppl A):37–38.
27. Deal CL, Schnitzer TJ, Lipstein E, et al. Treatment of arthritis with topical capsaicin: a double-blind trial. Clin Ther 1991;13:383–395.
28. Dieppe PA, Sathapatayavongs B, Jones HE, Bacon PA, Ring EF. Intra-articular steroids in osteoarthritis. Rheumatol Rehabil 1980;19:212–217.
29. Marshall KW. Viscosupplementation for osteoarthritis: current status, unresolved issues, and future directions. J Rheumatol 1998;25:2056–2058.

6

Marrow Stimulation and Microfracture for the Repair of Articular Cartilage Lesions

Daniel J. Solomon, MD, Riley J. Williams III, MD, and Russell F. Warren, MD

Summary

Small full-thickness chondral injuries of the knee can be treated by marrow stimulation techniques. In the United States, the technique used most frequently to address posttraumatic femoral cartilage defects is microfracture arthroplasty. This chapter reviews the history, underlying theory, technique, and outcomes of microfracture and other marrow stimulation techniques.

Key Words: Microfracture; cartilage; knee; defect.

INTRODUCTION

Articular cartilage lesions are one of the most common findings during knee surgery. Some estimates put the number of articular cartilage repair procedures at more than 385,000 a year in the United States. In an effort to better define the patient population that might benefit from articular cartilage repair techniques, Curl et al. retrospectively reviewed the findings in 31,516 arthroscopies. They noted a 63% incidence of knee cartilage lesions. Outerbridge grade IV chondral lesions in patients under age 40 accounted for 4% of all lesions noted at arthroscopy *(1)*. As long-term joint function is a primary objective in active patients, this young patient group represents those who would benefit most from treatment and repair of a cartilage injury.

Shelbourne et al. reviewed 125 patients with Outerbridge grade III or IV articular cartilage defects; these patients had no meniscal injury noted at the time of anterior cruciate ligament (ACL) reconstruction *(2)*. The mean size of the articular defects was 1.7 cm^2 (range 0.5–6.5 cm^2). The study matched these patients by age and sex with 125 patients in whom ACL reconstruction was performed during which no chondral or cartilage injuries were noted. Follow-up evaluation was performed at an average of 6.3 yr postoperatively. Although both groups had mean subjective scores greater than 92, the authors found that patients with cartilage defects had significantly lower subjective scores than the control group. Objectively, there were no differences between the two groups.

It is a clinical fact that a significant number of articular cartilage injuries remain undiscovered until such time that a surgical procedure is performed. Although magnetic resonance imaging (MRI) has been able to detect such injuries reliably for many years, this technology is not widespread. As such, most surgeons are unable to plan appropriately for the majority of these lesions as they are often incidentally found. Clearly, the inability to detect these lesions represents a clinical dilemma to the practicing orthopedist and in part represents a

From: *Cartilage Repair Strategies*
Edited by: Riley J. Williams © Humana Press Inc., Totowa, NJ

major reason why microfracture and other marrow stimulation methods of cartilage repair remain quite popular.

The difficulties of treating cartilage lesions have been appreciated for centuries. In 1743, Hunter stated: "It is universally allowed that ulcerated cartilage is a troublesome thing and that when destroyed, it is not recovered" *(3)*. Articular cartilage is an avascular, aneural structure that possesses a limited capacity for repair. As such, clinicians have sought methods by which the body's repair mechanism might be enhanced. Marrow stimulation, as it relates to cartilage repair, essentially describes the surgeon's attempt to recruit pluripotent marrow-based stem cells into an otherwise unhealed cartilage defect. Different techniques have been used to allow marrow elements below the subchondral plate to populate the affected area and "regenerate" cartilage.

Magnuson originally proposed open debridement and abrasion of the exposed bone surface in the osteoarthritic knee in 1941 *(4)*. In the 1950s, Pridie described another open method of resurfacing arthritic joints *(5)*. He described drilling through the eburnated, exposed bone in osteoarthritic knees as a means of promoting cartilage regeneration and gaining pain relief. Insall reported results from the Pridie procedure in 62 knees *(6)*. Forty patients reported less pain after the procedure, and 46 of 62 patients thought the procedure was a success. Insall re-emphasized the need for careful patient selection. He discussed that the procedure should be reserved for middle-aged, potentially active patients.

The described marrow stimulation techniques were originally performed as open procedures using an arthrotomy. In the early 1980s, these procedures were pursued with renewed interest as comparable arthroscopic techniques were developed. Historically, marrow stimulation techniques have been used for treatment of osteoarthritic knees. Johnson described good success with abrasion arthroplasty with strict adherence to exclusion criteria in patients who otherwise meet indications for total knee arthroplasty *(7,8)*. He noted that appropriate indications are critical in obtaining a good or excellent result. Other authors have not been able to duplicate these results, with some finding that the addition of abrasion arthroplasty to arthroscopic debridement led to inferior results compared to those patients treated with debridement alone.

Friedman et al. reviewed 1 year follow-up results of 73 patients who underwent abrasion arthroplasty *(9)*. Sixty percent had notable improvement, and only 6% were worse after procedure. Of the 15 patients under age 40 in their group, 86% were improved. Johnson's criticism of that study was that postoperative nonweight-bearing was encouraged but not mandated *(7)*. Friedman and colleagues noted that many of their patients had been noncompliant with their nonweight-bearing status after 3 to 4 weeks.

Bert and Maschka performed a retrospective review with a mean of 5 years follow-up for 59 patients who underwent arthroscopic debridement with abrasion arthroplasty compared to a group of 67 patients who had arthroscopic debridement alone *(10)*. In the abrasion group, they found 51% good or excellent results vs 66% good or excellent results in the debridement-only group. The authors suggested that both groups had unpredictable results, but the abrasion group appeared to deteriorate more rapidly.

Rand examined the role of arthroscopy in the osteoarthritic knee by reviewing 3 year postoperative results of 28 patients who had debridement with abrasion arthroplasty *(11)*. Only 39% of these patients thought they were improved, and 50% underwent total knee arthroplasty within 3 years. In his comparison group, who had debridement alone, 77% were considered improved.

In a histological study of failed cartilage repair procedures, Nehrer et al. reported on 12 patients who underwent abrasion arthroplasty an average of 21 months prior to undergoing revision surgery *(12)*. The authors noted that the joint surface was not restored in any of the 12 patients. Only 2% of the tissue retrieved had the appearance of healthy articular cartilage when stained with safranin O.

Johnson has emphasized that the arthroscopic abrasion arthroplasty procedure is palliative, not curative. He also suggested that the procedure be used as a salvage approach in patients seeking to avoid knee arthroplasty *(7)*. Following abrasion arthroplasty, the postoperative regimen requires patients to be non-weight bearing for 2 full months following surgery to avoid displacing the fibrin clot that forms on the abraded surface of the bone. In a review of his 2 and 5 year results, 76% of the patients had ongoing complaints; however, only 6% deteriorated to the point of having a total knee replacement. Johnson's criticism of the studies by Rand, Bert, and Friedman and their coauthors included that they did not have the same rigorous contraindications that he applied to patients undergoing the same procedure.

Hubbard found that there is a significant benefit of articular debridement compared to washout alone for grades III–IV Outerbridge changes of the medial femoral condyle *(13)*. In 76 knees with a mean follow-up of 4.4 years, knee debridement resulted in a mean improvement in the Lysholm score of 28 at 1 year and 21 at 5 years following surgery. The washout-only group had a mean improvement in the Lysholm score of 5 at 1 years and 4 at 5 years. Although marrow stimulation techniques were not used in this study, it does suggests a benefit from debridement of unstable cartilage encountered during arthroscopy.

Steadman and colleagues first described the microfracture method in the early 1980s. The technique was described for the treatment of posttraumatic full-thickness cartilage lesions as opposed to resurfacing of osteoarthritic knees. Important differences between microfracture and abrasion arthroplasty or drilling included the preservation of subchondral plate integrity and the avoidance of possible thermal necrosis. The microfracture method allows a marrow cell-rich fibrin clot to adhere to the exposed bony surface, thus facilitating a fibrocartilaginous repair. Steadman noted that proper postoperative management and rehabilitation, including use of continuous passive motion (CPM), are critical to obtaining an optimal result.

MARROW STIMULATION: HOW DOES IT WORK?

Articular cartilage is avascular. Thus, full-thickness cartilage injuries that do not involve bone have no intrinsic capacity to heal on their own. Violation of the subchondral plate promotes bleeding and the local migration of cells and other anabolic factors that might support the formation of repair tissue. Open marrow stimulation techniques that were developed by Magnuson and Pridie followed the concept that repair tissue emanated from the vascular bed deep to the sclerotic subchondral plate of a condylar lesion. Penetration of the subchondral bone was required to stimulate the formation of repair tissue; this penetration of bone was achieved by either drilling or burring. The method by which repair tissue formed in the area of cartilage injury was poorly understood. However, it is now appreciated that marrow stimulation techniques facilitate the local recruitment of marrow-based mesenchymal stem cells within a cartilage defect by the creation of vascular access channels. Following the creation of these channels, marrow blood containing fibrin, platelets, and marrow-based cells forms what Steadman and colleagues have termed a *superclot*. Within this clot, marrow-based stem cells populate the defect within the fibrin clot scaffold. It is believed that the pluripotent nature of these stem cells allows for the formation of reparative fibrocartilage via cellular differentiation along a chondral phenotype.

Shapiro et al. evaluated the repair tissue that formed after creating full-thickness chondral defects in rabbits *(14)*. Full-thickness chondral defects were created, and the subchondral bony plate was violated. Marrow-based mesenchymal cells repopulated the defect, proliferated, and later differentiated into repair tissue. Based on autoradiography after cellular labeling, chondrocytes from the adjacent intact articular cartilage did not migrate into the repair tissue. The repair tissue was demonstrated to be mostly fibrocartilage. Collagen fibrils did not integrate into the remaining native cartilage, suggesting a potential vulnerability to shear forces at the repair tissue-native tissue interface. This weak point was theorized to be the potential source of repair tissue degradation. Unfortunately, reparative fibrocartilage is composed mainly of type I collagen; structurally, fibrocartilage is much less resilient to compressive loads compared to articular cartilage, which is primarily composed of type II collagen. The resulting fibrocartilage has decreased resilience and stiffness and poor wear characteristics compared to hyaline cartilage.

The microfracture procedure is ideally suited to the treatment of isolated cartilage defects. Such defects are believed to cause pain and joint dysfunction because of altered joint reactive forces that are associated with the persistence of these lesions on the articular surface. Essentially, the joint is abnormal because some of the surface is missing; the microfracture procedure seeks to add tissue and resurface the joint in an isolated area. Filling such cartilage defects may decrease the forces on intact cartilage that exists at the edge or rim of the defect. In horses, Convery et al. found that defects in the weight-bearing portion of the femoral condyle, ranging from 6 mm^2 to 1 cm^2, resulted in increased defect rim stress concentration and chondral wear at the lesion rim *(15)*. Defects of 9, 15, and 21 mm diameter drilled to a depth equal to the diameter on the femoral surfaces led to perimeter chondral breakdown and progressive degeneration on the corresponding tibial surface. Dunn et al. found that the cartilage surrounding the defect had decreased compliance and developed characteristic histological changes *(16)*.

The goal of microfracture and marrow stimulation techniques is to restore as much normal architecture and structure as possible. Sgaglione stated that the "Holy Grail" for treatment of focal articular cartilage lesions will be a method that restores organized hyaline cartilage through a practical, minimally invasive approach that is minimally morbid not only perioperatively but also over an extended period of time *(17)*.

Alfredson, Lorentzon, and colleagues described marrow stimulation by drilling combined with autogenous periosteal patch transplantation with good results *(18,19)*. This technique is a hybrid of using a periosteal patch over the surface of a chondral defect treated with drilling or microfracture. Lorentzon and coworkers reported 17 excellent and 8 good results from 26 patients treated with this combined technique for chondral defects of the patella. The patients all used CPM postoperatively and were followed for a mean of 42 months *(19)*.

Future adjuncts to microfracture and marrow stimulation may include the addition of growth factors. A great deal of research is ongoing concerning the benefits of a variety of growth factors on chondrocyte maturation and development. We do not yet know the value of adding growth factors to the fibrin clot and mesenchymal milieu in vitro. Martinek and colleagues reviewed the use of gene therapy for augmentation of articular cartilage repair *(20)*. The benefit of a gene therapy approach would be steady upregulation of growth factor in the joint. There remain challenges in the control of regulation and, of course, which factors to

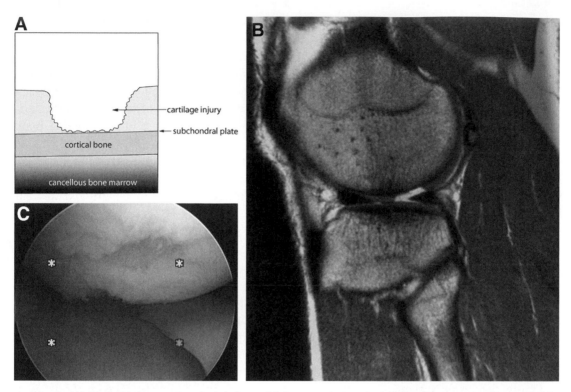

Fig. 1. (A) Full-thickness chondral defect with intact subchondral plate. **(B)** Preoperative magnetic resonance imaging showing full-thickness chondral lesion of the lateral femoral condyle. **(C)** Arthroscopic picture of full-thickness (Outerbridge grade IV) chondral injury to femoral condyle. (Illustration by Cynthia Bugwadia, Hospital for Special Surgery, Digital Media Center.)

regulate. The value of any growth factor therapy would be a potential increase in the proportion of type II to type I collagen, an increased number of viable chondrocytes, or creation of a more normal, hyaline-type layered architecture to the repair cartilage after microfracture.

INDICATIONS

Microfracture is a simple, single-stage procedure ideally suited for the first-line treatment of a small, well-contained, Outerbridge grade III or IV cartilage lesion (Fig. 1). Microfracture was originally developed as a method to treat posttraumatic articular cartilage injuries of the knee that had progressed to full-thickness defects. Its use has since expanded to treatment of unstable cartilage lesions that overlie subchondral bone and focal areas of degenerative joint disease. The technical simplicity of the procedure, cost-effectiveness, and relatively low patient morbidity make microfracture an invaluable tool for smaller full-thickness cartilage lesions detected preoperatively with MRI or found serendipitously during arthroscopy.

The size of the cartilage lesion best addressed with microfracture or other marrow stimulation techniques is controversial. There are few studies in the literature that compare different cartilage repair procedures; thus, we have few clinical data to guide us in the decision-making process. Animal and anatomic studies exist that address the critical lesion size for the treatment of a cartilage defect. Guettlar et al. reported a critical lesion diameter of 10 mm (0.79 cm^2) over which defect rim stresses increase significantly compared to smaller lesions *(21)*. The authors postulated that size of the femoral condyle and shear stress may also play a significant role in the progression of degenerative changes at the lesion site. Jackson et al. found progressive deterioration of osteochondral defects in defects that measured 6 mm diameter and depth in goats *(22)*. They described a "zone of influence" surrounding the lesion; collapse of the surrounding area of articular cartilage and subchondral bone was demonstrated by histology.

We typically employ the microfracture technique in symptomatic articular cartilage lesions of the femoral condyles and trochlea that measure less than 4 cm^2 with preserved subchondral bone. In patients with lower demand, microfracture can be utilized to treat larger lesions.

WORKUP

The detailed workup includes the following components: history, physical examination, and imaging studies.

The surgeon should ascertain the etiology and acuity of the cartilage injury. Patients with a preoperative duration of symptoms that is less than 12 months fare better following microfracture compared with individuals who have experienced pain in excess of 12 months prior to surgical repair *(23)*. Previous management, especially prior surgery, should be noted; arthroscopic photographs should also be inspected when available. This information aids in assessing the lesion's character and allows the surgeon insight into which methods were employed in trying to promote healing prior to his or her involvement. In lesions that were previously treated by microfracture or other cartilage procedure (osteochondral autograft transfer, autologous chondrocyte implantation), clinical improvement success is unlikely if microfracture is performed again. Successful microfracture becomes less likely if integrity of the subchondral plate has been previously violated.

The patient's demographics (age, gender, family history), general medical history, and lifestyle choices should be considered in the decision-making process in cartilage surgery. For example, patients less than 30 years old tend to have better clinical outcomes postoperatively following microfracture; thus, age should be considered during surgical indication for this technique. In addition, the presence of systemic disease (rheumatoid arthritis, Lyme disease) is a contraindication to the surgical repair of isolated cartilage lesions. Relevant information from the patient's history should be considered in all potential microfracture cases.

The patient's ability to comply with rehabilitation has a significant long-term impact on the success of cartilage repair procedures. Typically, patients must tolerate 6 weeks of nonweight bearing on the operated limb and use a CPM machine over the same time period after surgery. Patients should be aware of the postoperative limitations and expectations following the microfracture procedure to ensure optimal functional outcomes. Moreover, most cartilage repair cases take several months to "heal," and most studies report a return to high-level sports at a time that usually exceeds 6–8 months following surgery. Thus, patient expectation should be actively managed prior to surgery to ensure a smooth functional recovery.

Physical examination should begin with measurement of the patient's height and weight to determine their body mass index (BMI; patient weight in kilograms divided by patient height in meters). A BMI of more than 30 has been associated with poorer outcomes after microfracture compared to similarly treated patients with a BMI less than 30 *(23)*.

During the physical examination, body habitus and gait are assessed; clinical knee alignment should also be noted. The focused knee examination should test for knee tenderness (joint lines, patella facets); knee stability (ACL, posterior cruciate ligament, collateral ligaments); and range of motion. Ligamentous integrity is important as most cartilage procedures should be accompanied by ligament repair or reconstruction of deficient stabilizers of the knee joint. It is believed patients with ligamentous insufficiencies are susceptible to abnormal knee translation and the application of excessive shear forces on the cartilage surface. In addition to ligament insufficiency, meniscal integrity should be evaluated with both physical examination and imaging studies. Meniscal volume is an important predictor of clinical success in the patient with articular cartilage injury. All patients who are under consideration for chondral repair must have functional meniscal tissue present in the affected compartment as it has been demonstrated that increased localized joint forces occur with a decreasing percentage of meniscal tissue. Tenderness at the joint lines are usually associated with both chondral lesions of the condyles and meniscal repair; as such, imaging studies, especially MRI, are critical in completing the patient workup.

Radiological assessment should include the following knee views: standing anteroposterior view, standing posteroanterior 40° flexion view, lateral view, patellar view (Merchant's). Long alignment films (standing hip-knee-ankle anteroposterior view) should be obtained as well. The mechanical axis is measured on a straight line from the center of the femoral head to the center of the tibio-talar joint. All patients should be assessed for limb malalignment; osteotomy is considered for knees that extend beyond physiology tibio-femoral varus or valgus. The clinician should assess patellofemoral alignment in the case of patellar or trochlear lesions.

MRI provides an excellent noninvasive method of evaluating the chondral surfaces of the knee. Detailed MRI images are obtained using a cartilage-specific fast spin echo sequence *(24–28)*. The depth of the defect is estimated, and a modified radiographic Outerbridge scoring system is applied to these images. For traumatic lesions and osteochondral lesions, penetration of the tidemark and associated bone bruises can be identified. Lesion location and size can be estimated using multiplanar imaging. In addition, the adjacent and opposing surfaces can be evaluated for integrity. The specific characteristics of a chondral lesion are difficult to determine directly using radiography.

Fortunately, cartilage-sensitive MRI accurately provides the clinician with useful information. For example, whether there is containment of the cartilage injury can be determined using MRI. A well-circumscribed or "contained" lesion is necessary for a successful outcome following microfracture. Thus, it behooves the surgeon to understand this specific characteristic prior to planning the microfracture approach. This is yet another reason why cartilage-sensitive MRI is recommended prior to every planned cartilage repair case and is regarded as a powerful tool in preoperative planning in these patients.

MRI can be used postoperatively to evaluate the morphological feature of the repair tissue, including percentage of defect fill, repair tissue incorporation, fissuring, and bony overgrowth (Fig. 2). When postmicrofracture lesions are imaged postoperatively, MRI typically demonstrates a hyperintense signal in the repair tissue that is consistent with less-organized cartilage and increased water mobility in the cartilage matrix. MRI T2 mapping is a relatively new imaging technique that more extensively evaluates the cartilage collagen content of repaired lesions. T2 mapping uses the correlation between water content and T2 relaxation times to provide information about cartilage orientation, zonal structure and quality. In repair cartilage,

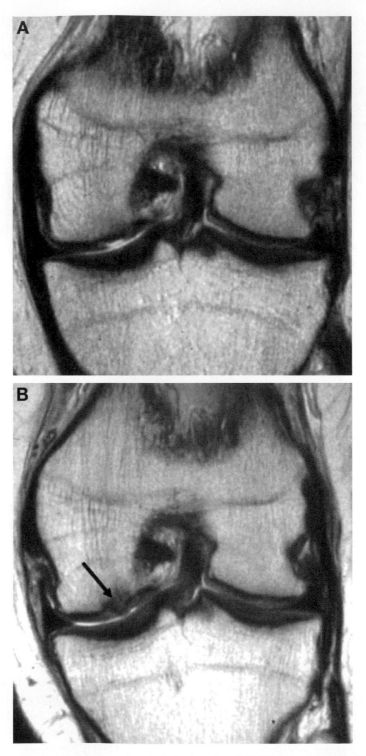

Fig. 2. (A) Magnetic resonance imaging (MRI) showing full-thickness chondral defect of femoral condyle. **(B)** Six months following microfracture, chondral surface filled in with fibrocartilage but bony overgrowth of subchondral plate (solid arrow) obvious with MRI. (Illustration by Cynthia Bugwadia, Hospital for Special Surgery, Digital Media Center.)

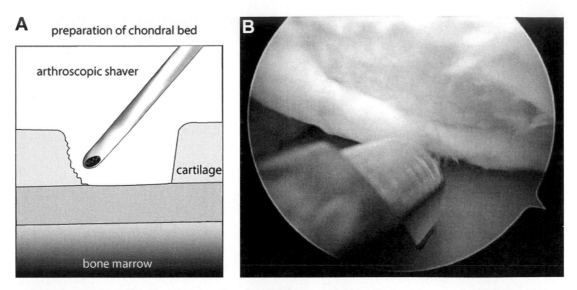

Fig. 3. (A) Illustration of arthroscopic preparation of chondral lesion for microfracture creating a "contained lesion" and debriding the calcified subchondral plate. **(B)** Arthroscopic image of motorized shaver used for chondral debridement prior to microfracture. (Illustration by Cynthia Bugwadia, Hospital for Special Surgery, Digital Media Center.)

there is typically a lack of the expected T2 stratification from the subchondral plate to the articular surface with T2 heterogeneity.

SURGICAL METHOD

Once a patient has been indicated for surgery, we apply the microfracture technique as described by Steadman et al. *(29–32)*. We apply a well-padded pneumatic tourniquet to the patient's upper thigh but do not typically inflate it. Following the administration of regional anesthesia (spinal or epidural block), the arthroscopy commences. A thorough ligamentous and arthroscopic examination of the knee is preformed; all surfaces are graded according the Outerbridge classification. Once the microfracture has been completed, blood and fat may obscure visualization. As such, we recommend performing other intra-articular procedures, such as meniscal debridement or repair and ACL reconstruction prior to the microfracture portion of the case.

Once the lesion has been identified, the area is cleared of all unstable and damaged cartilage. Fibrous tissue should be removed from the bony base of the defect. Care must be taken to avoid violation of the subchondral plate when performing any deep debridement. The cartilage surrounding the defect rim should be debrided with a shaver or arthroscopic knife to create a stable perpendicular edge of healthy cartilage (Fig. 3). We do not recommend aggressive use of a motorized burr for this debridement as there is a risk of removing excessive amounts of bone.

Arthroscopic awls are used to make multiple holes in the defect 3–4 mm apart to a depth of approx 5 mm. Care is taken to position and space the holes such that the subchondral bone bridges between the perforations remain intact, thus ensuring subchondral plate integrity. The rim of the lesion is treated first; the central holes are created last. Various angled awls can be utilized to assist in ensuring the holes are perpendicular to the joint surface (Fig. 4).

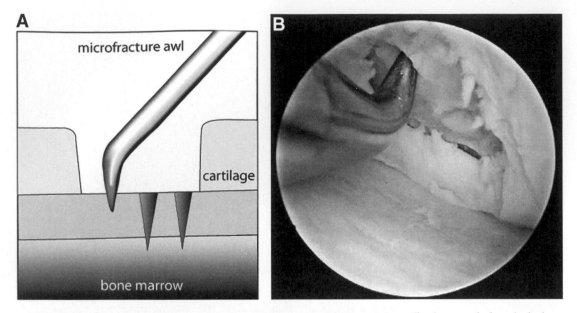

Fig. 4. (A) Illustration of microfracture technique. Awl is kept perpendicular to subchondral plate. **(B)** Arthroscopic image of microfracture awl. (Illustration by Cynthia Bugwadia, Hospital for Special Surgery, Digital Media Center.)

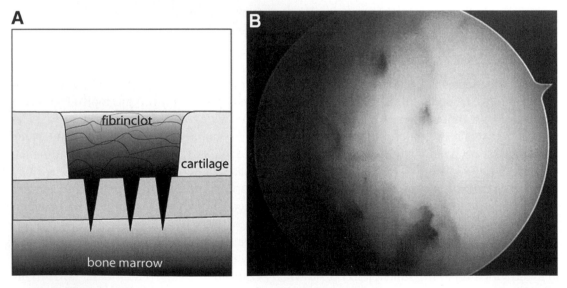

Fig. 5. (A) Defect fills with fibrin clot contained by prepared wall of intact cartilage around lesion. **(B)** Arthroscopic image of blood with marrow elements emanating from microfractures. (Illustration by Cynthia Bugwadia, Hospital for Special Surgery, Digital Media Center.)

Once the holes have been created, all excess bony debris is removed using a shaver. The arthroscopic pump pressure is decreased to visualize blood and fat droplets emanating from the holes, thus confirming the creation of vascular access channels within the defect. The tourniquet, if used, is deflated (Fig. 5). A drain should not be used as the success of the procedure relies on formation of a clot in the defect. Once bleeding has been confirmed within the defect, all instruments are removed. An intra-articular cocktail, if used, should not contain epinephrine.

REHABILITATION

Cartilage physiology is considered in the rehabilitation of patients who undergo the microfracture procedure. Chondrocytes are sensitive to pressure and deformation. CPM may help stimulate chondrocyte matrix production. Motion likely has a molding effect that results in the shaping of the newly formed repair tissue such that it conforms to the treated articular surface. Weight bearing, especially in the first 6 weeks after surgery, is detrimental, however. Potential propagation of the microfractures or collapse of the subchondral plate in the early stage is the risk of early weight bearing and should be avoided at all costs. Shear or excessive pressure in this early phase can flatten the repair cartilage or displace the mesenchymal cells and clot from the defect.

Following surgery, patients remain toe-touch weight bearing with crutches for at least 6 weeks; patients with larger lesions may be protected for 8 weeks. Once this protected weight-bearing interval is complete, weight bearing is gradually increased over the subsequent 2-week period until full weight bearing is tolerated. CPM is initiated in the recovery room and continued 6–8 hours a day for 6 weeks. Machine settings are started at 0–60° of knee motion and are increased as tolerated 10° per day until full range of motion is achieved. Cryotherapy is initiated in the recovery room and continues until all swelling and effusion are resolved. A femoral nerve block can be quite helpful for postoperative pain control. The use of anti-inflammatory medications is avoided if possible for 4 weeks following surgery.

Isometric exercises and dynamic quadriceps training start in supervised physical therapy during the first postoperative week. We institute water exercises at 2 weeks and allow patients to begin riding a stationary bicycle as soon as range of motion permits. Resistance exercises are started in physical therapy at 6 weeks. Pivoting and jumping are restricted until at least 4 months postoperatively. Patients are not allowed to run until 6 months following surgery and only at this time if their quadriceps and core pelvic strength allows. High-level sports are usually allowed around 8–12 months following surgery.

Our rehabilitation protocol is modified for patellar or trochlear lesions. After microfracture, the patient's knee is braced in extension. If there are no treated lesions of the weight-bearing tibial or femoral surfaces, then partial weight bearing is allowed at 1 week; full weight bearing is allowed at 2 weeks, with the brace locked in full extension. A CPM device is applied with the brace off for 6 hours a day for 6 weeks with a range from 0 to 80°; care is taken to avoid knee flexion beyond 80–90°.

CLINICAL FOLLOW-UP

As part of our institutional cartilage registry, all patients are evaluated prior to surgery and at 3, 6, 12, 24, and 48 months following surgery using validated functional outcome measures. Postoperative MRI with cartilage sequencing provides an excellent evaluation of the percentage of lesion fill and has the added advantage of evaluating the underlying subchondral plate with respect to integrity and overgrowth (Figs. 2, 6). Cartilage-sensitive MRI is obtained 3 months following microfracture to assess lesion fill.

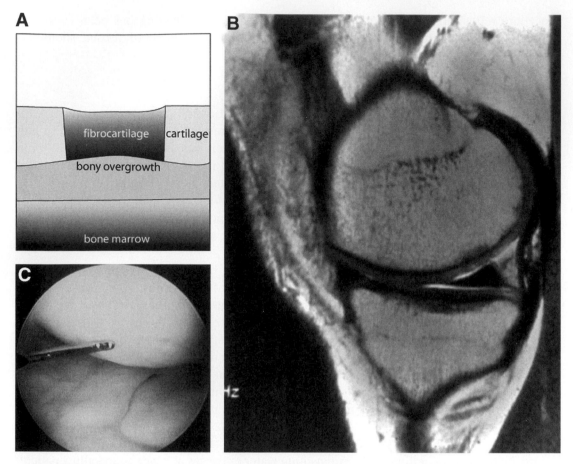

Fig. 6. (A) Final appearance with fibrocartilage fill of defect and mild bony overgrowth of subchondral plate. **(B)** Magnetic resonance imaging appearance of femoral condyle microfracture 4 mo postoperatively. **(C)** Arthroscopic appearance of healed medial femoral condyle lesion after microfracture. (Illustration by Cynthia Bugwadia, Hospital for Special Surgery, Digital Media Center.)

LITERATURE REVIEW

As the developer of the microfracture technique, Steadman and his colleagues have written extensively about this method of treating cartilage injuries. To study the healing response in articular cartilage after microfracture, Frisbee and colleagues used two equine models that studied the use of microfracture to treat articular cartilage lesions. In one study, microfractured knees were evaluated at 8 weeks postoperatively, and they were examined at 4 and 12 months in another study *(33,34)*.

In the 8-week study, the authors created a chondral defect of the femoral condyle in the same animal in different knees; half were treated with microfracture, and half were used as controls. An increase was noted in type II collagen messenger ribonucleic acid (mRNA) expression in repair tissue after microfracture compared to the control knees *(33)*. No significant difference in the expression of other matrix mRNA or protein levels, including type II collagen protein, was noted in the first 8 weeks after microfracture.

In their long-term study, Frisbee and coworkers had previously described enhancement of type II collagen protein after microfracture *(34)*. The authors suggested that the lack of type

II collagen protein in their 8-week equine model could be a reflection of sample collection times, measuring increased mRNA production that had not yet been matched by increased protein translation. In their earlier study, they found repair tissue after microfracture to have significantly more type II collagen than the control at 4 and 12 months following surgery.

The use of CPM is a critical adjunct to the success of marrow stimulation techniques. Salter's work in rabbits demonstrated a more rapid and complete metaplasia of healing tissue within articular cartilage defects when CPM was used compared to those animals that did not receive CPM following the creation of a cartilage defect *(35)*. Rodrigo et al. compared a group of patients who utilized postoperative CPM (6–8 hours/day, 8 weeks) after microfracture to a group of patients who were not able to comply with the postoperative CPM regimen *(36)*. Of their first 298 microfracture patients, 77 underwent second-look arthroscopy; these patients comprised the cohort for this study. Of the 77 patients, 46 were CPM compliant, and 31 were not CPM compliant. At arthroscopy, the cartilage repair tissue quality was visually graded (1 for poor, 5 for excellent); they found a mean cartilage grade for patients in the CPM group of 2.67 compared to a mean score of 1.67 in the non-CPM group. Of the patients in the non-CPM group, 45% had no improvement in cartilage repair grade after their microfracture procedure. Age, lesion size, or lesion location did not affect the cartilage repair score. The authors did not assess functional outcome in this study.

Blevins et al. assessed the functional outcome and lesion morphology in a group of 48 highly competitive athletes and 188 recreational athletes who underwent the microfracture procedure *(37)*. The largest improvement in mean functional scores occurred in the first postoperative year. Second-look arthroscopy was performed in 26 highly competitive and 54 recreational athletes. In the highly competitive group, 95% improved at least one cartilage repair grade compared with 65% in the recreational group. Of the highly competitive athletes, 77% returned to sport; 71% of the elite athletes reported achieving a level of play that was equal or superior to their preinjury level of competition, and 50% were still competing 3 years after microfracture.

In another study, Steadman and coworkers reported results using microfracture to treat chondral injuries in 25 National Football League players *(38)*. Nineteen of these athletes returned to play the season following their surgery. The average Lysholm score improved from a preoperative score of 52 to a postoperative score of 90 at an average of 4.5 years follow-up. Pain and the incidence of recurrent swelling decreased, and functional outcome also improved significantly in the majority of athletes.

Gobbi et al. also described use of microfracture to treat chondral lesions in athletes *(39)*. Fifty-three athletes, 26 professional and 27 recreational, with an average age of 38 years and mean follow-up of 6 years were included. The mean Lysholm scores improved from 57 preoperatively to 87 at final follow-up. Subjective ratings increased from a preoperative score of 40 (maximum score 100) to a postoperative score of 70 at final follow-up. Knee pain and swelling improved in 70% of patients. Functional testing was normal in 70% at final evaluation. The International Knee Documentation Committee (IKDC) score was normal or nearly normal in 70% of patients at final follow-up. The Tegner activity level was 3.2 before surgery; this number peaked at 6 at 2 years after surgery. The mean Tegner score ultimately declined to 5 at final follow-up evaluation. Strenuous sports activities increased following this trend, with improvement in 80% of patients at 2 years and gradually decreased to 55% of patients at final follow-up. Ten patients had repeat arthroscopy with tissue sampling. Histology in those samples revealed areas of fibromyxoid tissue with some differentiation and was described as "fibrocartilaginous hybrid tissue."

Steadman also reviewed longer-term outcomes of microfracture for isolated posttraumatic chondral lesions *(40)*. Seventy-one knees (mean patient age 30 years) with at least 7 years between surgery and the follow-up evaluation were included. The mean Lysholm score improved from 59 before surgery to 89 at final follow-up. Tegner activity level improved from 3 before surgery to 6 at final follow-up. Patient age over 35 years was determined to be a negative predictor of clinical success. Statistically, lesion size did not affect outcome. Using Western Ontario and McMaster University (WOMAC) pain scores, 23 knees were pain free at final follow-up; 38 had mild pain, and 10 had moderate pain. Overall, most improvement occurred in the first year after surgery, but improvement did continue for 2 to 3 years postoperatively. Little change was seen from year 2 to 7 regarding patients' ability to perform activities of daily living (ADLs), sports, and strenuous work.

In another study, Steadman and colleagues also reviewed outcome of microfracture arthroplasty for the treatment of isolated degenerative chondral lesions in patients aged 40–70 years at an average of 2.6 years of follow-up *(41)*. The mean Lysholm scores improved from 54 to 83; the mean Tegner activity score improved from 2.9 to 4.5 at final follow-up. Thirteen (16%) of the 81 patients in this cohort underwent manipulation after the microfracture procedure. Five patients (6.2%) had either revision microfracture or total knee arthroplasty within 3 years of the index microfracture. There was a trend to lower Lysholm scores in lesions larger than 400 mm^2 and in patients with lesions on adjacent articular surfaces.

Knutsen et al. compared autologous chondrocyte implantation with microfracture in a prospective randomized study of 80 patients *(42)*. Their well-designed study utilized a blinded independent observer and included arthroscopic and histological outcomes in addition to Lysholm, Tegner, and SF-36 subjective score. They found that, 2 years postoperatively, improvement in the microfracture group regarding Short Form (SF)-36 outcome was significantly better than that in the autologous chondrocyte implantation group. Younger and more active patients fared better in both groups. There was no difference in the arthroscopic or histological findings between the two groups.

PERSONAL EXPERIENCE

Mithoefer et al. reported on a prospective cohort of patients who underwent femoral condyle microfracture for isolated chondral injuries at Hospital for Special Surgery *(23)*. At an average follow up of 41 months, 66% of the 48 patients had good or excellent subjective results based on the IKDC and functional outcome. MRI was used to evaluate the lesion after microfracture and demonstrated good fill volume in 54% of lesions. All knees with good fill (>66% lesion fill) were shown to have significantly improved functional outcome. Bony overgrowth occurred in 25% of the microfractures, but it did not have any direct negative effect on outcome scores. However, poor lesion fill on follow-up MRI correlated with limited functional improvement and decreased functional scores after 24 months. Greater duration of preoperative symptoms led to worse outcomes. Of patients, 75% experienced a significant improvement in their ADL score if their preoperative symptom duration was less than 12 months compared with only 37% improvement if their symptoms were of longer duration. A BMI greater than 30 kg/m^2 was associated with poor clinical outcome and a relatively poor subjective rating scores. Gender, defect location, defect size, prior operations, and meniscectomy did not influence scores. The best results were observed in patients whose lesions had good fill volume on MRI, lower BMI, and shorter preoperative symptoms.

Good lesion fill was associated with improved ADL scores in 100% of patients. Improved ADL scores were less frequent with moderate (43%) and poor (33%) defect fill. Repair cartilage volume plays a critical role in the durability of knee functional improvements after microfracture repair.

REFERENCES

1. Curl WW, Krome J, Gordon ES, et al. Cartilage injuries: a review of 31,516 knee arthroscopies. Arthroscopy 1997;13:456–460.
2. Shelbourne KD, Jari S, Gray T. Outcome of untreated traumatic articular cartilage defects of the knee. J Bone Joint Surg 2003;85A(suppl 2):8–16.
3. Hunter W. On the structure and diseases of articulating cartilages. Philos Trans R Soc 1743;42(B):514–521.
4. Magnuson PB. Joint debridement: surgical treatment of degenerative arthritis. Surg Gynecol Obstet 1941;73:1–9.
5. Pridie KH. A method of resurfacing osteoarthritic knee joints. J Bone Joint Surg 1959;41B: 618–619.
6. Insall JN. The Pridie debridement operation for osteoarthritis of the knee. Clin Orthop 1974; 101:61–67.
7. Johnson LL. Arthroscopic abrasion arthroplasty: a review. Clin Orthop 2001;391(suppl):S306–S317.
8. Johnson LL. Arthroscopic abrasion arthroplasty historical and pathologic perspective: present status. Arthroscopy 1986;2:54–69.
9. Friedman MJ, Berasi C, Fox J, et al. Preliminary results with abrasion arthroplasty in the osteoarthritic knee. Clin Orthop 1984;182:200–205.
10. Bert JM, Maschka K. The arthroscopic treatment of unicompartment gonarthrosis: a 5-yr follow-up study of abrasion arthroplasty plus arthroscopic debridement and arthroscopic debridement alone. Arthroscopy 1989;5:25–32.
11. Rand JA. Role of arthroscopy in osteoarthritis of the knee. Arthroscopy 1991;7:358–363.
12. Nehrer S, Spector M, Minas T. Histological analysis of tissue after failed cartilage repair procedures. Clin Orthop 1999;365:149–162.
13. Hubbard M. Articular debridement vs washout of degeneration of the medial femoral condyle. J Bone Joint Surg. 1996;78B:217–219.
14. Shapiro F, Koide S, Glimcher MJ. Cell origin and differentiation in the repair if full thickness defects of articular cartilage. J Bone Joint Surg 1993;75A:532–553.
15. Convery FR, Akeson WH, Keown GH. The repair of large osteochondral defects. An experimental study in horses. Clin Orthop 1972;82:253–262.
16. Dunn WR, Mithoefer K, Prickett W, Warren R. An equine model for cartilage repair combining microfracture with and without fibrin clot supplementation. Unpublished manuscript; 2006.
17. Sgaglione NA. Decision-making and approach to articular cartilage surgery. Sports Med Arthrosc Rev 2003;11:192–201.
18. Alfredson H, Thorsen K, Lorentzon R. Treatment of tear of the anterior cruciate ligament combined with localized deep cartilage defects in the knee with ligament reconstruction and autologous periosteum transplantation. Knee Surg Sports Traumatol Arthrosc 1999;7:69–74.
19. Lorentzon R, Alfredson H, Hildingsson C. Treatment of deep cartilage defects of patella with periosteal transplantation. Knee Surg Sports Traumatol Arthrosc 1998;6:202–208.
20. Martinek V, Ueblacker P, Imhoff AB. Current concepts of gene therapy and cartilage repair. J Bone Joint Surg 2003;85B:782–788.
21. Guettlar JH, Demetropoulos CK, Yang KH, et al. Osteochondral defects in the human knee: influence of defect size on cartilage rim stress and load redistribution to surrounding cartilage. Am J Sports Med 2004;32:1451–1458.
22. Jackson D, Lalor P, Aberman H, et al. Spontaneous repair of full thickness defects of articular cartilage in a goal model. J Bone Joint Surg 2001;83A:53–64.

23. Mithoefer K, Williams RJ, Warren RF, et al. Prospective evaluation of the microfracture technique for treatment of articular cartilage lesions of the knee. J Bone Joint Surg Am 2005; 87(9): 1911–1920.
24. Potter H, Linklater J, Allen AA, et al. Magnetic resonance imaging of articular cartilage in the knee: an evaluation with use of fast-spin echo imaging. J Bone Joint Surg 1998;80A:1276–1284.
25. McCauley T, Distler D. Magnetic resonance imaging of articular cartilage of the knee. J Am Acad Orthop Surg 2001;9:2–8.
26. Sonin AH, Pensy RA, Mulligan ME, et al. Grading articular cartilage of the knee using fast spin-echo proton density-weighted MR imaging without fat suppression. AJR Am J Roentgenol 2002;179:1159–1166.
27. Wada Y, Watanabe A, Yamashita T, et al. Evaluation of articular cartilage with 3D-SPGR MRI after autologous chondrocyte implantation. J Orthop Sci 2003;8:514–517.
28. Brown WE, Potter HG, Marx RG, et al. Magnetic resonance imaging appearance of cartilage repair in the knee. Clin Orthop 2004;422:214–223.
29. Steadman JR, Rodkey WG, Singleton SB, et al. Microfracture technique for full-thickness chondral defects: technique and clinical results . Operative Tech Orthop 1997;7:300–304.
30. Steadman JR, Rodkey WG, Rodrigo JJ. Microfracture: surgical technique and rehabilitation to treat chondral defects. Clin Orthop 2001;391(suppl):S362–S369.
31. Steadman JR, Rodkey WG, Briggs KK. Microfracture to treat full-thickness chondral defects: surgical technique, rehabilitation, and outcomes. J Knee Surg 2002;15:170–1706.
32. Bartz RL, Steadman JR, Rodkey WG. The technique of microfracture of full-thickness chondral lesions and postoperative rehabilitation. Tech Knee Surg 2004;3:198–203.
33. Frisbee DD, Oxford JT, Southwood L, et al. Early events in cartilage repair after subchondral bone microfracture. Clin Orthop 2003;407:215–227.
34. Frisbee DD, Trotter GW, Powers BE, et al. Arthroscopic subchondral bone plate microfracture technique augments healing of large osteochondral defects in the radial carpal bone and medial femoral condyle of horses. J Vet Surg 1999;28:242–255.
35. Salter RB. The biologic concept of continuous passive motion of synovial joints. The first 18 yr of basic research and its clinical application. Clin Orthop 1989;242:12–25.
36. Rodrigo JJ, Steadman JR, Sillman J, et al. Improvement of full-thickness chondral defect healing in the human knee after debridement and microfracture using continuous passive motion. Am J Knee Surg 1994;7:109–116.
37. Blevins FT, Steadman JR, Rodrigo JJ, et al. Treatment of articular cartilage defects in athletes: an analysis of functional outcome and lesion appearance. Orthopedics 1998;21:761–768.
38. Steadman JR, Miller BS, Karas SG, et al. The microfracture technique in the treatment of full-thickness chondral lesions of the knee in National Football League players. J Knee Surg 2003;16:83–86.
39. Gobbi A, Nunag P, Malinowski K. Treatment of full thickness chondral lesions of the knees with microfracture in a group of athletes. Knee Surg Sports Traum Arthrosc 2004; May 10 [epub ahead of print].
40. Steadman JR, Briggs KK, Rodrigo JJ, et al. Outcomes of microfracture for traumatic chondral defects of the knee: average 11-year follow-up. Arthroscopy 2003;19:477–484.
41. Miller BS, Steadman JR, Briggs KK, et al. Patient satisfaction and outcome after microfracture of the degenerative knee. J Knee Surg 2004;17:13–17.
42. Knutsen G, Engebretsen L, Ludvigsen T, et al. A randomized trial of chondrocyte implantation compared with MFX in the knee. J Bone Joint Surg 2004;86A:455–464.

7

Cartilage Repair With Chitosan–Glycerol Phosphate-Stabilized Blood Clots

Michael D. Buschmann, PhD, Caroline D. Hoemann, PhD, Mark B. Hurtig, DVM, and Matthew S. Shive, PhD

Summary

A new biomaterial for cartilage repair has been developed and investigated in animal studies and in a clinical cohort. The biomaterial is a physiological solution of chitosan (a natural polysaccharide containing glucosamine residues) in a buffer containing glycerol phosphate (GP). The soluble and physiological characteristics of this polymer solution permit its combination with freshly drawn autologous whole blood to form a hybrid polymer-blood mixture that can be applied to cartilage and bone surfaces, to which it adheres and solidifies as a polymer-stabilized clot. Histology and electron microscopy analysis of in vitro-generated chitosan-GP/blood clots revealed the chitosan component to be dispersed among the blood components, to interact closely with platelets, and to impede platelet-mediated clot contraction, thereby maintaining a voluminous bioactive and adhesive clot at the site of application. Experiments in microdrilled cartilage lesions in adult rabbits comparing chitosan-GP/blood clots to controls (microdrilled only) highlighted the ability of chitosan-GP/blood clots to recruit more host cells and to increase subchondral vascularization and bone-remodeling activity during acute and intermediate stages of repair. This led to the establishment of more hyaline repair cartilage that was integrated with a porous subchondral bone plate. Microfractured cartilage defects in adult sheep treated with chitosan-GP/blood clots resulted in a statistically significant increase in tissue fill with a greater proportion of hyaline cartilage compared to controls (microfracture only). Patients with femoral condyle cartilage lesions have received chitosan-GP/blood implants to resurface articular cartilage as part of a compassionate use program for medical devices. Results to date suggest safety and clinical benefit of this approach that is free from both donor site morbidity and suture damage to healthy adjacent cartilage. This single-intervention approach is now the subject of a multicenter, randomized comparative clinical trial designed and initiated to investigate cartilage repair resulting from treatment with chitosan-GP and microfracture vs microfracture alone.

Key Words: Cartilage repair; chitosan; microfracture; osteoarthritis.

DEVELOPMENT OF FUNCTIONAL PROPERTIES OF HYALINE ARTICULAR CARTILAGE

Structure of Adult Articular Cartilage

Adult articular cartilage is composed of three stratified layers with distinct morphological characteristics *(1)*: the superficial, transitional, and radial zones. The superficial zone includes the articulating surface and contains chondrocytes with a discoidal morphology, a tangential orientation of collagen fibrils, and specific extracellular matrix (ECM) components, including

From: *Cartilage Repair Strategies*
Edited by: Riley J. Williams © Humana Press Inc., Totowa, NJ

superficial zone protein *(2)*. The extraordinary lubrication properties of the articular surface depend on load-induced exudation of fluid from the highly hydrated ECM *(3)* in addition to molecular lubrication arising from ECM and synovial fluid components at this interface *(4)*. The transitional zone, lying below the superficial zone, contains chondrocytes with a rounder morphology and displays a more isotropic orientation of collagen. The bulk of adult articular cartilage lies in the deepest, or radial, zone, so named to depict the radiating pattern of vertically oriented collagen fibrils emanating from the calcified cartilage layer just below the articular cartilage. The polygonally shaped chondrocytes of the radial zone are organized in vertical columns.

Below the radial zone lies the layer of calcified cartilage that interdigitates with the subchondral bone plate, the latter containing small vascularized osteons protruding into the calcified zone *(5)*. This cortical subchondral bone plate then melds with marrow-rich cancellous bone.

Although these general morphological characteristics of adult articular cartilage are conserved across species and between different joint surfaces, the proportion of each zone and each zone's detailed structures vary with age, species, and site. As an example, the articular cartilage of the central load-bearing region of the medial condyle in young adults is approx 2.4 mm thick with superficial:transitional:radial proportions of 10:10:80% and lies on top of a calcified cartilage layer that is 130 μm thick and a subchondral bone plate that is only 190 μm thick *(6)*.

Biomechanics of Adult Articular Cartilage

Biomechanical properties of articular cartilage are the result of a synergistic interaction between the three primary components of the ECM: collagen type II, the proteoglycan aggrecan, and the interstitial electrolyte fluid. The distance between adjacent glycosaminoglycan chains on aggrecan at the concentrations found in articular cartilage (~50 mg/mL) is only about 4 nm *(7)*, creating a very high resistance to the passage of interstitial fluid *(8)*, which comprises nearly 80% of the extracellular volume. Thus, a vertical compressive load exerted on articular cartilage could reduce cartilage height by expanding it laterally without creating relative flow of fluid with respect to aggrecan. However, the integrated structure of a healthy collagen network effectively resists tissue expansion, thereby trapping the proteoglycan in place, which in turn resists exudation of interstitial fluid and builds up a large hydrodynamic pressure of interstitial water. In this way, load in the articular cartilage of diarthroidial joints is primarily carried by interstitial water, but in a manner that depends on the presence of a high concentration of aggrecan entrapped by a dense and crosslinked collagen network.

Mathematical models of these load-bearing phenomena that separately account for the properties of these three components (proteoglycan, collagen, water) *(9–15)* have suggested that the primary role of the collagen network is to resist lateral expansion and retain proteoglycan because it is the fluid component that is the principle bearer of compressive load. Thus, a long-standing paradox in the biomechanics of adult articular cartilage has been the mechanical role and state of stress of vertically oriented collagen in the radial zone because collagen is typically oriented along the axis of tensile loading and extension, as in tendons and ligaments, rather than along the lines of compression, as in the radial zone of articular cartilage. This issue may be partly resolved by considering the developmental growth processes that gave rise to the stratified structure of adult articular cartilage. Such processes may also be critically important when designing strategies to repair cartilage lesions and achieve the functional structure of hyaline articular cartilage.

Development of Articular Cartilage

A resemblance between the stratification seen in adult articular cartilage *(1)* and the zonal organization in the cartilaginous growth plate *(16)* can be recognized. In the growth plate, flattened cells in the reserve zone are on top of columns of chondrocytes in the proliferating and hypertrophic zones, which in turn rest on a layer of calcified cartilage and bone containing a high density of blood vessels, similar to the zones found in adult articular cartilage. Appositional longitudinal bone growth is achieved in the growth plate by cellular hypertrophy and matrix synthesis in the columnar proliferating and hypertrophic zones *(17)*.

Although the development of articular cartilage has not been studied in as great detail as has the growth plate, the morphological similarity of these two structures is striking, and evidence has been presented for a similar appositional growth process in the development of articular cartilage of marsupials *(18)* and mammals (E. B. Hunziker, personnel communication, 2005). Stem cell progenitors have also been identified in the superficial zone of young articular cartilage *(19)*, similar to reserve stem cells found in the top zone of the cartilaginous growth plate. Most importantly, the growth and differentiation process of articular cartilage and the cartilaginous growth plate eventually diverge so that a functional layer of hyaline cartilage remains at the articulating surface while the growth plate closes at skeletal maturity. This divergence in development would appear to be the result of local microenvironmental stimuli involving gradients of diffusible morphogenetic factors and mechanical load-bearing signals.

In view of these developmental processes, the vertical orientation of collagen and columnar organization of chondrocytes in the radial zone of articular cartilage may be seen as a consequence of appositional growth of proliferating and hypertrophic chondrocyte columns where these cells secrete and assemble collagen in vertically oriented longitudinal septa during growth and development, as in the growth plate *(17)*. This radial zone structure remains in the adult and provides for biomechanical integration of a functional osteochondral unit by anchoring the uncalcified articular cartilage to the calcified cartilage layer, possibly in a manner that limits interfacial shear stress. Cartilage repair strategies that target the regeneration of this integrated and stratified hyaline articular structure could aim to facilitate the above-described natural processes of articular cartilage growth at the subchondral base of a surgically prepared lesion.

STRATEGIES FOR CARTILAGE REPAIR

Cell and Tissue Implantation

All experimental evidence to date suggests that resident chondrocytes are incapable of mounting an effective repair response, possibly because of limited matrix synthesis and proliferative capacity and their encapsulation in a nonmigratory ECM *(20–22)*. One approach to address this inherent deficiency is to deliver exogenous chondrocytes or tissue constructs that have been grown in vitro to mimic the composition and properties of cartilage. Although this approach is reasonable, it has encountered some significant difficulties in reaching clinical success.

Cell delivery into a chondral defect without penetration of subchondral bone, as is suggested for autologous chondrocyte implantation (ACI), is an attempt to re-create a functional osteochondral unit in a manner that does not resemble the naturally occurring developmental processes described above. It may not be possible for a relatively low number of chondrocytes placed on top of an intact subchondral bone plate to create a layer of progenitor stem cells surrounded by vascular supply and appropriate morphogenetic signals to induce appositional growth that leads to hyaline articular cartilage that is well integrated with its osseous base. Indeed, most animal studies examining the role and fate of implanted autologous chondrocytes have not provided strong evidence for the residence and contribution of these implanted cells toward the structure of the resulting repair tissue *(23–25)*. In clinical practice, the subchondral bone is also often breached to bleeding marrow *(26–28)*, thus allowing access to subchondral marrow elements that have the capacity to differentiate down the osteochondral lineage. It is also interesting to note that histomorphologic features of biopsies retrieved from repair cartilage from ACI qualified as successful or hyaline may often be suggestive of subchondral bone-derived repair cartilage *(27,29–33)*, described in more detail in the next section. To model the actual clinical practice of ACI, large animal studies have intentionally breached subchondral bone *(34)* and even provided microfracture holes *(35)*. The results of these studies and others *(36–38)* appear to suggest that implanted autologous chondrocytes may provoke a subchondral bone reaction but do not directly contribute to structural repair of cartilage lesions.

The implantation of in vitro-engineered tissue constructs may also be an appealing option *(39,40)*; however, the likelihood that they possess the correct compositional, structural, and biomechanical characteristics specific to the site of implantation is low, suggesting that extensive in vivo remodeling would be required. One alternative is preimplantation mechanical conditioning; however, even with these time-consuming approaches, the mechanical properties of such tissues are a fraction of those of native cartilage *(41)*. It is also not clear how such constructs could be effectively anchored with a vertical collagenous structure to the subchondral plate or to an implantable bone biomaterial *(42)*, barring their resorption and subsequent replacement by repair tissue originating from marrow below the base of the defect.

Bone Marrow Stimulation

The bone marrow stimulation family of surgical techniques includes Pridie drilling *(43)*, abrasion arthroplasty *(44)*, and microfracture *(45)*. These methods share the common feature of intentionally injuring subchondral bone below the cartilage lesion to induce wound repair and tissue regrowth. These surgical methods have gained partial acceptance over the years because clinical results have varied significantly between different practitioners and patient groups. However, a number of animal studies in multiple species have clearly demonstrated the intrinsic ability of injured subchondral bone to repair itself and to generate chondral repair tissue, albeit a tissue lacking hyaline articular structure and with limited reproducibility.

A randomized comparative clinical study found that microfracture was superior to ACI in terms of subjective clinical outcomes at 2 yr posttreatment, and that biopsy histological appearances were similar in the two groups *(31)*. A mixed retrospective/prospective study using magnetic resonance imaging to compare 5-yr outcomes of ACI and microfracture found that although microfracture led to slightly less lesion filling with uncharacterized tissue, it was associated with a much lower rate of reoperation compared to ACI (10 vs 60%) *(46)*. Given this low level of morbidity of microfracture and an acceptable level of clinical success, microfracture remains the primary first choice in many treatment algorithms for lesions of limited size (less than 2 cm^2) *(26,47)*.

Unfortunately, historical widespread and nonstandardized use of microfracture has resulted in uncontrolled and inconsistent surgical technique, follow-up measures, and physiotherapy programs, and consequently there remains a lack of understanding regarding why microfracture appears successful for some patients and surgeons and not for others. Furthermore, despite intrinsic differences between microfracture and the older and less-favored methods of Pridie drilling and abrasion arthroplasty, there have been no controlled animal studies or clinical studies directly comparing these approaches to identify which features or consequences of these different methods influence their success.

Animal studies of spontaneous repair of osteochondral lesions have determined that the manner in which the cartilage lesion is surgically prepared can greatly influence the repair response. Skeletally mature animals must be used in these studies because bone marrow-derived repair is clearly much more efficacious in young animals than in older ones *(48–52)*. Detailed studies in an abraded equine model *(53)* and in drilled rabbit trochlea *(49,54–57)* have identified the following sequence of events in the reparative process: hematoma formation in the subchondral space, proliferation and migration of inflammatory and stromal cells from the cancellous marrow into the fibrin clot, transformation of the fibrin clot into a vascularized provisional and cellular granulation tissue, bone remodeling, and frequently the induction of growth plate-like structures at foci within granulation tissue. These latter structures then grow in a manner similar to that described in which zones of proliferation, hypertrophy, calcification, vascular invasion, and endochondral bone formation can be identified.

In reported successful cases for which bone marrow stimulation has resulted in a hyaline-like articular surface, it would appear that this process was sufficient in restoring articular cartilage, whereas in others it was not. Previous animal and clinical studies have identified several surgically controlled factors that critically influence the success of bone marrow stimulation procedures: (1) size of the lesion *(58–61)*; (2) depth of the lesion and damage to viable subchondral bone *(62,63)*; (3) presence of the calcified cartilage layer (*see* next paragraph); (4) the number, size, and depth of channels accessing deep marrow *(49,56)*; and (5) postoperative articulation and load bearing *(64)*. Location of the lesion can also be a critical determinant of success *(53,65)*.

It is important to emphasize that calcified cartilage is an effective barrier to marrow-derived repair, as has been shown in several studies and species *(35,38,53,66–70)*. Thus, although removal of all calcified cartilage from cartilage lesions may maximize spontaneous repair, evidence strongly suggests that excessive debridement that impinges too deep into subchondral bone can result in lack of repair *(59)*, subchondral cysts *(62)*, and ultimately poor clinical outcome, as in abrasion arthroplasty that was performed too aggressively *(63)*. Hence, retention or restoration of subchondral bone support is a requisite for cartilage repair.

The Blood Clot in Cartilage Repair

The residence and stability of the marrow-derived blood clot in the chondral zone and subchondral zone of the debrided cartilage lesion after bone marrow stimulation is not ensured and has been rarely examined. The central hemostatic component in blood is the platelet, an anuclear, discoid-shaped cell (2-μm diameter) containing growth factor-rich (platelet-derived growth factor [PDGF], transforming growth factor-β) α-granules, a contractile cytoskeleton, and multiple integrin-binding sites and cell-signaling pathways *(71)*. On exposure to subendothelial structures such as collagen, platelets adhere and bind to each other to form an aggregated plug that rapidly contracts and secretes its granular components to stimulate fibrin formation, acute inflammation, and wound repair *(72)*.

The loss of clot volume during clot retraction induced by the platelet actin-myosin contractile apparatus is impressive because more than half of the original volume can be lost within a few hours by serum exudation during this contractile phase *(73)*. Such clot retraction

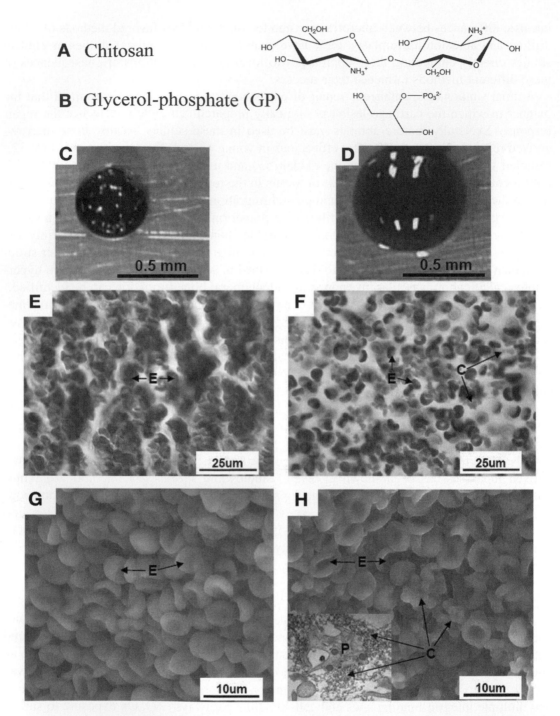

Fig. 1. Physiological chitosan-glycerol phosphate solutions mixed with freshly drawn blood produce adherent solidifying implants. Chitosan is a cationic polymer of glucosamine that is partly acetylated (**A**). Buffering chitosan with glycerol phosphate (**B**) produces solutions of chitosan-GP that have near-neutral pH and physiological osmolarity. Mixing 1 vol chitosan-GP solution with 3 vol freshly drawn blood produces a hybrid polymer/blood mixture that adheres to tissue surfaces, solidifies within 15 min, but does not retract (**D**) over time as with a regular blood clot (**C**). Photos in **C** (blood only) and **D** (chitosan-GP/blood) were taken 1 hr postsolidification, showing a significant

is advantageous in dermal wounds, for which rapid closure can be achieved by drawing opposing wound edges together. However, retraction in a cartilage lesion in which the clot is only integrated to the bone bed will simply result in detachment from cartilaginous surfaces and shrinkage, forming compact clot residues adhered to sites of bleeding bone such as microfracture holes. Indeed, the few studies examining clot stability and residence following abrasion and drilling have confirmed this expectation *(36,54,57,69,74)*. Consequently, a critical aspect to examine and control in bone marrow-derived cartilage repair is the quantity and quality of the resulting blood clot present in the cartilage lesion. These observations suggest that, to improve existing bone marrow stimulation procedures, a voluminous, adherent, and physically stabilized blood clot should reside above a debrided cartilage lesion containing multiple access channels to deep trabecular marrow.

CHITOSAN-GLYCEROL PHOSPHATE/BLOOD CLOTS IN CARTILAGE REPAIR

Structure and Properties of Chitosan-Glycerol Phosphate/Blood Clots

One approach to stabilizing the blood clot in the cartilage lesion is to disperse a soluble polymer scaffold throughout uncoagulated whole blood. The ideal polymer should be soluble at physiological pH and osmolarity, be nontoxic to maintain biological viability of clot components, and would resorb in a reasonable time frame. The polymer should also permit or promote coagulation rather than inhibit it, simultaneously reinforce the clot and impede clot retraction, and adhere to cartilaginous and osseous surfaces.

A polymer solution with these unique properties was developed by dissolving chitosan in an aqueous glycerol phosphate (GP) buffer *(75)*. Chitosan is a linear polysaccharide containing glucosamine and *N*-acetyl-glucosamine residues (Fig. 1A) and is derived by deacetylation of chitin, a major component in the shells of crustaceans *(76)*. Chitosan has been researched extensively in biomedical fields because of its abundance, biodegradability, biocompatibility, low toxicity, and adhesiveness to tissues *(77)*. Previous studies have also shown chitosan to stimulate repair of dermal *(78)*, corneal *(79)*, and bone *(80)* lesions and to amplify mitogenic responses to PDGF *(81)*. In addition, chitosan can be hemostatic because of its ability to chain erythrocytes and activate platelets *(82–84)*. Degradation and clearance of chitosan is effectively accomplished by enzymatic degradation *(85–87)* followed by elimination as low molecular weight fragments (<10 kDa) in urine *(88)*.

A major technical limitation in the biomedical application of high molecular weight chitosan has been its insolubility at physiological pH. Developments have overcome this limitation using GP as a buffer *(89,90)*. GP can titrate chitosan to neutral pH (6.8) and near isotonicity while maintaining chitosan in a soluble state rather than as precipitated particulates as was previously the case. Mixing chitosan-GP with freshly drawn whole blood

---

Fig. 1. *(Continued)* (>50%) loss of clot volume for blood alone vs a negligible loss of volume for chitosan-GP/blood. Histological sections of these clots reveal a packed mass of erythrocytes (indicated by E in the figure) for blood alone **(E)** vs an expanded viable clot with erythrocytes separated by a chitosan-containing component (C) for chitosan-GP/blood **(F)**. Environmental scanning electron micrographs of hydrated clots show the packed mass of erythrocytes for blood alone **(G)** and reveal a chitosan-containing component is interlaced throughout the clot mass as small aggregates of approx 2-μm diameter spheres **(H)**. A transmission electron micrograph **(H inset)** indicates chitosan in close apposition to a platelet (P) that is not yet degranulated.

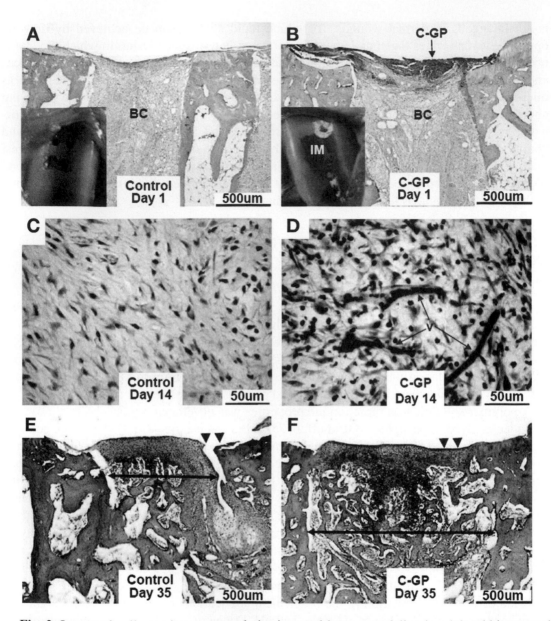

Fig. 2. Increased cell recruitment, vascularization, and bone remodeling in adult rabbits treated with chitosan-GP/blood implants. The 3.5 × 4.5 mm cartilage defects were created using flat scalpel blades in the trochlea of 8- to 15-month-old New Zeeland white rabbits. Four 0.9-mm diameter holes were then drilled 4 mm deep into the subchondral bone to initiate bleeding (**A inset**). Histological analysis of acute defects suggested that about half of the calcified cartilage between the drill holes was intact. A physiological solution of chitosan (1.7% w/v) in glycerol phosphate buffer (135 m*M*) at pH 6.8 was mixed with 3 vol of freshly drawn autologous blood and deposited onto the defect in one knee, where it adhered and solidified (**B inset**). The contralateral knee was similarly operated as a control without the chitosan-GP/blood implant. At 1 d postoperative sacrifice, Safranin O/Fast Green-stained sections taken along the central axis of a drill hole (**A**), (**B**) showed a blood clot (BC) filling the drill hole in the control knee (**A**) and the chitosan-GP/blood (C-GP) implant interfacing with this blood clot in the treated knee (**B**). The subsequent repair response characterized at 14 d postoperative (**C**), (**D**) revealed a granulation tissue in the chitosan-GP/ blood-implanted knee that was

(chitosan-GP to blood ratio of 1:3) produces a chitosan-GP/blood clot that does not retract (Fig. 1D) compared to a whole blood clot alone (Fig. 1C). This noncontractile clot property is specific for chitosan-GP/blood mixtures and is not found for other polysaccharides, including hyaluronic acid *(73)*. The hemostatic activity of chitosan also slightly accelerates coagulation of chitosan-GP/blood clots compared to whole blood, solidifying in approx 7–10 min *(73)*. Histological sections of these clots reveal an expanded structure for chitosan-GP/ blood clots (Fig. 1F) compared to whole blood clots (Fig. 1E), explained through environmental scanning electron microscopy, by which the chitosan component is seen dispersed throughout the blood as small aggregates of approx 2-μm diameter spheres (Fig. 1H). Transmission electron microscopy demonstrates close apposition of chitosan to platelet membranes (Fig. 1H inset), suggesting that chitosan may impede platelet-mediated clot contraction by physically disrupting binding of fibrinogen to platelets. Interestingly, some of the chitosan-associated platelets are not yet degranulated (Fig. 1H inset), a state that may provide for an extended period of release of α-granule contents, including PDGF and transforming growth factor-β.

Modulation of Acute Events in Cartilage Repair by Chitosan-Glycerol Phosphate/Blood Clots

A small animal model of cartilage repair was used to examine the acute events in bone marrow-derived cartilage repair and their modulation by the presence of chitosan-GP/blood clots. Adult (8- to 15-mo-old) New Zealand white rabbits ($n = 49$) were bilaterally operated, and uncalcified cartilage was carefully scraped from a 3.5×4.5 mm^2 region on each trochlea. These rectangular defects then received four drill holes (0.9-mm diameter) each to a depth of approx 4 mm (Fig. 2A inset). Although the calcified layer may impede repair tissue formation, its removal in preliminary experiments in this small animal model resulted in frequent osteolysis and subchondral cyst formation, and thus it was partly retained.

Autologous blood was freshly drawn from the rabbit's ear and combined at a ratio of 3 parts blood to 1 part chitosan-GP. Approximately 25 μL of chitosan-GP/blood was applied to alternating right or left trochlear defect and allowed to solidify for 8 min (Fig. 2B inset) before closing the knee. The other trochlear defect was allowed to bleed freely and represented a bone marrow stimulation control.

Animals were sacrificed at fixed times ranging from 1 d to 56 d postsurgery, and knees were fixed and decalcified, and sections were generated in paraffin, plastic, and cryosections for histological examination. Staining with Safranin O/Fast Green was used to identify hyaline tissue and chitosan *(91)*; Gomori's trichrome specifically stained erythrocytes, permitting an appreciation of angiogenic activity and vascularization events.

The chitosan-GP/blood clot was present in 23 of 24 animals sacrificed between day 1 and 14 postoperative, but chitosan was no longer detected after 35 d, indicating an approx 1-mo residence time. Interestingly, this residence time was similar to an optimal residence time for different biomaterials, identified in a rabbit study employing deeper (1.5-mm) osteochondral

---

Fig. 2. *(Continued)* more cellular and more vascular (v = capillary vessels) than control (**D** vs **C**). At 35 d postoperative, a differentiating chondral repair tissue can be observed above vascularized subchondral bone in both control (**E**) and treated (**F**) knees. The knee treated with the chitosan-GP/blood implant revealed increased subchondral bone remodeling compared to control, resulting in a wider zone of new vascularized bone (arrows in **F** vs **E**), which has permitted greater articular resurfacing with adherent repair tissue (arrowheads).

defects *(92)*. On day1, chitosan-GP was identified as a dark staining material that filled chondral portions of the defect (Fig. 2B) more than the fibrin clot in the control (Fig. 2A) and interfaced with the blood clot in the drill holes (Fig. 2B). The marrow stimulation-only control followed the previously described sequence of proliferation and migration of inflammatory and stromal cells from the cancellous marrow into the fibrin network (days 3–14), transformation of the fibrin clot into a vascularized provisional and cellular granulation tissue (days 7–21), bone formation and remodeling (days 7–21), and induction of growth plate-like structures at foci in deeper zones of the drill holes (days 14–35), which eventually produced bone filling in the osseous portion of the defect and an irregular resurfacing of the articular surface with a mixture of fibrocartilage interspersed with more hyaline-like tissue in certain regions.

Differences in the biological events within the defect region were observed as early as 1 d postoperative comparing chitosan-GP-treated defects to control and continued throughout the study. Defects treated with chitosan-GP also followed the above-described generic reparative sequence of events but with the following distinct modifications: Chitosan-GP was found to (1) increase cell migration into the drill holes (Fig. 2D vs 2C); (2) increase vascularization in the defect that included both large vessels deep in the defect invading growth plate-like foci, as well as small vessels in more superficial regions (Fig. 2D), which could increase anabolic capacity, progenitor cell recruitment, and proliferation in this region; (3) increase intramembranous bone formation (i.e., without a cartilaginous precursor) in deeper regions of the drill holes and spatially displace growth plate-like foci to be closer to the chondral zone; and (4) increase the volume of remodeled subchondral bone (Fig. 2F vs 2E), which in turn increased the regeneration of tissue with good attachment to subchondral bone (arrows in Fig. 2F vs detachment in Fig. 2E). These observations were quantified using unbiased stereological methods and are presented in further detail elsewhere *(54)*.

Animals sacrificed at the latest time-point in this series of studies of 56 d *(93)* showed that treatment with chitosan-GP significantly increased the percentage of the cross-sectional area of defects that was covered between the drill holes with attached and integrated repair tissue (76% chitosan-GP vs 39% control) and the amount of repair tissue that stained intensely for collagen type II (51% chitosan-GP vs 11% control). Furthermore, histological scoring at 56 d using the O'Driscoll scale *(64)* revealed that chitosan-GP treatment led to significantly greater hyaline morphology, toluidine blue staining intensity, and cellularity for repair tissue in the chondral zone, both between the drill holes and over the drill holes. Finally, the porosity of subchondral bone plate, assessed stereologically, was nearly doubled in chitosan-GP defects vs control defects, a likely consequence of increased vascularization and bone remodeling found at earlier times as described.

Taken together, these observations demonstrate that chitosan-GP/blood implants adhere to cartilage defects containing access channels to subchondral bone and reside for approx 1 mo. During this time, with reference to marrow stimulation controls, treatment with chitosan-GP/blood increases cell recruitment, transient vascularization, and bone remodeling, which later results in greater resurfacing of the cartilage lesion with tissue of improved hyaline quality that is well integrated with a porous subchondral bone.

Improvement in Fill and Hyaline Quality of Cartilage Repair by Chitosan-Glycerol Phosphate/Blood Clots in Microfractured Adult Sheep Articular Cartilage Defects

The ability of chitosan-GP/blood implants to improve the repair of cartilage defects vs a microfracture control group was assessed in an adult (3- to 6-yr-old) ovine model (further details are presented in ref. *69*). Unilateral arthrotomy was performed in each animal, and two 1-cm^2 chondral defects were created, one in the central load-bearing region of the medial condyle and the other on the lateral distal facet of the trochlea. Although an attempt was made to remove the entire layer of calcified cartilage without damaging subchondral bone, histological analysis of acutely prepared defects showed that about 50% of the defect surface was still covered with calcified cartilage, a reflection of the current practical difficulty in accurately debriding the calcified zone without impinging on subchondral bone. These defects were then microfractured using an awl and mallet to evenly place 14–20 holes, 1.5 mm in diameter and 3 mm deep, starting at the periphery and moving inward, respecting 2- to 3-mm spacing between adjacent holes (Fig. 3A). Sheep were then randomly chosen to receive microfracture treatment only or to further receive a chitosan-GP/blood clot prepared in a similar manner to that described with freshly drawn autologous blood (Fig. 3B). Twenty-four sheep were operated; 4 were sacrificed within 2 h of joint closure to examine acute defects and implant residency, 6 (3 chitosan-GP and 3 control) were sacrificed after 3 mo of healing, and 14 (8 chitosan-GP and 6 control) were sacrificed after 6 mo of healing.

The sheep that were sacrificed within 2 h of joint closure revealed that a greater amount of chitosan-GP/blood filled the defect compared to microfracture only. Trochlear defects were more uniformly filled than condylar defects because of their concave vs convex curvature, respectively, and the nature of the opposing surface where trochlear defects face a smooth patella and condylar defects face the meniscus, the tibial plateau, and a fat pad that is quite prominent in sheep. Histological processing and analysis of these defects also revealed greater adherence of chitosan-GP/blood to both cartilagenous and osseus surfaces, including calcified cartilage, compared to the blood clot in the microfracture-only group. The limited numbers of animals sacrificed at 3 mo provided only a glimpse into the repair processes that occur in large animals but confirmed their similarity to the events described in rabbits, including the identification of growth plate-like structures arising in foci of the granulation tissue and resembling articular cartilage developmental processes as described above.

In the best case observed at this time-point, the chondral defect was uniformly covered with repair tissue after 3 mo of healing (Fig. 3C) in a chitosan-GP/blood-treated defect. Histological examination of this defect revealed an immature tissue in which a superficial undifferentiated granulation tissue (GT in Fig. 3C^1) rested above hypertrophic cartilage (HC in Fig. 3C^1), which was found above calcified cartilage (CC in Fig. 3C^1), which in turn was supported by an osseous base undergoing vascular invasion. Another region from this block viewed histologically also showed growth plate-like structures, but rather than presenting a uniform synchronous development across the surface (as in Fig. 3C^1), two distinct foci were observed (Fig. 3C^2) with growth that appeared to be independently mediated, possibly by signaling gradients (indicated by open arrows in Fig. 3C^2) generated between large vessels (V in Fig. 3C^2) below the calcified zone and smaller vessels (v in Fig. 3C^2) in the superficial granulation tissue. The more homogeneous and uniform structure in Fig. 3C^1 may partly be the result of finer distribution of smaller vessels in the superficial granulation tissue that was occasionally discerned at high magnification.

In the best-case repair observed at 6 mo, also seen following chitosan-GP treatment, the cut face of the decalcified block (Fig. 3D) revealed thicker repair tissue than at 3 mo (Fig. 3D). Vascular structures were often identified below regions of robust cartilage

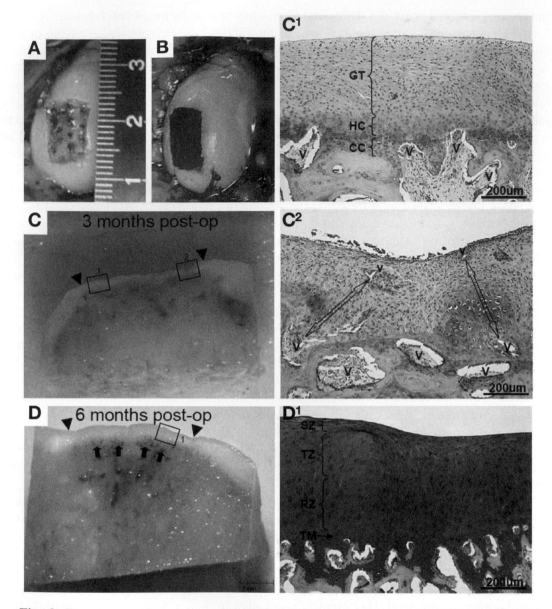

Fig. 3. Best-case cartilage repair in adult sheep treated with chitosan-GP/blood implants. Cartilage defects (1 cm²) were created in the medial condyle (**A**) using a surgical chisel and curette to remove all noncalcified cartilage and at least 50% of the calcified cartilage as assessed histologically on acutely prepared defects. The defects were then microfractured using an awl to evenly place 14–20 holes, each 1.5-mm diameter and 3 mm deep, which subsequently bled. A physiological solution of chitosan (1.7% w/v) in glycerol phosphate buffer (135 m*M*) at pH 6.8 was mixed with 3 vol freshly drawn blood and deposited onto the defect, where it adhered and solidified (**B**). A sacrifice at 3 mo postoperative revealed a uniform resurfacing of repair tissue on decalcified blocks (**C**; arrowheads indicate initial defect margins). A Safranin O/Fast Green-stained section from this block (**C¹**) revealed an immature repair tissue composed of a differentiating granulation tissue (GT) above hypertrophic chondrocytes (HC) that are above calcified cartilage (CC) invaded by bone marrow—derived blood vessels (V). A different region from this block (**C²**) shows two similar nascent growth plate-like structures (open double-headed arrows) that appear to be

repair (arrows in Fig. 3D). Histological analysis of this defect revealed a remarkably hyaline articular cartilage (Fig. 3D[1]) in which all three stratified layers (superficial, transitional, and radial) could be identified above a re-established tidemark and a porous subchondral bone plate. Differences compared to the original hyaline articular cartilage surrounding this site included nonuniform thickness, possibly arising because of foci lacking complete coordination as seen at 3 mo (Fig. 3C[2]), and a less-regular subchondral bone structure. These observations suggest that a coordinated and robust establishment of these growth foci at the base of a cartilage lesion can lead to a uniform layer of fully regenerated articular cartilage.

Several quantitative and unbiased estimators of cartilage repair quantity and quality were used to statistically compare chitosan-GP-treated defects ($n = 8$) to microfracture-only defects ($n = 6$). Two systematically sampled sections from each block were histomorphometrically analyzed for the volume of tissue filling the defect. By normalizing to the same site in the unoperated contralateral knee, the percentage fill variable was determined and resulted in greater tissue fill in chitosan-GP defects vs control defects (52 vs 31%) in condyle sites.

This repair tissue was also examined for hyaline quality by quantitatively assessing the volume of repair tissue that stained with Safranin O (% hyaline), revealing significantly greater hyalinity of this more voluminous repair seen with chitosan-GP treatment compared to control (86 vs 71%) in condyle sites. Hyaline quality was further confirmed by biochemical analysis of repair tissue biopsies in which glycosaminoglycan content of chitosan-GP-treated defects was almost two times that in the microfracture-only control (49 ± 14 mg/g vs 27 ± 16 mg/g) and equaled that of the unoperated contralateral sites, a remarkable result never previously reported in adult large-animal studies of cartilage repair. Subsequent multivariate statistical analysis using the two independent variables (% fill and % hyaline) as repeated measures demonstrated that chitosan-GP treatment significantly improved repair in defects of both the condyle and the trochlea ($p > 0.05$). In addition, an important reduction in the incidence and severity of subchondral cysts to chitosan-GP treatment was found; cysts were identified in five of six control condyles but in only three of eight chitosan-GP-treated defects. Taken together with the information obtained from the acute small-animal studies and the intermediate 3-mo large-animal sacrifices, it can be concluded that chitosan-GP/blood clots improve the quantity and quality of repair cartilage by amplifying bone marrow-derived repair processes that display some similarity to the developmental growth of articular cartilage.

CLINICAL EXPERIENCE WITH CHITOSAN-GLYCEROL PHOSPHATE/BLOOD CLOTS

Thirty-three human subjects were treated with chitosan-GP from August 2003 to December 2004 under Health Canada's Special Access Programme for medical devices,

---

Fig. 3. *(Continued)* morphogenetically driven by bone marrow-derived blood vessels (V) and smaller vessels (v) still present in the granulation tissue. A decalcified block from a 6-mo postoperative sacrifice **(D)** revealed uniform cartilage resurfacing that was thicker than at 3 mo. Good cartilage resurfacing was frequently associated with fine and dense subchondral vascularization (filled arrows in **D**). A Safranin O/Fast. Green-stained section **(D[1])** from this block revealed relatively mature articular cartilage containing superficial (SZ) transitional (TZ) and radial (RZ) zones with a reestablished tidemark (TM) above an actively remodeling bone bed.

Table 1
BST-CarGel (Chitosan-GP) Clinical Experience[a] Characteristics and Indications of Treated Patients

Gender	n	Average age (yr), mean ± SD (range)	Average femoral condyle lesion size (cm²), mean ± SD (range)	Tibia[b]
M	22	53.2 ± 9.8 (35–70)	4.3 ± 3.3 (0.5–12)	10
F	11	55.0 ± 9.1 (44–66)	4.3 ± 2.8 (0.5–8.75)	6

[a]Not a clinical study. Permission was granted by Health Canada on a case-by-case basis under the Special Access Programme for medical devices.

[b]Number with concomitant tibial lesion treated with microfracture only.

which is designed to enable compassionate use. Notably, treatment occurred on a case-by-case basis and by law was not considered a clinical study. In particular, the absence of a control group as well as the wide-ranging characteristics of the treated patients and lesions impede rigorous interpretation of outcomes.

Symptomatic, singular femoral cartilage lesions of grade 3/4 or 4 were arthroscopically debrided by removing unstable or damaged cartilage in addition to the calcified cartilage layer but without impinging subchondral bone. Vertical margins were created, and evenly spaced microfracture holes were then produced throughout the prepared lesion. Treated lesions encompassed the spectrum of both acute (traumatic) and chronic (degenerative) types and ranged in size from 0.5 to 12 cm², with a mean area of 4.3 cm² for both males and females (Table 1). In 16 cases, opposing tibial lesions were debrided and microfractured only. Osteochondritis dissecans and an exposed subchondral cyst each accounted for the treatment of 1 patient. Chitosan-GP was delivered by arthroscopy for 22 patients and by miniarthrotomy for 11 patients. Because knee stability is critical for effective cartilage repair, concomitant anterior cruciate ligament reconstruction preceded treatment with chitosan-GP in 2 patients.

All patients were directly observed for 24 h postoperatively, and 31 of 33 patients remained in a private clinic for 5 d to facilitate physiotherapy. A standardized physiotherapy program was implemented for 12 wk, which required patients to be non-weight bearing with crutches for at least 6 wk while undergoing assisted passive motion 3–5 times per week. Progressive weight bearing increased from touch down to 100% over the next several weeks according to clinical status and function. Stationary cycling was initiated when range of motion exceeded 110°, accompanied by standard strengthening and proprioception exercises. Safety was assessed through general and knee-related medical exams, as well as with blood analyses. In addition, self-administered questionnaires were given preoperatively and again post-operatively after 3, 6, and 12 mo. With the exception of the first 4 patients who filled out Knee Injury and Osteoarthritis Outcome, all patients completed the Western Ontario and McMaster University (WOMAC) Osteoarthritis Index.

Safety of chitosan-GP treatment was demonstrated because no uncharacteristic observations were made during physical exams or blood analyses for all patients. After 12 mo postoperatively, WOMAC scores for pain, stiffness, and function improved substantially compared with preoperative baseline scores in chitosan-GP-treated patients (Fig. 4). Although considered anecdotal and short term, the uniformity of the WOMAC data suggests a true clinical benefit arising from chitosan-GP treatment. Ongoing follow-up at 2 yr is confirming this

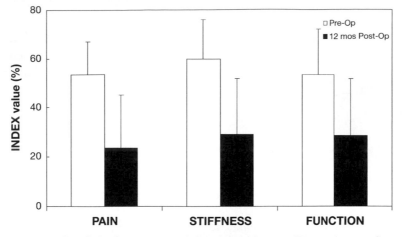

Fig. 4. Improvement in clinical symptoms following chitosan-GP treatment of cartilage lesions. Self-administered WOMAC questionnaires filled 12 mo postoperatively demonstrated substantial improvement over preoperative baseline. The WOMAC index is a validated health status instrument consisting of 24 questions that probe clinically and patient-relevant symptoms in the areas of pain, stiffness, and physical function *(94)*. Improvement is represented by a decrease in value. Data represent mean plus standard deviation, $n = 9$.

clinical benefit in 2 patients, whose prognoses prior to chitosan-GP treatment were to have total knee arthroplasties.

A multicenter, randomized comparative clinical trial has been designed and initiated to investigate cartilage repair resulting from treatment with chitosan-GP and microfracture vs microfracture alone. Nevertheless, the cohort of patients treated within the framework of Health Canada's Special Access Programme for medical devices demonstrates the potential of chitosan-GP to resurface cartilage lesions that may arise from variable etiologies within a substantially varied patient population. Furthermore, requiring only a single intervention, chitosan-GP treatment falls within currently accepted clinical practice and represents a novel and versatile treatment modality for both small and large lesions. Detailed clinical discussion and surgical specific, including lesion preparation, chitosan-GP preparation, and delivery techniques have recently been described elsewhere *(95)*.

FUTURE PERSPECTIVES

The troublesome nature of cartilage repair identified many centuries ago has continued to vex the orthopedic clinical and research communities in spite of intense efforts to improve repair and devise new procedures of cartilage resurfacing. Advances in the past decades are nonetheless significant in advancing our knowledge and capacity to intervene prior to joint destruction and replacement and eventually to regenerate hyaline articular cartilage. The strategy of harnessing, controlling, and amplifying extrinsic cartilage repair from the subchondral bone is a particularly promising avenue for further development because these processes can be activated when the subchondral bone plate is penetrated. A functional repair of the articular surface can result from this approach depending on appropriate patient selection, surgical technique, and application of materials such as chitosan-GP to promote repair. Some challenges remaining to be addressed in this area include refining both the surgical techniques and the implantable materials to maximize successful cartilage regeneration and to adapt specifically to patient needs as a function of age, joint, lesion site, lesion size, and concomitant pathologies.

ACKNOWLEDGMENTS

Financial support was provided by the Canadian Arthritis Network (CAN), the Canadian Institutes of Health Research (CIHR), and BioSyntech Canada Inc. Assistance from Drs. Anik Chevrier, Jun Sun, Evgeny Rossomacha, Monica Iliescu, Marc McKee, Pierre Ranger, and Nicholas Duval is greatly appreciated.

REFERENCES

1. Schenk RK, Eggli PS, Hunziker EB. Articular cartilage morphology. In Kuettner KE, Schleyerbach R, Hascall VC, eds., Articular Cartilage Biochemistry. New York: Raven Press; 1986;3–23.
2. Schumacher BL, Block JA, Schmid TM, Aydelotte MB, Kuettner KE. A novel proteoglycan synthesized and secreted by chondrocytes of the superficial zone of articular cartilage. Arch Biochem Biophys 1994;311:144–152.
3. McCutchen CW. Lubrication of joints. In Sokoloff L, ed., The Joints and Synovial Fluid. London: Academic Press; 1980;438–483.
4. Hills BA. Boundary lubrication in vivo. Proc Inst Mech Eng [H] 2000;214:83–94.
5. Hunziker EB. Articular cartilage structure in human and experimental animal models. In Kuettner KE, Schleyerbach R, Hascall VC, eds., Articular Cartilage and Osteoarthritis. New York: Raven Press; 1992;183–199.
6. Hunziker EB, Quinn TM, Hauselmann HJ. Quantitative structural organization of normal adult human articular cartilage. Osteoarthritis Cartilage 2002;10:564–572.
7. Buschmann MD, Grodzinsky AJ. A molecular model of proteoglycan-associated electrostatic forces in cartilage mechanics. J Biomech Eng 1995;117:179–192.
8. Eisenberg SR, Grodzinsky AJ. Electrokinetic micromodel of extracellular-matrix and other polyelectrolyte networks. Physicochemical. Hydrodynamics 1988;10:517–539.
9. Cohen B, Lai WM, Mow VC. A transversely isotropic biphasic model for unconfined compression of growth plate and chondroepiphysis. J Biomech Eng 1998;120:491–496.
10. Fortin M, Soulhat J, Shirazi-Adl A, Hunziker EB, Buschmann MD. Unconfined compression of articular cartilage: nonlinear behavior and comparison with a fibril-reinforced biphasic model. J Biomech Eng 2000;122:1–6.
11. Korhonen RK, Laasanen MS, Toyras J, Lappalainen R, Helminen HJ, Jurvelin JS. Fibril reinforced poroelastic model predicts specifically mechanical behavior of normal, proteoglycan depleted and collagen degraded articular cartilage. J Biomech 2003;36:1373–1379.
12. Li LP, Shirazi-Adl A, Buschmann MD. Alterations in mechanical behaviour of articular cartilage due to changes in depth varying material properties—a nonhomogeneous poroelastic model study. Comput Methods Biomech Biomed Eng 2002;5:45–52.
13. Li LP, Soulhat J, Buschmann MD, Shirazi-Adl A. Nonlinear analysis of cartilage in unconfined ramp compression using a fibril reinforced poroelastic model. Clin Biomech 1999;1–10.
14. Soltz MA, Ateshian GA. A conewise linear elasticity mixture model for the analysis of tension-compression nonlinearity in articular cartilage. J Biomech Eng 2000;122:576–586.
15. Soulhat J, Buschmann MD, Shirazi-Adl A. A fibril-network-reinforced biphasic model of cartilage in unconfined compression. J Biomech Eng 1999;121:340–347.
16. Poole AR. The growth plate : cellular physiology, cartilage assembly and mineralisation. In Hall B, Newman S, eds., Cartilage: Molecular Aspects. Boca Raton, FL: CRC Press; 1991;179–213.
17. Hunziker EB. Growth plate structure and function. Pathol Immunopathol Res 1988;7:9–13.
18. Hayes AJ, MacPherson S, Morrison H, Dowthwaite G, Archer CW. The development of articular cartilage: evidence for an appositional growth mechanism. Anat Embryol (Berl) 2001;203:469–479.
19. Dowthwaite GP, Bishop JC, Redman SN, et al. The surface of articular cartilage contains a progenitor cell population. J Cell Sci 2004;117:889–897.
20. Buckwalter JA, Mankin HJ. Articular cartilage repair and transplantation. Arthritis Rheum 1998;41:1331–1342.

21. Mankin HJ. The reaction of articular cartilage to injury and osteoarthritis (first of two parts). N Engl J Med 1974;291:1285–1292.

22. Mankin HJ. The reaction of articular cartilage to injury and osteoarthritis (second of two parts). N Engl J Med 1974;291:1335–1340.

23. Dell'Accio F, Vanlauwe J, Bellemans J, Neys J, De Bari C, Luyten FP. Expanded phenotypically stable chondrocytes persist in the repair tissue and contribute to cartilage matrix formation and structural integration in a goat model of autologous chondrocyte implantation. J Orthop Res 2003;21:123–131.

24. Grande DA, Pitman MI, Peterson L, Menche D, Klein M. The repair of experimentally produced defects in rabbit articular cartilage by autologous chondrocyte transplantation. J Orthop Res 1989;7:208–218.

25. Hunziker EB. Articular cartilage repair: basic science and clinical progress. A review of the current status and prospects. Osteoarthritis Cartilage 2002;10:432–463.

26. Alford JW, Cole BJ. Cartilage restoration, part 2: techniques, outcomes, and future directions. Am J Sports Med 2005;33:443–460.

27. Bartlett W, Skinner JA, Gooding CR, et al. Autologous chondrocyte implantation vs matrix-induced autologous chondrocyte implantation for osteochondral defects of the knee: a prospective, randomised study. J Bone Joint Surg Br 2005;87:640–645.

28. Briggs TW, Mahroof S, David LA, Flannelly J, Pringle J, Bayliss M. Histological evaluation of chondral defects after autologous chondrocyte implantation of the knee. J Bone Joint Surg Br 2003;85:1077–1083.

29. Henderson IJ, Tuy B, Connell D, Oakes B, Hettwer WH. Prospective clinical study of autologous chondrocyte implantation and correlation with MRI at 3 and 12 months. J Bone Joint Surg Br 2003;85:1060–1066.

30. Horas U, Pelinkovic D, Herr G, Aigner T, Schnettler R. Autologous chondrocyte implantation and osteochondral cylinder transplantation in cartilage repair of the knee joint. A prospective, comparative trial. J Bone Joint Surg Am 2003;85-A:185–192.

31. Knutsen G, Engebretsen L, Ludvigsen TC, et al. Autologous chondrocyte implantation compared with microfracture in the knee. A randomized trial. J Bone Joint Surg Am 2004;86-A:455–464.

32. Nehrer S, Spector M, Minas T. Histologic analysis of tissue after failed cartilage repair procedures. Clin Orthop 1999;365:149–162.

33. Roberts S, McCall IW, Darby AJ, et al. Autologous chondrocyte implantation for cartilage repair: monitoring its success by magnetic resonance imaging and histology. Arthritis Res Ther 2003;5:R60–R73.

34. Russlies M, Behrens P, Ehlers EM, et al. Periosteum stimulates subchondral bone densification in autologous chondrocyte transplantation in a sheep model. Cell Tissue Res 2005;319:133–142.

35. Dorotka R, Bindreiter U, Macfelda K, Windberger U, Nehrer S. Marrow stimulation and chondrocyte transplantation using a collagen matrix for cartilage repair. Osteoarthritis Cartilage 2005;13:655–664.

36. Breinan HA, Minas T, Hsu HP, Nehrer S, Sledge CB, Spector M. Effect of cultured autologous chondrocytes on repair of chondral defects in a canine model. J Bone Joint Surg Am 1997;79:1439–1451.

37. Nehrer S, Breinan HA, Ramappa A, et al. Chondrocyte-seeded collagen matrices implanted in a chondral defect in a canine model. Biomaterials 1998;19:2313–2328.

38. Vasara AI, Hyttinen MM, Lammi MJ, et al. Subchondral bone reaction associated with chondral defect and attempted cartilage repair in goats. Calcif Tissue Int 2004;74:107–114.

39. Buschmann MD, Gluzband YA, Grodzinsky AJ, Kimura JH, Hunziker EB. Chondrocytes in agarose culture synthesize a mechanically functional extracellular matrix. J Orthop Res 1992;10:745–758.

40. Martin I, Obradovic B, Treppo S, et al. Modulation of the mechanical properties of tissue engineered cartilage. Biorheology 2000;37:141–147.

41. Waldman SD, Spiteri CG, Grynpas MD, Pilliar RM, Kandel RA. Long-term intermittent compressive stimulation improves the composition and mechanical properties of tissue-engineered cartilage. Tissue Eng 2004;10:1323–1331.
42. Tanaka T, Komaki H, Chazono M, Fujii K. Use of a biphasic graft constructed with chondrocytes overlying a beta-tricalcium phosphate block in the treatment of rabbit osteochondral defects. Tissue Eng 2005;11:331–339.
43. Insall JN. Intra-articular surgery for degenerative arthritis of the knee. A report of the work of the late K. H. Pridie. J Bone Joint Surg Br 1967;49:211–228.
44. Johnson LL. Arthroscopic abrasion arthroplasty historical and pathologic perspective: present status. Arthroscopy 1986;2:54–69.
45. Steadman JR, Rodkey WG, Singleton SB, Briggs KK. Microfracture technique for full-thickness chondral defects: technique and clinical results. Operative techniques in orthopaedics. 1997;7:300–304.
46. Browne JE, Anderson AF, Arciero R, et al. Clinical outcome of autologous chondrocyte implantation at 5 yr in US subjects. Clin Orthop Relat Res 2005;436:237–245.
47. Fox JA, Kalsi RS, Cole BJ. Update on articular cartilage restoration. Tech Knee Surg 2003;2:2–17.
48. Lu C, Miclau T, Hu D, et al. Cellular basis for age-related changes in fracture repair. J Orthop Res 2005;23:1300–1307.
49. Meachim G, Roberts C. Repair of the joint surface from subarticular tissue in the rabbit knee. J Anat 1971;109:317–327.
50. O'Driscoll SW, Keeley FW, Salter RB. The chondrogenic potential of free autogenous periosteal grafts for biological resurfacing of major full-thickness defects in joint surfaces under the influence of continuous passive motion. An experimental investigation in the rabbit. J Bone Joint Surg Am 1986;68:1017–1035.
51. Wei X, Messner K. Maturation-dependent durability of spontaneous cartilage repair in rabbit knee joint. J Biomed Mater Res 1999;46:539–548.
52. Yamamoto T, Wakitani S, Imoto K, et al. Fibroblast growth factor-2 promotes the repair of partial thickness defects of articular cartilage in immature rabbits but not in mature rabbits. Osteoarthritis Cartilage 2004;12:636–641.
53. Hurtig MB, Fretz PB, Doige CE, Schnurr DL. Effects of lesion size and location on equine articular cartilage repair. Can J Vet Res 1988;52:137–146.
54. Chevrier A, Hoemann CD, Sun J, Buschmann MD. Chitosan-glycerol phosphate/blood implants increase cell recruitment, transient vascularization and subchondral bone remodeling in drilled cartilage defects. Osteoarthritis Cartilage 2007;15:316–327.
55. Chevrier A, Sun J, Hoemann CD, Buschmann MD. Early reparative events in adult rabbits with drilled chondral defects treated with an injectable chitosan-glycerol phosphate implant. Trans Int Soc Cartilage Repair. 2004; Gent, Belgium, May 26–29.
56. Mitchell N, Shepard N. The resurfacing of adult rabbit articular cartilage by multiple perforations through the subchondral bone. J Bone Joint Surg Am 1976;58:230–233.
57. Shapiro F, Koide S, Glimcher MJ. Cell origin and differentiation in the repair of full-thickness defects of articular cartilage. J Bone Joint Surg Am 1993;75A:532–553.
58. Convery FR, Akeson WH, Keown GH. The repair of large osteochondral defects. An experimental study in horses. Clin Orthop Relat Res 1972;82:253–262.
59. Jackson DW, Lalor PA, Aberman HM, Simon TM. Spontaneous repair of full-thickness defects of articular cartilage in a goat model. A preliminary study. J Bone Joint Surg Am 2001; 83-A:53–64.
60. Mandelbaum BR, Browne JE, Fu F, et al. Articular cartilage lesions of the knee. Am J Sports Med 1998;26:853–861.
61. Otsuka Y, Mizuta H, Takagi K, et al. Requirement of fibroblast growth factor signaling for regeneration of epiphyseal morphology in rabbit full-thickness defects of articular cartilage. Dev Growth Differ 1997;39:143–156.

62. Howard RD, McIlwraith CW, Trotter GW, et al. Long-term fate and effects of exercise on sternal cartilage autografts used for repair of large osteochondral defects in horses. Am J Vet Res 1994;55:1158–1167.
63. Johnson LL. Arthroscopic abrasion arthroplasty: a review. Clin Orthop 2001;S306–S317.
64. O'Driscoll SW, Keeley FW, Salter RB. Durability of regenerated articular cartilage produced by free autogenous periosteal grafts in major full-thickness defects in joint surfaces under the influence of continuous passive motion. A follow-up report at one year. J Bone Joint Surg Am 1988;70:595–606.
65. Brown TD, Pope DF, Hale JE, Buckwalter JA, Brand RA. Effects of osteochondral defect size on cartilage contact stress. J Orthop Res 1991;9:559–567.
66. Frisbie DD, Oxford JT, Southwood L, et al. Early events in cartilage repair after subchondral bone microfracture. Clin Orthop 2003;215–227.
67. Frisbie DD, Trotter GW, Powers BE, et al. Arthroscopic subchondral bone plate microfracture technique augments healing of large chondral defects in the radial carpal bone and medial femoral condyle of horses. Vet Surg 1999;28:242–255.
68. Hanie EA, Sullins KE, Powers BE, Nelson PR. Healing of full-thickness cartilage compared with full-thickness cartilage and subchondral bone defects in the equine third carpal bone. Equine Vet J 1992;24:382 386.
69. Hoemann CD, Hurtig M, Rossomacha E, et al. Chitosan-glycerol phosphate/blood implants improve hyaline cartilage repair in ovine microfracture defects. J Bone Joint Surg Am 2005;87:2671–2686.
70. Vachon A, Bramlage LR, Gabel AA, Weisbrode S. Evaluation of the repair process of cartilage defects of the equine third carpal bone with and without subchondral bone perforation. Am J Vet Res 1986;47:2637–2645.
71. Colman RW, Hirsh J, Marder VJ, Clowes AW, George FN. Hemostasis and Thrombosis: Basic Principles and Clinical Practice. New York: Lippincott Williams and Wilkins; 2001.
72. Morgenstern E, Ruf A, Patscheke H. Ultrastructure of the interaction between human platelets and polymerizing fibrin within the first minutes of clot formation. Blood Coagul Fibrinolysis 1990;1:543–546.
73. Hoemann CD, Sun J, McKee MD, et al. Rabbit hyaline cartilage repair after marrow stimulation depends on the surgical approach and a chitosan-GP stabilised *in-situ* blood clot. Trans Orthop Res Soc 2005;30:1372.
74. Johnson LL. Characteristics of the immediate postarthroscopic blood clot formation in the knee joint. Arthroscopy 1991;7:14–23.
75. Chenite A, Chaput C, Wang D, et al. Novel injectable neutral solutions of chitosan form biodegradable gels *in situ*. Biomaterials 2000;21:2155–2161.
76. Skjak-Braek G, Anthonsen T, Sandford P. Chitin and Chitosan. New York: Elsevier Applied Science; 1989.
77. Shigemasa Y, Minami S. Applications of chitin and chitosan for biomaterials. Biotechnol Genet Eng Rev 1996;13:383–420.
78. Cho YW, Cho YN, Chung SH, Yoo G, Ko SW. Water-soluble chitin as a wound healing accelerator. Biomaterials 1999;20:2139–2145.
79. Sall KN, Kreter JK, Keates RH. The effect of chitosan on corneal wound healing. Ann Ophthalmol 1987;19:31–33.
80. Di Martino A, Sittinger M, Risbud MV. Chitosan: a versatile biopolymer for orthopaedic tissue-engineering. Biomaterials 2005;26:5983–5990.
81. Inui H, Tsujikubo M, Hirano S. Low molecular weight chitosan stimulation of mitogenic response to platelet-derived growth factor in vascular smooth muscle cells. Biosci Biotechnol Biochem 1995;59:2111–2114.
82. Chou T-C, Fu E, Wu C-J, Yeh J-H. Chitosan enhances platelet adhesion and aggregation. Biochem Biophys Res Commun 2003;302:480–483.
83. Malette WG, Quigley HJ, Gaines RD, Johnson ND, Rainer WG. Chitosan: a new hemostatic. Ann Thorac Surg 1983;36:55–58.

84. Rao SB, Sharma CP. Use of chitosan as a biomaterial: studies on its safety and hemostatic potential. J Biomed Mater Res 1997;34:21–28.
85. Aerts JMFG, Boot RG, Renkema GH, et al. Chitotriosidase: a human macrophage chitinase that is a marker for Gaucher disease manifestation. Chitin Enzymol Proc Int Symp Chitin Enzymol 1996;1:3–10.
86. Muzzarelli RA. Human enzymatic activities related to the therapeutic administration of chitin derivatives. Cell Mol Life Sci 1997;53:131–140.
87. Varum KM, Myhr MM, Hjerde RJ, Smidsrod O. In vitro degradation rates of partially N-acetylated chitosans in human serum. Carbohydr Res 1997;299:99–101.
88. Onishi H, Machida Y. Biodegradation and distribution of water-soluble chitosan in mice. Biomaterials 1998;20:175–182.
89. Chenite A, Buschmann M, Wang D, Chaput C, Kandani N. Rheological characterisation of thermogelling chitosan/glycerol-phosphate solutions. 2001;46:39–47.
90. Hoemann CD, Sun J, Legare A, McKee MD, Buschmann MD. Tissue engineering of cartilage using an injectable and adhesive chitosan-based cell-delivery vehicle. Osteoarthritis Cartilage 2005;13:318–329.
91. Rossomacha E, Hoemann CD, Shive M. Simple methods for staining chitosan in biotechnological applications. J Histotechnol 2004;27:1–6.
92. Solchaga LA, Temenoff JS, Gao J, Mikos AG, Caplan AI, Goldberg VM. Repair of osteochondral defects with hyaluronan- and polyester-based scaffolds. Osteoarthritis Cartilage 2005;13:297–309.
93. Hoemann CD, Sun J, McKee MD, et al. Chitosan-glycerol phosphate/blood implants elicit hyaline cartilage repair integrated with porous subchondral bone in microdrilled rabbit defects. Osteoarthritis Cartilage. 2007;15:78–89.
94. Bellamy N, Buchanan WW, Goldsmith CH, Campbell J, Stitt LW. Validation study of WOMAC: a health status instrument for measuring clinically important patient relevant outcomes to antirheumatic drug therapy in patients with osteoarthritis of the hip or knee. J Rheumatol 1988;15:1833–1840.
95. Shive MS, Hoemann CD, Restrepo A, et al. BST-CarGel: in situ chondroinduction for cartrilage repair. Oper Tech Orthop 2006;16:271–278.

8

Autologous Osteochondral Transplantation

**Anthony Miniaci, MD, Clinton Jambor, MD,
and Frank A. Petrigliano, MD**

Summary

Focal cartilage defects of knee constitute a challenging clinical problem for the orthopedic surgeon. These injuries typically occur in active patients, can result in debilitating pain, and have a limited capacity for spontaneous healing. Autologous osteochondral transplantation has been advocated as a treatment for focal cartilage defects, as this surgical technique can restore hyaline cartilage architecture and, to some degree, the structural support of underlying subchondral bone. The short- and intermediate-term outcomes following this procedure are encouraging. This chapter serves to review the indications, surgical technique, and rehabilitation protocol for autologous osteochondral transplantation of the knee and provide a comparison of its clinical results to other cartilage restoration procedures.

Key Words: Autologous osteochondral transplantation; mosaicplasty.

INTRODUCTION

The main function of articular cartilage is to transfer loads across adjacent joint surfaces, reduce friction within the joint, and transfer stresses to the underlying subchondral bone *(1)*. The treatment of chondral injuries of the weight-bearing joints is a challenging and common problem for the orthopedic surgeon *(2,3)*. Unlike other tissues within the body, cartilage is unique in that it is unable to produce an adequate healing response *(4)*.

Previous attempts to treat symptomatic cartilage lesions have had limited success. Techniques such as abrasion chondroplasty and microfracture attempt to stimulate the intrinsic healing response by recruiting pluripotent mesenchymal cells from the bone marrow *(5)*. These procedures lead to the formation of fibrocartilage scar tissue *(6–8)* with inferior biomechanical and biochemical properties compared to that of the hyaline articular cartilage *(9–13)*. Other cartilage repair methods, such as autologous chondrocyte transplantation, following which many authors have reported the formation of hyaline cartilage *(14,15)*, have also been found to promote the creation of cartilage repair tissue that possesses characteristics of fibrocartilage both histologically and with electron microscopy from specimens biopsied on follow-up arthroscopies *(16)*.

Osteochondral autograft transplantation is a well-established technique in the treatment of chondral and osteochondral defects. Also known as *mosaicplasty*, this method was first described by Yamashita et al. *(17)* and later popularized by Hangody et al. *(18)*. The procedure involves harvesting small, cylindrical, osteochondral plugs from the comparatively non-weight-bearing periphery of the patellofemoral joint or margin of the intercondylar notch and transplanting them into an area of cartilage damage. Through the utilization of numerous cylinders, it is possible to maintain the radius of curvature of the affected cartilage surface and potentially maintain overall articular congruence *(19)*.

It has been demonstrated in both canine and equine models that (1) the transplanted hyaline cartilage demonstrates consistent survival, and (2) the press-fit graft undergoes osseous incorporation into the recipient subchondral bone while the transplanted cartilage experiences lateral integration with surrounding hyaline cartilage via fibrocartilage elaborated by the osseous base of the defect *(20,21)*. This viable transplanted hyaline cartilage has the benefit of providing immediate functionality at the time of implantation. These findings have prompted basic science research directed at improving the technique of osteochondral allograft transplantation and clinical research to characterize further its clinical role relative to existing cartilage repair procedures *(22,23)*.

Autologous osteochondral transplantation is performed as a one-stage procedure, can be performed open or arthroscopically, and is relatively inexpensive. The main cost is the initial outlay for the specialized surgical instrumentation. Because it is an autologous transplant, the procedure carries no risk of disease transmission or graft-host incompatibility. When used in carefully selected patients, the results of osteochondral autograft transplantation are favorable in comparison to other surgical techniques.

INDICATIONS

The indications for mosaicplasty in the knee are focal unipolar cartilage defects measuring 1–5 cm². Lesions less than 1 cm² tend to be asymptomatic. With larger lesions, greater than 5 cm², autologous osteochondral grafting is limited because of the amount of donor tissue available for harvesting. Even defects with bone loss can be reconstructed with this procedure. However, the technique is limited to lesions with bone loss of depths less than 10 mm.

DIAGNOSIS AND CLINICAL EVALUATION

The clinical presentation of patients with cartilage injuries is often nonspecific. Patients frequently complain of pain and may have episodes of mechanical symptoms, including locking and catching. Physical exam often reveals an effusion and joint line tenderness. The knee joint should be evaluated for any other ligamentous or meniscal pathology and a thorough assessment of limb alignment and patellofemoral tracking is crucial. Lower limb alignment pathology should be corrected either prior to or in conjunction with a mosaicplasty procedure.

Imaging studies are an important part of the preoperative workup. A series of weight-bearing radiographs is initially performed. For the knee, we prefer to obtain anteroposterior, lateral, Rosenburg *(24)*, and patellar views to evaluate better the load-bearing areas of the femoral condyle and patella for signs of early degenerative arthritis. Axial alignment can be measured on standing full-length lower extremity radiographs.

Magnetic resonance imaging (MRI) is helpful in identifying the location, size, depth, and extent of chondral lesions preoperatively. The most sensitive imaging study to evaluate chondral injury is an MRI with T_1-weighted fat-suppressed three-dimensional gradient echo sequences *(25)*. Previous studies have demonstrated an 81–93% sensitivity, 94–97% specificity, and 91–97% accuracy for the detection of chondral defects *(26–28)*. Chondral damage is demonstrated by an altered contour as opposed to simply a change in signal intensity.

SURGICAL METHOD

Once the decision has been made to proceed with the mosaicplasty procedure, the following surgical method is employed. After anesthesia and preoperative antibiotics are administered, a tourniquet is placed on the upper thigh. Both lower extremities are prepped and draped in case additional bone plugs need to be harvested from the contralateral knee. Osteochondral autografting may be performed either entirely arthroscopically or open through an arthrotomy.

It is extremely important to inform patients preoperatively of the potential need to harvest plugs from the contralateral knee, especially when operating on larger defects. The patient must also understand that, even if an arthroscopic procedure is selected, a formal arthrotomy may be required to gain access to the lesion and harvest sites. Fortunately, patellar eversion is seldom necessary during the harvest or implantation of osteochondral plugs for lesions of the femoral condyles or trochlea.

Joint Access/Portal Placement

Portal placement is vital to gain perpendicular access to the harvest and defect sites. A spinal needle inserted through the skin into the joint may help when placing portal incisions. Vertical portal incisions are preferred; these portals facilitate the harvest procedures by allowing chisel placement that is perpendicular to the articular surface. In addition, if the need arises to perform an arthrotomy, the portals can simply be extended. The anterolateral and anteromedial portals are made 1 cm laterally and medially, respectively, to the patellar tendon. This portal positioning aids in accessing the lateral and medial borders of the trochlea for harvesting bone plugs. Approximately nine to twelve 4.5-mm plugs may be harvested from each knee with this technique.

Graft Harvest

A thorough evaluation of the chondral lesion is performed arthroscopically. The defect is probed, and its size, stability, and accessibility are assessed. The overlying damaged and loose cartilage is then debrided down to the calcified layer with a shaver.

The number, diameter, and position of the graft cylinders that will be required to fill the defect can be determined by placing the harvesting punch or the delivery chisel over the lesion. Commercial sizing guides are also available and can be used to estimate the number of plugs that will be necessary to fill the cartilage defect. Using the sharpened end of the punch, small marks can be created to template out the lesion. Plugs with a diameter of 3–5 mm are generally used. Smaller plugs have been shown to be too fragile, whereas larger plugs may be associated with degenerative changes at both the harvest site and on its opposing chondral surface *(29)*.

When resurfacing condylar defects, grafts should be harvested from the margins of the lateral and medial condyles above the sulcus terminalis *(30,31)*. Lesions in the trochlear groove are resurfaced with bone plugs harvested from the intercondylar notch. Grafts from this area are best suited for trochlear reconstruction as both of these surfaces are concave. Harvest sites should be place no closer than 2–3 mm apart. Donor sites placed too close together can cause the bone tunnels to intersect. This can lead to collapse of the overlying bone or result in an unexpectedly short plug harvest from the donor area. Manually driven harvesting punches are preferred. Power trephination has been shown to result in decreased chondrocyte survival rates because of thermal necrosis *(32)*.

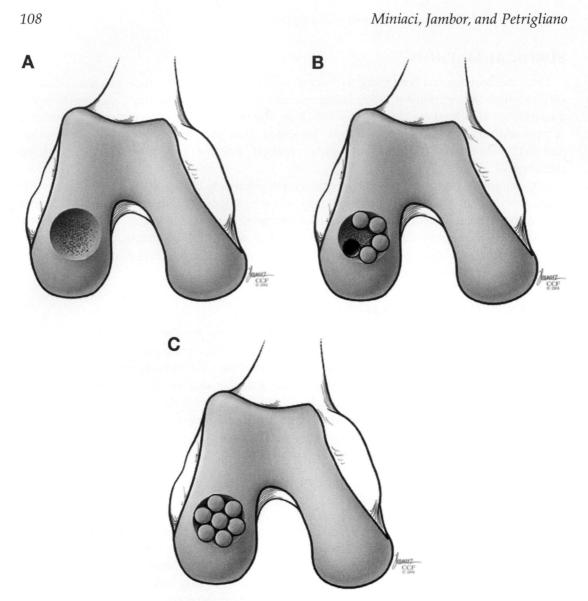

Fig. 1. Osteochondral graft insertion sequence: **(A)** Osteochondral defect on femoral condyle; **(B)** peripheral plugs are placed in lesion first; **(C)** central plug placed after peripheral plugs are seated.

The harvesting chisel is inserted perpendicular to the articular surface and is advanced with a mallet to the desired depth, usually about 15–20 mm total depth. Longer plugs are harvested when attempting to reconstruct defects with bone loss greater than 10 mm deep. Preoperative planning with MRI is important to determine depth of the lesion and amount of bone loss to be corrected. For stable plugs, one needs to have at least half of the plug buried in bone. Therefore, for a 15-mm bone defect a 30-mm plug is necessary. The grafts are then removed, measured, and placed in a saline-soaked sponge on the back table. The recipient site is then prepared.

Preparation and Implantation of the Recipient Site

Graft insertion necessitates several steps. After the exact location of the recipient plug is selected, the insertion angle is determined using either a spinal needle or the graft insertion

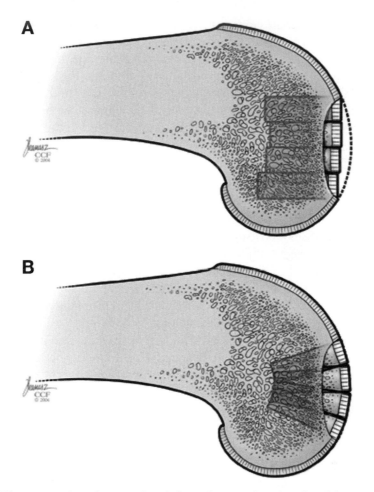

Fig. 2. (A) When central grafts are placed first, they tend to be placed in a recessed position, creating a flattened contour. **(B)** Proper graft placement.

tool. This step is critical and ensures that the osteochondral plugs will be inserted perpendicular to the joint surface. The appropriate size drill is advanced to the proper depth and removed while alignment is maintained at all times with the drill sleeve. The hole is then dilated with a tunnel dilator, and the bone plug is placed into the insertion tool. If the cartilage on the harvested plug or the cartilage surrounding the recipient site is at an obliquity, then the graft should be properly oriented within the inserter prior to placement to best match the contour of the surrounding cartilage and joint surface anatomy. If possible, graft insertion should be carried out with the inflow pump turned off. Osteochondral grafts tend to swell in saline. This can cause a size mismatch between the harvested graft and the recipient tunnel, possibly leading to graft breakage during insertion. In addition, turning off the inflow during insertion also prevents the graft from accidentally being expelled from the insertion tool because of fluid pressure. This step is crucial if performing this procedure arthroscopically.

The graft is inserted by gentle manual pressure. Excessive force can injure the chondrocytes. Forces greater than 15 mPa in adults or 7.5 mPa in youths will result in damage to the articular cartilage *(33)*. Therefore, we do not recommend using a mallet to place the osteochondral plug.

To approximate the appropriate contour better, peripheral plugs should be placed in the lesion prior to inserting the more central ones (Fig. 1A,C). Central plugs are usually seated higher than the surrounding peripheral plugs. If the central plugs are inserted first, then they tend to be placed in a recessed position, creating a flattened contour (Fig. 2A,B). This eventually leads to fibrocartilage overgrowth, rendering the transplanted hyalin cartilage ineffectual.

The grafts should be seated with their base firmly set against the bottom of the drill hole and have good side-to-side contact. After all the grafts are placed, the knee is put through a range of motion, and the stability of the grafts is assessed. Wounds are closed in a standard fashion, and a compressive dressing is applied.

POSTOPERATIVE REHABILITATION

Postoperatively patients are placed in a hinged knee brace set at 0–90°. The next day, therapy is initiated, stressing range-of-motion exercises and isometric quadriceps strengthening. An emphasis is placed on regaining range of motion and reducing the postoperative effusion. A graduated exercise program is advanced as the patient becomes more comfortable. Patients are permitted touch down weight bearing for the first 6 wk. Although we are not sure whether weight-bearing status affects the final results, basic science studies noted that pistoning of unstable plugs caused cyst formation beneath the plugs. Obtaining stable plugs at the time of implantation is of foremost importance; however, we do use touch down weight bearing as an added precaution.

On evaluation at 6 wk postoperatively, if patients are found to be relatively comfortable and their radiographs are satisfactory, we allow progressive weight bearing as tolerated. Patients are permitted to return to sports when there is minimal effusion and nearly full range of motion and quadriceps strength is approx 80% of the contralateral leg.

OUR EXPERIENCE

The main indications for surgery with the mosaicplasty technique are focal osteochondral defects that are secondary to either trauma or osteochondritis dissecans (OCD). The location of the defect is important in terms of long-term prognosis. The locations best suited for treatment are on the femoral condyles. Mosaicplasty performed on either the medial or lateral femoral condyle has demonstrated good results. Tibial plateau lesions are usually asymmetric arthritic lesions and rarely a focal chondral or osteochondral defect. We have not had much experience treating tibial plateau lesions with autologous osteochondral grafting.

We have performed a number of cases in the patellofemoral joint. Obtaining proper plug orientation and angulation on the patella and trochlear groove is technically demanding. At this point, mosaicplasty in the patellofemoral joint cannot be performed arthroscopically and requires an arthrotomy. Reconstructing kissing lesions in the patellofemoral joint is especially difficult because the plugs can catch as the patella tracks within the trochlear groove. The results of mosaicplasty in the patellofemoral joint are fair but are not as successful as those on the femoral condyles.

Lesions that are secondary to OCD can also be treated with the mosaicplasty technique. These lesions can be categorized as either fragment missing or fragment intact.

When the osteochondral fragment is missing, the surgeon is faced with a reconstructive problem. The cartilage and bony defects must be reconstructed while ensuring that the plugs are inserted at the proper level to restore the normal joint contour. We have had good success with these, especially with OCD lesions of the patella and the femoral condyle.

OCD lesions with the fragment still intact or with a fragment that can be returned to the defect may be stabilized with autologous osteochondral plugs (Fig. 3A,B). All of the fixation principles

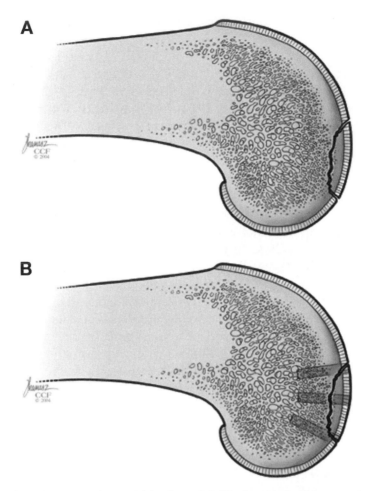

Fig. 3. Illustration demonstrating stabilization of OCD fragment with osteochondral plugs. **(A)** Cross-sectional lateral view of *in situ* OCD fragment. **(B)** Cross-sectional lateral view of OCD stabilized with osteochondral plugs.

that are required for proper healing of an OCD fragment are provided by the bone plugs. The mosaicplasty technique allows you to drill across the fragment and into the base of the lesion, stimulating a blood supply; it provides stable fixation because of the interference fit, and it bone grafts the bottom of defect, with the bone plugs extending across the lesion. We have had excellent success in healing all of these defects, never having one that has not healed to date *(33)*.

CLINICAL OUTCOMES

The successful clinical application of osteochondral autograft transplantation in the treatment of chondral lesions of the knee has been well described. In 2004, Hangody and Fules reported on their 10-yr experience with mosaicplasty. This review of 831 patients included 597 femoral condyle procedures, 188 patellofemoral joint procedures, and 25 tibial plateau procedures. Clinical outcome measures demonstrated good-to-excellent results in 92% of patients with femoral condylar implantations, 87% of tibial implantations, and 79% of patellofemoral implantations. Long-term donor site morbidity was noted in 3% of patients. Of the 83 patients who were followed with serial arthroscopy, 69 had good gliding surfaces, histological evidence of survival of the transplanted hyaline cartilage, and fibrocartilage coverage of the donor sites *(34)*.

In another retrospective review, Jakob et al. evaluated 110 patients treated with multiple autologous osteochondral plugs for repair of articular cartilage defects. Fifty-two consecutive patients underwent mosaicplasty for chondral defects of the knee. At 2 yr following surgery, an increased level of knee function was found in 86% of patients, with improvement noted in 92% of patients at latest follow-up *(19)*. Overall repair assessment at second-look arthroscopy revealed cartilage that was graded as nearly normal, and histological examinations revealed that the transplanted cartilage retained its hyaline character, corroborating similar findings in studies evaluating the quality of transplanted cartilage *(34,35)*.

Chow et al. evaluated a series of 33 patients with full-thickness, symptomatic, cartilage lesions of the femoral condyles treated with arthroscopic autologous osteochondral transplantation. At a mean follow-up of 45 mo, significant improvements in mean Lysholm knee scores were noted, with good or excellent outcome accomplished in 83% of knees *(35)*. Histology revealed normal hyaline cartilage in the 9 patients found to have complete healing, and articular congruency was noted in 92% of patients who underwent MRI.

Few randomized controlled trials exist to compare the outcomes of autologous osteochondral transplantation to other cartilage repair techniques. Horas et al. commented on outcomes in 40 patients with traumatic articular cartilage lesions of the femoral condyle who were randomly treated with either open osteochondral autograft transplantation or autologous chondrocyte implantation (ACI). As measured by postoperative Lysholm scores, osteochondral transplantation was associated with faster recovery at 6, 12, and 24 mo compared to ACI *(36)*. Histological evaluation of biopsy specimens revealed a preponderance of fibrocartilage in the transplant regions of the ACI group; the biopsies obtained from patients treated with osteochondral autograft transplantation demonstrated a persistent interface between the transplant and surrounding cartilage. The authors concluded that both treatments resulted in a decrease in symptoms at 2 yr; however, improvements in the ACI group lagged behind those treated with osteochondral transplantation. These results contrast those of a previous prospective clinical trial, in which Bentley et al. followed 100 patients randomized to undergo ACI or osteochondral autograft procedures for symptomatic articular cartilage lesions of the knee. At a mean follow-up of 19 mo, functional assessment demonstrated 88% excellent or good results after ACI compared with 69% after osteochondral allograft transplantation *(37)*.

Gudas et al. compared the outcomes of arthroscopic osteochondral allograft transplantation and microfracture procedures for the treatment of articular cartilage defects of the femoral condyles in young competitive athletes at a mean follow-up of 37 mo. Both groups demonstrated significant clinical postoperative improvement; however, the allograft group showed significantly better results as determined by functional and objective outcome measures *(36)*. Second-look arthroscopy demonstrated better macroscopic repair grades in the osteochondral allograft group, and histological evaluation also demonstrated better cartilage quality. Moreover, 93% of the patients in the autograft group returned to preinjury activity level vs 52% of those patients in the microfracture group *(38)*.

Collectively, these studies illustrate the short-term success of osteochondral allograft transplantation in treating focal, symptomatic, chondral lesions of the knee. However, few prospective studies exist to compare the results of osteochondral autografting with other established therapies, and the existing comparisons have yielded inconsistent conclusions. Although mosaicplasty procedures may provide satisfactory short-term results, the structural and functional longevity of this procedure remain unknown. Moreover, there is minimal evidence establishing appropriate selection criteria for this procedure, including ideal patient age, size of chondral defect, or duration of symptoms. Further randomized studies are required to delineate the aforementioned criteria and characterize the long-term outcomes of patients who undergo autologous osteochondral transplantation for cartilage defects of the knee.

REFERENCES

1. Hasler EM, Herzog W, Wu JZ, et al. Articular cartilage biomechanics: theoretical models, material properties, and biosynthetic response. Crit Rev Biomed Eng 1999;27:415–488.
2. Noyes FR, Bassett RW, Grood ES, Butler DL. Arthroscopy in acute traumatic hemarthrosis of the knee. Incidence of anterior cruciate ligament tears and other injuries. J Bone Joint Surgery Am 1980;62:687–695, 757.
3. Curl WW, Krome J, Gordon ES, Rushing J, Paterson-Smith B, Poehling GG. Cartilage injuries: a review of 31,516 knee arthroscopies. Arthroscopy 1997;13:456–460.
4. IIunter W. Of the structure and disease of articulating cartilages. 1743. Clin Orthop 1995; 317:3–6.
5. Kim HK, Moran ME, Salter RB. The potential for regeneration of articular cartilage defects created by chondral shaving and subchondral abrasion. An experimental investigation in rabbits. J Bone Joint Surg Am 1991;73:1301–1315.
6. Campell CJ. The healing of cartilage defects. Clin Orthop 1969;64:45–63.
7. Insall J. The Pridie debridement operation for osteoarthritis of the knee. Clin Orthop 1974; 101:61–67.
8. Pridie KH. A method of resurfacing osteoarthritic knee joints. J Bone Joint Surg 1959; 41B:618–619.
9. Mitchell N, Shepard N. The resurfacing of adult rabbit articular cartilage by multiple perforations through the subchondral bone. J Bone Joint Surg 1976;58A:230–233.
10. Buchwalter JA, Rosenberg LC, Hunkziter EB. Articular cartilage, structure, response to injury and methods of facilitating repair. In Ewing JW, ed., Articular Cartilage and Knee Joint Function. Basic Science and Arthroscopy. New York: Raven Press; 1990:19–56.
11. Mandelbaum BR, Browne JE, Fu F, et al. Articular cartilage lesions of the knee. Am J Sports Med 1998;26:853–861.
12. Mankin HJ. The response of articular cartilage to mechanical injury. J Bone Joint Surg Am 1982;64:460–466.
13. Furukawa T, Eyre DR, Koide S, Glimcher MJ. Biomechanical studies on repair. Cartilage resurfacing experimental defects in the rabbit knee. J Bone Joint Surg Am. 1980;62:79–89.
14. Brittberg M, Lindahl A, Nilsson A, Ohlsson C, Isaksson O, Peterson L. Treatment of deep cartilage defects in the knee with autologous chondrocyte transplantation. N Engl J Med 1994; 331:889–895.
15. Grande DA, Pitman MI, Peterson L, Menche D, Klein M. The repair of experimentally produced defects in rabbit articular cartilage by autologous chondrocyte transplantation. J Orthop Res 1989;7:208–218.
16. Horas U, Pelinkovic D, Herr G, Aigner T, Schnettler R. Autologous chondrocyte implantation and osteochondral cylinder transplantation in cartilage repair of the knee joint. A prospective, comparative trial. J Bone Joint Surg Am 2003;85-A:185–192.
17. Yamashita F, Sacked K, Suzy F, Taka S. The transplantation of an autogenic osteochondral fragment for osteochondritis of the knee. Clin Orthop 1985;210:43–50.
18. Hangody L, Kish G, Karate Z, Serb I, Udvarhelyi I. Arthroscopic autogenous osteochondral mosaicplasty for the treatment of femoral condylar articular defects. A preliminary report. Knee Surg Sports Traumatol Arthrosc 1997;5:262–267.
19. Jakob RP, Franz T, Gautier E, Mainil-Varlet P. Autologous osteochondral grafting in the knee: indication, results, and reflections. Clin Orthop Relat Res 2002:170–184.

20. Bodo G, Kaposi A, Hangody L, et al. The surgical technique and the age of horse both influence the outcome of mosaicplasty in a cadaver stifle model. Acta Vet Hung 2001;49:111–116.
21. Feczko P, Hangody L, Varga J, et al. Experimental results of donor site filling for autologous osteochondral mosaicplasty. Arthroscopy 2003;19:755–761.
22. Evans P, Miniaci A, Hurtig M. Manual Punch vs power harvesting of osteochondral grafts. Arthroscopy 2004;20:306–310.
23. Pearce SG, Hurtig MB, Clarnette R, Kalra M, Cowan B, Miniaci A. An investigation of two techniques for optimizing joint surface congruency using multiple cylindrical autografts. J Arthrosc 2000;1:50–55.
24. Rosenburg TD, Paulos LE, Parker RD, et al. The 45° posteroanterior flexion weight bearing radiograph of the knee. J Bone Joint Surg Am 1988;70A:1479–1483.
25. Chung CB, Frank LR, Resnick D, Cartilage imaging techniques: current clinical applications and state of the art imaging. Clin Orthop 2001;391S:S370–S378.
26. Disler DG, McCauley TR, Kelman CG, et al. Fat-suppressed three-dimensional spoiled gradient-echo MR imaging of hyaline cartilage defects in the knee: comparison with standard MR imaging and arthroscopy. AJR Am J Roentgenol 1996;167:127–132.
27. Recht MP, Piraino DW, Paletta GA, Schils JP, Belhobek GH. Accuracy of fat- three-dimensional spoiled gradient-echo FLASH MR imaging in the detection of patellofemoral articular cartilage abnormalities. Radiology 1996;198:209–212.
28. Disler DG, McCauley TR, Wirth CR, Fuchs MD. Detection of knee hyaline cartilage defects using fat-suppressed three-dimensional spoiled gradient echo MR imaging: comparison with standard MR imaging and correlation with arthroscopy. AJR Am J Roentgenol 1995;165: 377–382.
29. Miniaci A. The effect of graft size and number on outcome of mosaic arthroplasty resurfacing: an experimental model in sheep. Proc Int Soc Arthrosc Knee Surg Orthop Sports Med 2001; 5:169.
30. Ahmed CS, Cohen ZA, Levine WN, Ateshian GA, Mow VC. Biomechanical and topographic considerations for autologous osteochondral grafting in the knee. Am J Sports Med 2001; 29:201–206.
31. Bartz RL, Kamaric E, Noble PC, Lintner D, Bocell J. Topographic matching of selected donor and recipient sites for osteochondral autografting of the articular surfaces of the femoral condyles. Am J Sports Med 2001;29:207–212.
32. Miniaci A, Evans P, Hurtig MB. Harvesting techniques for osteochondral transplantation. Proc Int Soc Arthrosc Knee Surg Orthop Sports Med 1999;86:147.
33. Hand C, Lobo J, White L, Miniaci A. Osteochondral autografting resurfacing. Sports Med Arthrosc Rev 2003;11:245–263.
34. Hangody L, Fules P. Autologous osteochondral mosaicplasty for the treatment of full-thickness defects of weight-bearing joints: 10 years of experimental and clinical experience. J Bone Joint Surg Am 2003;85-A(suppl 2):25–32.
35. Chow JC, Hantes ME, Houle JB, Zalavras CG. Arthroscopic autogenous osteochondral transplantation for treating knee cartilage defects: a 2- to 5-year follow-up study. Arthroscopy 2004; 20:681–690.
36. Horas U, Pelinkovic D, Herr G, Aigner T, Schnettler R. Autologous chondrocyte implantation and osteochondral cylinder transplantation in cartilage repair of the knee joint. A prospective, comparative trial. J Bone Joint Surg Am 2003;85-A:185–192.
37. Bentley G, Biant LC, Carrington RW, et al. A prospective, randomised comparison of autologous chondrocyte implantation vs mosaicplasty for osteochondral defects in the knee. J Bone Joint Surg Br 2003;85:223–230.
38. Gudas R, Kalesinskas RJ, Kimtys V, et al. A prospective randomized clinical study of mosaic osteochondral autologous transplantation vs microfracture for the treatment of osteochondral defects in the knee joint in young athletes. Arthroscopy 2005;21:1066–1075.

9

Articular Cartilage Resurfacing Using Synthetic Resorbable Scaffolds

Riley J. Williams III, MD
and Gabriele G. Niederauer, PhD

INTRODUCTION

Cartilage repair is a challenging clinical problem because once adult cartilage sustains damage, whether traumatic or pathological, an irreversible, degenerative process can occur *(1)*. The resulting defects may lead to osteoarthritis *(2–4)*. Attempts to repair articular cartilage have included implantation of artificial matrices, growth factors, perichondrium, periosteum, and transplanted cells *(5)*, but to date no reliable, reproducible approach has been identified. Furthermore, repair tissue frequently lacks the physical structure and mechanical properties necessary to ensure long-term efficacy *(6)*. It is reasonable to hypothesize that the inferior mechanical properties of the repair tissue are partially caused by inadequate support during healing.

The use of biodegradable scaffolds for articular cartilage repair has been investigated by numerous researchers *(7–21)*. In an ideal mechanical environment, the stiffness of the implant matches that of the surrounding tissue as closely as possible. Such modulus matching would help the implant, repair tissue, and surrounding cartilage experience an equal and uniform stress distribution on loading. Bioresorbable scaffolds have the obvious advantage over permanent implants in that complete regeneration of articular cartilage can occur without the inhibition of residual foreign material. Such scaffolds can be used either alone or as delivery vehicles for cells, mitogens, or growth factors. The physical and mechanical scaffold properties can profoundly affect the healing response of the articular cartilage, especially when placed in a weight-bearing environment *(22–24)*. Furthermore, the proper mechanical environment for chondrocytes and their matrix is essential to obtain a structurally and biochemically appropriate tissue *(25–27)*.

Repair of osteochondral defects involves two types of distinct tissues: articular cartilage and subchondral bone. In designing a multiphase implant, the healing of the underlying subchondral area of the defect site is critical to support the overlying neocartilage regenerate. Over the last decades, bioactive glasses, calcium phosphates, and similar ceramics for bone repair have been shown to bond to bone and accelerate bone healing *(28–31)*. However, for subchondral bone repair in rabbit and goat osteochondral defects, bioactive glass and hydroxyapatite have yielded mixed results. Suominen et al. *(32)* treated 4×4 mm osteochondral defects in rabbit femurs with bioactive glass, hydroxyapatite, and hydroxyapatite-glass and reported the formation

From: *Cartilage Repair Strategies*
Edited by: Riley J. Williams © Humana Press Inc., Totowa, NJ

of lamellar subchondral bone with restoration of hyalinelike cartilage surface after 12 weeks. On the other hand, van Susante et al. *(33)* attempted to restore 10-mm cartilage defects in goat femurs with chondrocytes suspended in fibrin glue on top of hydroxyapatite cylinders. Because of inadequate fixation of the implant, fibrocartilaginous repair tissue resulted.

Polylactide-*co*-glycolides (PLGs) are often chosen for tissue engineering applications because their degradation can be tailored; however, in a highly porous configuration, their mechanical properties may be limited *(34–37)*. One method to enhance the strength of such scaffolds is to utilize reinforcement materials similar to the concept of rebar in concrete. Slivka et al. showed that incorporating chopped polyglycolic acid fibers improves the structural integrity of the scaffold during the initial weeks of healing, and native cartilage architecture can be approximated by preferentially aligning the fibers *(38)*. Porous 75:25 poly (D,L-lactide-*co*-glycolide) scaffolds reinforced with polyglycolide (PGA) fibers were prepared with mechanical properties tailored for use in articular cartilage repair. Compression testing was performed to investigate the influence of physiological testing conditions, manufacturing method, anisotropic properties caused by predominant fiber orientation, amounts of fiber reinforcement (0 to 20 wt%), and viscoelasticity via a range of strain rates. Using the same testing modality, the mechanical properties of the scaffolds were compared with pig and goat articular cartilage. The compressive modulus and yield strength proportionally increased with increasing fiber reinforcement up to 20%. The compressive modulus of the nonreinforced scaffolds was most similar to the pig and goat articular cartilage when compared using similar testing conditions and modality, but the improved yield strength of the stiffer scaffolds with fiber reinforcement could provide needed structural support for in vivo loads. Implantation of these fiber-reinforced scaffolds loaded with chondrocytes in a non-load-bearing, ectopic site confirmed their ability to form cartilage throughout the construct *(39)*.

PRECLINICAL STUDIES WITH SYNTHETIC SCAFFOLDS

The assessment of implant devices for replacing, repairing, or regenerating articular cartilage has been performed in various animal models, including rabbit *(40–50)*, dog *(50–52)*, pig *(53)*, sheep *(54–56)*, goat *(22,24,33,57–65)*, and horse *(66–70)*. In choosing the appropriate animal model, several considerations were taken into account, including joint size, anatomical location, cartilage thickness, and defect size.

Investigators have also explored the addition of bioactives to enhance the healing of cartilage defects. Bradica et al. *(40)* reported use of a multiphase device of polylactic acid (PLA) and collagen for osteochondral defect repair. Implants had an articular cartilage fabric of a type I collagen sponge and a subchondral bone construct composed of D,D-L,L-PLA with a cancellous bonelike architecture containing hyaluronic acid. The interface was a copolymer film of PLA and glycolic acid, acting as a barrier to fluids but allowing cell migration. The articular cartilage fabric contained recombinant human bone morphogenetic protein (rhBMP)-2 at 200 µg or 75/100 µL, with 5 µg/100 µL in the subchondral bone construct. Condylar defects (3 mm in diameter) were created in 54 rabbits, and implants were press-fit into place. Control implants contained saline, with additional unimplanted controls. Femurs were harvested at 24 weeks. BMP-charged devices induced a higher percentage of cartilage repair than did untreated defects, although differences in overall repair were not statistically significant.

Numerous cartilage repair products feature autologous cartilage harvest, chondrocyte expansion, and cell implantation and are currently available in the United States and Europe. In the United States, the indications for such products are large chondral lesions, which are

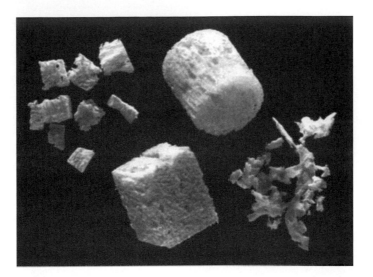

Fig. 1. TruRepair™ family of resorbable scaffolds (Smith and Nephew Endoscopy, San Antonio, TX)

often salvage cases; typically, these cases are quite costly. Therefore, a single-stage approach that would facilitate delivery of reparative cells to a cartilage defect would be ideal.

Lu et al. *(65)* have shown that cartilage tissue fragments from an intraoperative cartilage harvest can be a viable cell source in the treatment of cartilage injuries. These studies have shown that harvested cartilage can be minced into small pieces and distributed onto bioresorbable scaffolds (made of polycaprolactone-*co*-glycolide or copolymer of PGA and polylactide). These scaffolds can be anchored into the cartilage defect. This procedure was used to treat 7-mm full-thickness cartilage defects in the trochlear groove of skeletally mature sheep. After 6 mo, tissues were harvested, and visual evaluation showed that the defects healed better when treated with cartilage fragment-loaded implants.

The safety and performance characteristics of the TruFit™ CB implant (cartilage/bone) have been shown in numerous preclinical tests conducted by OsteoBiologics Inc. (OBI). The most relevant studies have been carried out in a goat model (femoral condyle and trochlea). Because goats provide a relatively large joint size, good cartilage thickness (~0.9–1.2 mm), ease of handling, and ready availability, this model has been used for numerous preclinical testing procedures *(22,24,33,57–65)*. Because the goat model provides a reasonable testing environment for human application, we have compared goat and human knee sizes. The average human medial condyle widths *(71)* were reported to be 1.66–1.84 times larger than the average medial condyle width of the goats utilized for the OBI studies. Similarly, the human femur widths *(71)* were 1.56–1.80 times larger than the average femur width of the goats utilized for the OBI studies.

The TruFit CB implant is composed of PLG copolymer, calcium sulfate, PGA fibers, and surfactant. The TruFit CB implant is formulated to be a porous, resorbable scaffold (Fig. 1) that allows ingrowth of new healing tissue and is ideal for filling cylindrical drill holes in osteochondral locations. The bilayer design of the TruFit CB provides both a cartilage and a bone phase, each designed to provide the appropriate mechanical properties for the adjacent tissue (Fig. 2). Accordingly, the top cartilage phase is softer and malleable enough to be contoured to the joint curvature. The TruFit CB has received the CE Mark for bone and

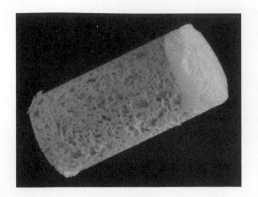

Fig. 2. TruFit CB (cartilage/bone) implant featured multiple layers designed to physically and mechanically match those of the adjacent articular cartilage and underlying bone.

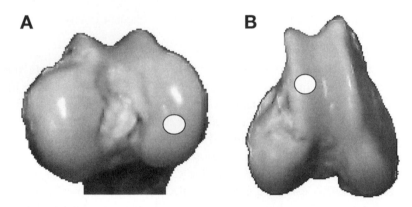

Fig. 3. Cranial view (**A**) and anterior view (**B**) of the femoral surfaces of the right knee joint. Defect sites were placed at the medial locations of the condyles and patellar groove. Sites on the left knee were at mirrored locations.

cartilage repair, enabling the TruFit CB to be marketed and distributed throughout the European community.

The objective of a recent TruFit CB Plug preclinical study was to examine the healing in adult goats of an osteochondral defect in the knee joint filled with a novel, resorbable tissue scaffold. Implants were prepared using poly(D,L-lactide-co-glycolide, 85:15) as the base material. PGA fibers were added to tailor the mechanical properties, and surfactant was added to make the implant surface more hydrophilic. Calcium sulfate was incorporated into the bone phase to enhance bone ingrowth. Cylindrical implants, 5×5 mm with a porosity of 75%, were press-fit into osteochondral defects of the medial femoral condyle and lateral trochlear groove of 12 Spanish goats (Fig. 3). Defect sites were treated and allowed to heal for 6 weeks (6 goats), 6 months (3 goats), and 12 months (3 goats). At euthanasia, subjective evaluations and evaluation of quantitative stiffness properties were performed. Histological sections were taken at approximately the center of the defect and stained with toluidine blue and Goldner's trichrome and immunohistochemically stained for type II collagen. Sections were blindly evaluated to assess tissue healing.

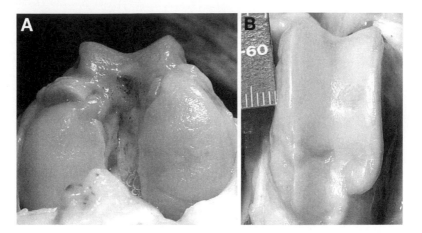

Fig. 4. Gross images of joint surface at 12 months: (**A**) femoral condyle; (**B**) trochlear groove.

All animals tolerated the surgeries well and returned to normal activity immediately. Evaluations at necropsy indicated no abnormalities of the joints, such as inflammation or abrasion of the opposing articulating surface. Visual observations showed that the new tissue integrated well with the native cartilage, that the surface of the repair site was fairly smooth, and that the defects were almost entirely filled (Fig. 4). The stiffness of the repair tissue ranged from 93 to 101% of the value for healthy cartilage, indicating that the biomechanical properties of the neocartilage were very similar to those of normal cartilage and significantly bcttcr than for fibrocartilage.

Overall qualitative evaluations of the histological slides showed that all groups had a high percentage of hyaline cartilage and good bony restoration (Fig. 5). Healing of the osteochondral defect continued to improve from the 6 weeks to the 12-month end point. Integration of healed tissue showed excellent bonding with the native cartilage, and the repair cartilage thickness was very close to that of adjacent cartilage, with no significant differences noted in the two treatment sites. In comparison to historical empty controls *(58)*, the scaffold provided mechanical support for the tissue to heal and prevent collapse of the adjacent defect walls.

The current investigation demonstrates that osteochondral defect donor sites in the knee joint can be successfully treated with multilayer, resorbable implants. The biologically friendly properties of the scaffold allow infiltration of key biologic elements, such as blood, proteins, and cells. The scaffolds go through staged resorption: The calcium sulfate dissolves in the first 3 months, and the polymer resorbs over a 9-month period. Staged resorption enables the tissue to replace the scaffold in a controlled manner. The osteoconductive phase containing calcium sulfate supports bone formation and remodeling; the top polymeric phase supports soft tissue formation and remodeling. Gross observations at all time-points demonstrated no significant cratering or osteophytosis, indicating a stable articulating joint. The osteochondral defect was stable throughout the course of this study, and there was minimal cartilage flow, which supports the lack of a zone of influence. The 12-month histological slides show the scaffolds to be completely replaced by cancellous bone in the subchondral bone region and show hyaline cartilage in the overlying region (Fig. 5).

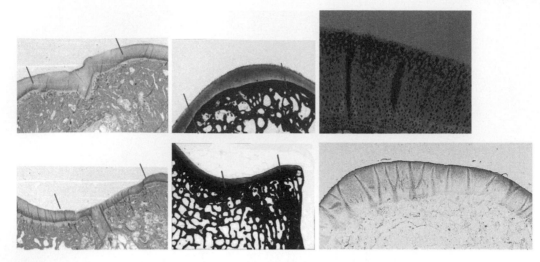

Fig. 5. Histological appearances of femoral condyle (bottom row) and trochlear groove (top row). Hatch marks show original lesion size. First column illustrates Goldner's TriChrome-stained sections of healing at 6 months. Column 2 demonstrates toluidine blue-stained sections at 12 months. Column 3, top, is 12-month up-close section stained with Safranin O/Fast Green. Column 3, bottom, shows the presence of type II collagen via immunohistochemical staining.

CLINICAL CASE WITH A SYNTHETIC RESORBABLE SCAFFOLD

History

A healthy 17-year-old player on a National Collegiate Athletic Association Division 1 lacrosse team presented to a sports medicine clinic with a knee injury. The patient was playing lacrosse when he experienced sharp pain in his left knee. The knee gave way and immediately became swollen; he was then unable to bear weight. Radiographs of the knee were negative for fracture or abnormality. On examination, the patient's active range of motion was limited (0 to 110° of flexion). The only physical exam parameter of note was tenderness on the medial and lateral facets of the patella. There was a large effusion.

Magnetic Resonance Imaging

A cartilage-sensitive magnetic resonance imaging (MRI) sequence, was used to assess the knee condition. Specifically, a fast spin echo sequence developed by Potter et al. *(72)* was utilized to detect possible chondral and underlying bone damage. Sagittal and axial views of the trochlea were captured and analyzed. MRI showed an osteochondral defect in the medial trochlea (Fig. 6), caused by a displaced osteochondritis dissecans (OCD) lesion, with full-thickness cartilage and bone loss measuring approx 10–11 mm. No other abnormalities were found on MRI.

Surgical Procedure

Based on the patient's symptoms and MRI findings, plans were made to proceed with arthroscopic evaluation and treatment of the OCD defect. Approximately 1 month after initial examination, diagnostic knee arthroscopy was performed using a two-portal technique. The knee joint was inspected, and one isolated, conical, trochlear osteochondral defect was found (Figs. 7 and 8). A large, loose body was removed from the medial gutter; this fragment

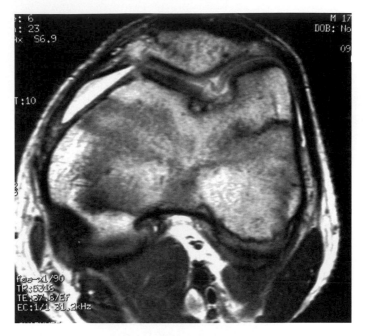

Fig. 6. Preoperative MRI.

represented the destabilized cartilage fragment (Fig. 9) that originated from the trochlear defect. A limited lateral parapatellar arthrotomy was used to approach the defect. A tourniquet was used after exsanguination of the leg. A sizing guide was used to determine the diameter of the lesion, which was found to be 9 mm in its widest dimension, superiorly. To prepare the OCD site for a bone graft substitute plug, a tubular harvester was used to remove the bone, and a cylindrical site with a depth of 10 mm was created. The defect was inspected to make sure no debris was present. To prepare the implant for insertion into the site, the TruFit delivery device (9 mm) was used to measure the depth of the defect, and the extra length of the implant was trimmed. A 9-mm Trufit Plug was implanted and impacted to a depth flush with the adjacent native cartilage (Fig. 10). The tourniquet was released; wounds were irrigated and closed.

Postoperative Observations/Evaluations

Postoperatively for the first week, cryotherapy and toe-touch weight bearing was prescribed; the operated knee was placed into a long-leg postoperative brace. Continuous passive motion was initiated immediately for 6 hours per day and continued for 6 weeks. After 1 week, weight bearing to tolerance with the brace locked in extension was recommended. For physiotherapy, the patient participated in an outpatient regimen from week 2–8. The patient was evaluated 1 week, 6 weeks, 3 months, and 12 months after surgery.

MRI Images

The MRI at 3 months (Fig. 11) displays the treated site flush in appearance with surrounding interface. Top phase material is slightly more hyperintense (axial images) than the native cartilage. The implant is stable in its implanted press-fit position. Minimal integration with surrounding bone is observed at this point, with a low signal intensity rim of demarcation. Congruent reconstruction of the articular surface is noted.

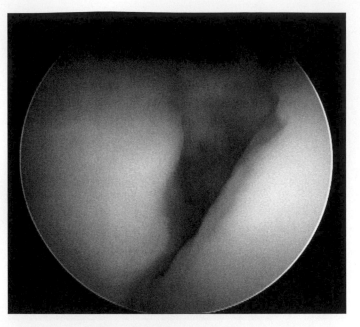

Fig. 7. Trochlear OCD defect.

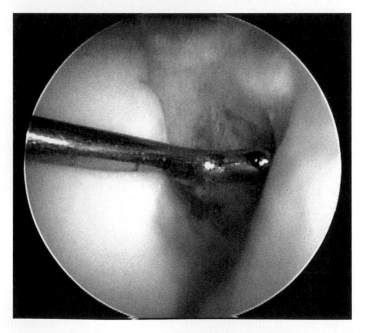

Fig. 8. Trochlear OCD defect on probing.

An MRI at 12 months (Fig. 12) shows progressive integration of the subchondral repair material filling the defect and no exposed bone. Trabecular bone incorporation into the plug in the defect margins was observed. Slight hyperintensity was noted in the top phase of the treated site when compared to the native articular cartilage, but no discernible fissures were noted at the interface with the native cartilage.

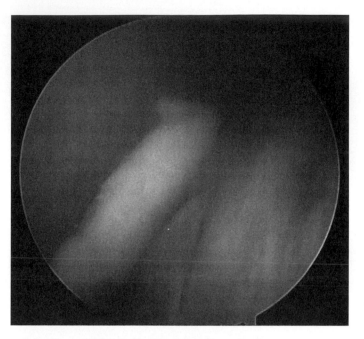

Fig. 9. Cartilaginous loose body.

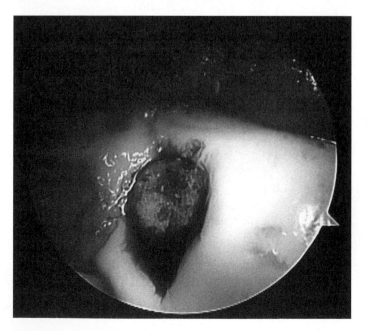

Fig. 10. TruFit plug positioned in the trochlear OCD defect. Note the infiltration of marrow/blood into the implant.

Subsequent quantitative T_2 mapping obtained at 12 months (Fig. 13) shows prolonged T_2 values in the subchondral region, with heterogeneous repair cartilage over the articular surface. The MRI appearance of synthetic tissue repair such as the TruFit plugs is slightly different when compared to either osteochondral allografts or autologous osteochondral plugs. The PLG

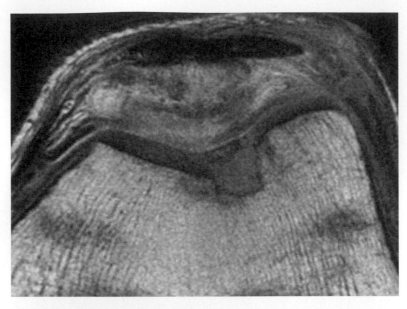

Fig. 11. Cartilage-sensitive MRI 3-month status postimplantation.

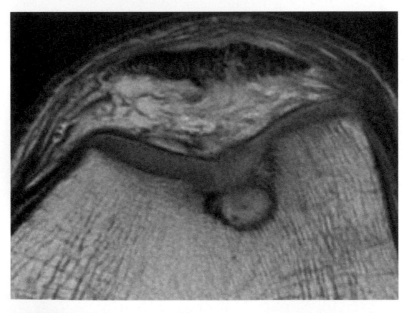

Fig. 12. Cartilage-sensitive MRI 12-month status postimplantation.

copolymer and calcium sulfate typically appear hypointense to native medullary bone on water-sensitive sequences, often with a delayed bone marrow edema pattern on fat suppression compared to traditional osteochondral grafting techniques.

Conclusions

At the latest follow-up (18 months postimplantation), the patient was asymptomatic (full activity with no complaints of pain and no effusions). The athlete continues to play lacrosse

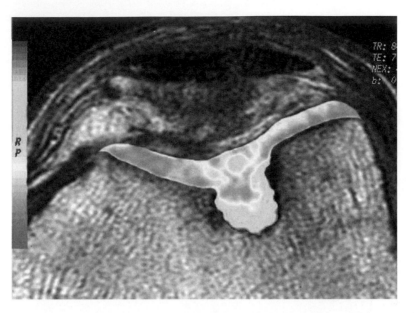

Fig. 13. Cartilage-sensitive MRI 12-month status postimplantation with T_2 mapping.

at the same level. The TruFit plug provides a viable alternative to autologous or allogenic transplantation for treating osteochondral defect sites of the trochlea. Because the TruFit plug offers a malleable implant, it is ideal for trochlear contouring.

TREATMENT OPTIONS

Surgical Technique

The TruKor® instruments (Smith and Nephew Endoscopy, San Antonio, TX) are provided in the following four sizes: 5 (Green), 7 (Red), 9 (Blue) and 11 (Purple) mm. The appropriate color is determined by measuring the maximum defect size with a ruler or sizer and selecting a size that completely covers the defect. Once size is determined, the appropriate TruKor instrument size is used throughout the procedure. The obturator, which aids insertion of the drill sleeve into the surgical site, is inserted into the handle end of the drill sleeve.

Once the drill sleeve has been placed within the surgical site, the obturator is removed from the drill sleeve, and the drill sleeve cap is inserted into the handle end of the drill sleeve. The drill sleeve cap seals the surgical access port to keep fluids from streaming out and provides a striking surface for the mallet. The TruKor drill sleeve is then placed over the selected site (Fig. 14), ensuring that the drill sleeve is seated perpendicular to the surface containing the defect. To seat the drill sleeve, it is gently pressed into the tissue, and a mallet is used to strike the drill sleeve cap and drive the drill sleeve into the bone to a depth of 5–15 mm (reference depth markings on sleeve) (Fig. 15). Once the desired depth has been attained, the drill sleeve is maintained in the bone, and the drill sleeve cap is removed from the drill sleeve (Fig. 16).

The drill is used to remove tissue from the affected area manually or with the assistance of power. Continue rotating clockwise until the drill contacts the stop on the drill sleeve and make one additional rotation to ensure tissue is removed completely. The drill should be kept within the drill sleeve and remove both together (Fig. 17). The surgical site is inspected to ensure that all tissue within the defect has been removed and flush if necessary. The site is now ready to receive the TruFit implant as described next.

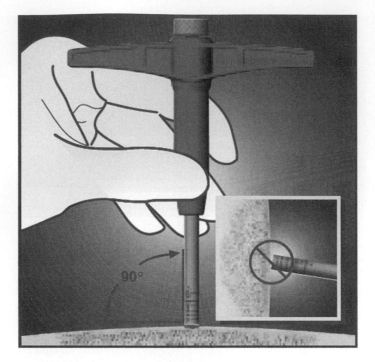

Fig. 14. Drill sleeve is placed perpendicular to defect.

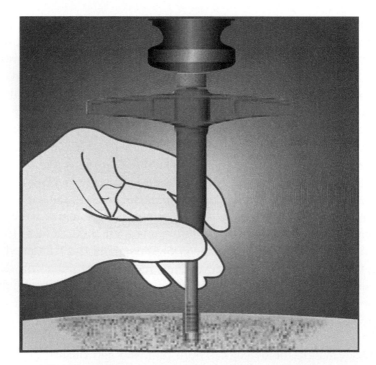

Fig. 15. Mallet is used to insert drill sleeve into bone.

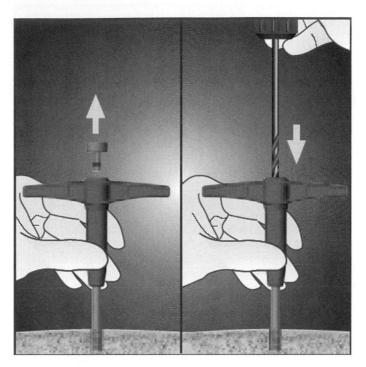

Fig. 16. Drill cap is removed and drill inserted.

TruFit Surgical Technique

The TruFit® (Smith and Nephew Endoscopy, San Antonio, TX) is provided as a kit containing one of each of the following: a cylindrical implant, a delivery device (outer sleeve and measuring tamp), and a trimming knife (Fig. 18). To assemble the TruFit Delivery Device, the measuring tamp is inserted into the outer sleeve in the direction of the arrow on the outer sleeve until contact with the preloaded implant is made. At this point, the implant should not extend beyond the delivery device. The measuring tamp of the delivery device is inserted into the defect, ensuring it contacts the bottom of the defect (Fig. 19).

The outer sleeve is slid down until the lip of the outer sleeve is snugly placed against the tissue surface (this automatically adjusts the implant to the correct position for trimming). The delivery device is then carefully removed from the surgical site (Fig. 20). The outer sleeve is firmly gripped at the window to secure the implant during cutting (Fig. 21). Using the lip of the delivery device as a guide, the notched end of the implant is cut with the trimming knife using a firm downward motion. Once the implant has been cut to a relatively flat surface, the delivery device is used to insert the implant into the defect (Fig. 22) by slightly advancing the implant beyond the tip of the outer sleeve and carefully seating the implant in the defect.

The implant is press-fit into the defect by pushing on the measuring tamp manually or lightly tamping with a mallet (Fig. 23). The delivery device is removed from the surgical site, and implant placement is inspected. If the implant needs further adjustment or contouring, then the measuring tamp is separated from the outer sleeve and used to impact the implant (Fig. 24). The final placement of the implant should be flush with the adjacent surface.

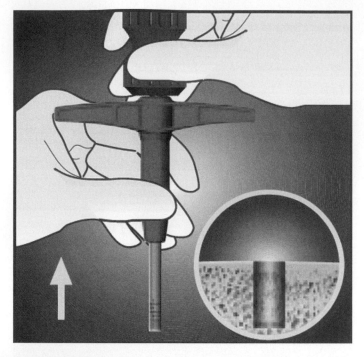

Fig. 17. Drill is turned until it reaches the hard stop on the shoulder. Drill sleeve and drill are removed together.

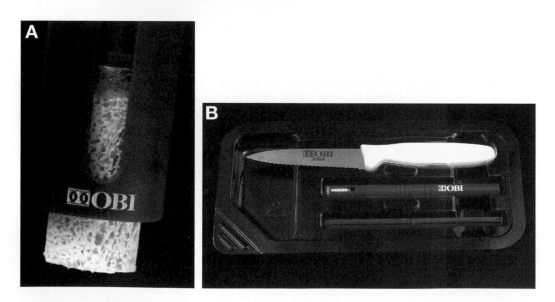

Fig. 18. (A) TruFit implant; **(B)** TruFit Kit containing a preloaded delivery device with implant and a trimming knife.

BENEFICIAL ROLE OF THE SCAFFOLDS

The TruFit CB Plug implant is intended to serve as a scaffold for cellular and matrix ingrowth in osteochondral defect repair such as bone or cartilage, thus helping the body heal itself. The device is a resorbable scaffold for use in the treatment of acute focal articular

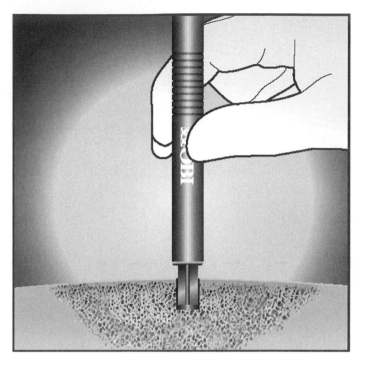

Fig. 19. Tamp is inserted into the defect site.

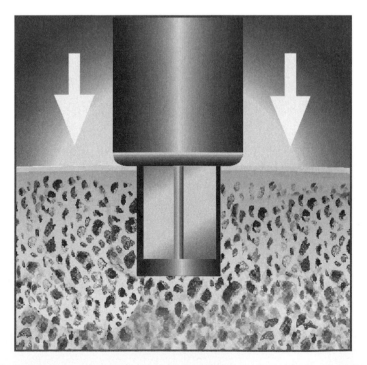

Fig. 20. Outer sleeve is slid down until it makes contact with the tissue surface.

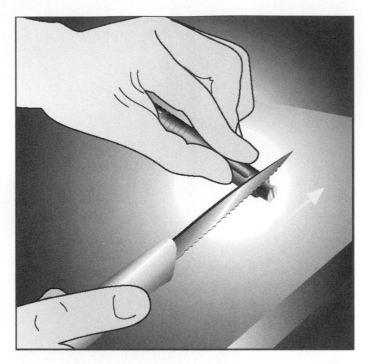

Fig. 21. Outer sleeve is gripped at the windowed end of the outer sleeve, and excess implant is cut using the trimming knife.

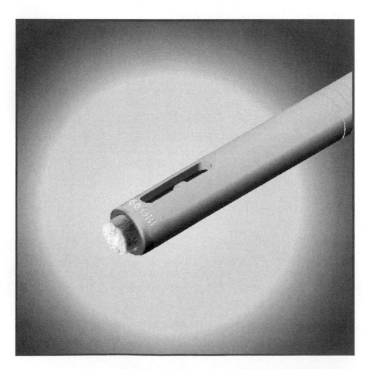

Fig. 22. Implant is slightly advanced to visualize.

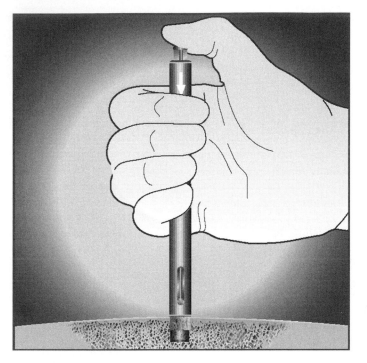

Fig. 23. Implant is inserted into the defect and tamp suppressed to place the implant into the defect.

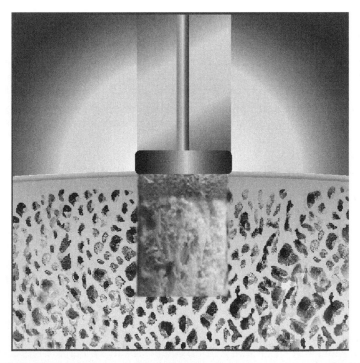

Fig. 24. If implant is proud, then tamp may be used to contour to seat the implant flush with surrounding cartilage.

cartilage or osteochondral defects. The clinical results to date suggest that the implant can provide a means for tissue restoration. The restored cartilage is very smooth and homogeneous and well integrated with the adjacent cartilage. Maintenance of the radius of curvature is achieved with no fissuring or any evidence of a "zone of influence" from the defect site.

REFERENCES

1. Mankin HJ. The response of articular cartilage to mechanical injury. J Bone Joint Surg 1982; 64A:460–466.
2. Alford J, Cole B. Cartilage restoration, part 1 basic science, historical perspective, patient evaluation, and treatment options. Am J Sports Med 2005;33:295–306.
3. Alford J, Cole B. Cartilage restoration, part 2 techniques, outcomes, and future directions. Am J Sports Med 2005;33:443–460.
4. Buckwalter JA, Mankin HJ. Articular cartilage: degeneration and osteoarthritis, repair, regeneration, and transplantation. In: Cannon WD Jr, ed., American Academy of Orthopaedic Surgery Instructional Course Lectures. 47th ed. Rosemont, IL: American Academy of Orthopaedic Surgeons; 1998:487–504.
5. Sgaglione NA. The future of cartilage restoration. J Knee Surg 2004;17:1–9.
6. Suh J-K, Aroen A, Muzzonigro TS, Disilvestro M, Fu FH. Injury and repair of articular cartilage: related scientific issues. Operative Tech Orthop 1997;7:270–278.
7. Freed LE, Vunjak-Novakovic G, Biron RJ, et al. Biodegradable polymer scaffolds for tissue engineering. Bio/Technology 1994;12:689–693.
8. Freed LE, Grande DA, Lingbin Z, Emmanual J, Marquis JC, Langer R. Joint resurfacing using allograft chondrocytes and synthetic biodegradable polymer scaffolds. J Biomed Mater Res 1994;28:891–899.
9. Ma PX, Schloo B, Mooney D, Langer R. Development of biomechanical properties and morphogenesis of in vitro tissue engineered cartilage. J Biomed Mater Res 1995;29:1587–1595.
10. Cima LG, Vacanti JP, Vacanti CA, Ingber DE, Mooney D, Langer R. Tissue engineering by cell transplantation using degradable polymer substrates. J Biomech Eng 1991;113: 143–151.
11. Grande DA, Halberstadt C, Naughton G, Schwartz RE, Manji R. Evaluation of matrix scaffolds for tissue engineering of articular cartilage grafts. J Biomed Mater Res 1997;34: 211–220.
12. Sittinger M, Reitzel D, Dauner M, et al. Resorbable polyesters in cartilage engineering: affinity and biocompatibility of polymer fiber structures to chondrocytes. J Biomed Mater Res Appl Biomater 1996;33:57–63.
13. Bujia J, Sittinger M, Minuth WW, Hammer C, Burmester G, Kastenbauer E. Engineering of cartilage tissue using bioresorbable polymer fleeces and perfusion culture. Acta Otolaryngol 1995; 115:307–310.
14. Sittinger M, Bujia J, Minuth WW, Hammer C, Burmester G. Engineering of cartilage tissue using bioresorbable polymer carriers in perfusion culture. Biomaterials 1994;15:451–456.
15. Freed LE, Marquis JC, Nohria A, Emmanual J, Mikos AG, Langer R. Neocartilage formation in vitro and in vivo using cells cultured on synthetic biodegradable polymers. J Biomed Mater Res 1993;27:11–23.
16. Mikos AG, Bao Y, Cima LG, Ingber DE, Vacanti JP, Langer R. Preparation of poly(glycolic acid) bonded fiber structures for cell attachment and transplantation. J Biomed Mater Res 1993; 27:183–189.
17. Vacanti CA, Upton J. Tissue-engineered morphogenesis of cartilage and bone by means of cell transplantation using synthetic biodegradable polymer matrices. Clin Plast Surg 1994; 21:445–462.
18. Dunkelman N, Zimber MP, LeBaron RG, Pavelec R, Kwan M, Purchio AF. Cartilage production by rabbit articular chondrocytes on polyglycolic acid scaffolds in a closed bioreactor system. Biotechnol Bioeng 1995;46:299–305.

19. Langer R, Vacanti JP, Vacanti CA, Atala A, Freed LE, Vunjak-Novakovic G. Tissue engineering: biomedical applications. Tissue Eng 1995;1:151–161.
20. Nehrer S, Breinan H, Ramappa A, et al. Matrix collagen type and pore size influence behaviour of seeded canine chondrocytes. Biomaterials 1997;18:769–776.
21. Nehrer S, Breinan HA, Ramappa A, et al. Chondrocyte-seeded collagen matrices implanted in a chondral defect in a canine model. Biomaterials 1998;19:2313–2328.
22. van Susante JLC, Buma P, Homminga GN, Van den Berg WB, Veth RPH. Chondrocyte-seeded hydroxyapaptite for repair of large articular cartilage defects. A pilot study in the goat. Biomaterials 1998;19:2367–2374.
23. Singhal AR, Agrawal CM, Athanasiou K. Salient degradation features of a 50:50 PLA/PGA scaffold for tissue engineering. Tissue Eng 1996;2:197–206.
24. Athanasiou K, Korvick DL, Schenck RC. Biodegradable implants for the treatment of osteochondral defects in a goat model. Tissue Eng 1997;3:39–49.
25. Vunjak-Novakovic G, Martin I, Obradovic B, et al. Bioreactor cultivation conditions modulate the composition and mechanical properties of tissue-engineered cartilage. J Orthop Res 1999; 17:130–138.
26. Quinn TM, Grodzinsky AJ, Buschmann MD, Kim YJ, Hunziker EB. Mechanical compression alters proteoglycan deposition and matrix deformation around individual cells in cartilage explants. J Cell Sci 1998;111:573–583.
27. Jones WR, Ting-Beall HP, Lee GM, Kelley SS, Hochmuth RM, Guilak F. Alterations in the Young's modulus and volumetric properties of chondrocytes isolated from normal and osteoarthritic human cartilage. J Biomech 1999;32:119–127.
28. Hulbert S, Bokos JC, Hench LL, Wilson J, Heimke G. Ceramics in clinical applications, past, present, and future. In Vinvenzini P, ed. High Tech Ceramics. Amsterdam: Elsevier Science Publishers; 1987:3–27.
29. Hench LL. Bioactive implants. Chem Industry 1995;14:547–550.
30. Jarcho M. Biomaterial aspects of calcium phosphates: properties and applications. Dent Clin North Am 1986;30:25–47.
31. de Groot K, Tencer A, Waite P, Nichols J, Kay J. Significance of the porosity and physical chemistry of calcium phosphate ceramics. Ann New York Acad Sci 1988;523:272–277.
32. Suominen E, Aho AJ, Vedel E, Kangasniemi I, Uusipaikka E, Yli-Urpo A. Subchondral bone and cartilage repair with bioactive glasses, hydroxyapatite, and hydroxyapaptite-glass composite. J Biomed Mater Res 1996;32:543–551.
33. van Susante JLC, Buma P, Schuman L, Homminga GN, Van den Berg WB, Veth RPH. Resurfacing potential of heterologous chondrocytes suspended in fibrin glue in large full-thickness defects of femoral articular cartilage: an experimental study in the goat. Biomaterials 1999;20:1167–1175.
34. Klompmaker J, Jansen HWB, Veth RPH, deGroot JH, Nijenhuis AJ, Pennings AJ. Porous polymer implant for repair of meniscal lesions: a preliminary study in dogs. Biomaterials 1991; 12:810–816.
35. Harris LD, Kim B-S, Mooney DJ. Open pore biodegradable matrices formed with gas foaming. J Biomed Mater Res 1998;42:396–402.
36. Slivka MA, Leatherbury NC, Kieswetter K, Niederauer GG. Porous, resorbable, fiber-reinforced scaffolds tailored for articular cartilage repair. Tissue Eng 2001;7:767–780.
37. Slivka MA, Leatherbury NC, Kieswetter K, Niederauer GG. Mechanical properties of resorbably scaffolds for articular cartilage repair. Poster presented at the 17th Southern Biomedical Engineering Conference, 1998, San Antonio, TX, p. 20.
38. Slivka MA, Leatherbury NC, Kieswetter K, Niederauer GG. In Vitro Compression Testing of Fiber-Reinforced, Bioabsorbable, Porous Implants. West Conshohocken, PA: American Society for Testing and Materials; 2000:124–135.
39. Lohmann CH, Schwartz Z, Niederauer GG, Carnes DL Jr, Dean DD, Boyan BD. Pretreatment with platelet derived growth factor-BB modulates the ability of costochondral resting zone

chondrocytes incorporated into PLA/PGA scaffolds to form new cartilage in vivo. Biomaterials 2000;21:49–61.

40. Bradica G, Frenkel SR, Brekke J, et al. Osteochondral defect repair in the rabbit using a multi-phasic implant and rhBMP-2. Paper presented at: American Academy of Orthopaedic Surgeons 2005 Annual Meeting; February 23, 2005, Washington, DC.

41. Salter RB, Simmonds DF, Malcolm BW, Rumble EJ, MacMichael D, Clements ND. The biological effect of continuous passive motion on the healing of full-thickness defects in articular cartilage. J Bone Joint Surg 1980;62:1232–1251.

42. Shimizu C, Coutts RD, Healey RM, Kubo T, Hirasawa Y, Amiel D. Method of histomorphometric assessment of glycosaminoglycans in articular cartilage. J Orthop Res 1997;15: 670–674.

43. O'Driscoll SW, Keeley FW, Salter RB. The chondrogenic potential of free autogenous periosteal grafts for biological resurfacing of major full-thickness defects in joint surfaces under the influence of continuous passive motion. J Bone Joint Surg 1986;68:1017–1035.

44. Shapiro F, Koide S, Glimcher MJ. Cell origin and differentiation in the repair of full-thickness defects of articular cartilage. J Bone Joint Surg 1993;75:532–553.

45. Frenkel SR, Toolan BC, Menche D, Pitman MI, Pachence JM. Chondrocyte transplantation using a collagen bilayer matrix for cartilage repair. J Bone Joint Surg Br 1997;79-B:831–836.

46. Frenkel SR, Chen GG, McCord G, Macon N, Morris E. The effect of BMP-2 in a collagen bilayer implant for articular cartilage repair in a rabbit model. April, New Orleans, Louisiana: Society for Biomaterials; Trnasactions 1997 p. 24.

47. Sellers RS, Peluso D, Morris E. The effect of recombinant human bone morphogenetic protein-2 (rhBMP-2). on the healing of full-thickness defects of articular cartilage. J Bone Joint Surg Am 1997;79-A:1452–1463.

48. Grande DA, Pitman MI, Peterson L, Menche D, Klein M. The repair of experimentally produced defects in rabbit articular cartilage by autologous chondrocyte transplantation. J Orthop Res 1989;7:208–218.

49. Upton J, Sohn SA, Glowacki J. Neocartilage derived from transplanted perichondrium: What is it? J Am Soc Plastic Reconstr Surg 1981;68:166–174.

50. Klompmaker J, Jansen HWB, Veth RPH, Nielsen HkL, de Groot JH, Pennings AJ. Porous polymer implants for repair of full-thickness defects of articular cartilage: an experimental study in rabbit and dog. Biomaterials 1992;13:625–634.

51. Hale JE, Rudert MJ, Brown TD. Indentation assessment of biphasic mechanical property deficits in size-dependent osteochondral defect repair. J Biomech 1993;26:1319–1325.

52. Breinan H, Martin SD, Hsu HP, Spector M. Healing of canine articular cartilage defects treated with microfracture, a type-II collagen matrix, or cultured autologous chondrocytes. J Orthop Res 2000;18:781–789.

53. Hunziker EB, Rosenberg LC. Repair of partial-thickness defects in articular cartilage: cell recruitment from the synovial membrane. J Bone Joint Surg Am 1996;78-A:721–733.

54. Homminga GN, Bulstra SK, Kuijer R, Van der Linden AJ. Repair of sheep articular cartilage defects with a rabbit costal perichondrial graft. Acta Orthop Scand 1991;62:415–418.

55. Schreiber R, Ilten-Kirby B, Dunkelman N, et al. Repair of osteochondral defects with allogeneic tissue engineered cartilage implants. Clin Orthop 1999;367S:382–395.

56. Hurtig MB, Novak K, McPherson R, et al. Osteochondral dowel transplantation for repair of focal defects in the knee: an outcome study using an ovine model. Vet Surg 1998;27:5–16.

57. Jackson DW, Halbrecht JL, Proctor C, Van Sickle D, Simon TM. Assessment of donor cell and matrix survival in fresh articular cartilage allograft in a goat model. J Orthop Res 1996; 14:255–264.

58. Jackson DW, Lalor PA, Aberman H, Simon TM. Spontaneous repair of full-thickness defects of articular cartilage in a goat model. J Bone Joint Surg 2001;83A:53–64.

59. Butnariu-Ephrat M, Robinson D, Mendes DG, Halperin N, Nevo Z. Resurfacing of goat articular cartilage by chondrocytes derived from bone marrow. Clin Orthop 1996;330:234–243.

60. Shahgaldi BF, Amis AA, Heatley FW, McDowell J, Bentley G. Repair of cartilage lesions using biological implants. J Bone Joint Surg Br 1991;73-B:57–64.
61. Niederauer GG, Slivka MA, Leatherbury NC, et al. Evaluation of multiphase implants for repair of focal osteochondral defects in goats. Biomaterials 2000;21:2561–2574.
62. Huibregtse BA, Samuels JA, O'Callaghan MW. Development of a cartilage defect model of the knee in the goat for autologous chondrocyte implantation research. Transactions of the Orthopaedic Research Society meeting; February 1, 1999; Anaheim, CA.
63. Volenec FJ, Pohl J, Bain S, Jackson D, Simon T, Aberman H. A novel collagen-hyaluronate implant promotes healing of full thickness defects in the articular cartilage of goats. Trans Orthop Res Soc 2002;451, Dallas, TX.
64. Schwartz H, Plouhar P, Gahunia H, et al. Site related differences in the healing of osteochondral defects in the goat knee. Trans Orthop Res Soc 2002;909, Dallas, TX.
65. Lu Y, Dhanaraj S, Wang Z, Kong W, Bradley D, Binette F. A novel intra-operative approach to treat full thickness articular cartilage defects with chondrocyte loaded implants. Transactions of the Washington, DC, Feb 21–23: 51st Annual Meeting of the Orthopedic Research Society Post No. 1363; 2005.
66. Hendrickson DA, Nixon AJ, Grande DA, et al. Chondrocyte-fibrin matrix transplants for resurfacing extensive articular cartilage defects. J Orthop Res 1994;12:485–497.
67. Sams AE, Nixon AJ. Chondrocyte-laden collagen scaffolds for resurfacing extensive articular cartilage defects. Osteoarthritis Cartilage 1995;3:47–59.
68. Convery FR, Akeson WH, Keown GH. The repair of large osteochondral defects. Clin Orthop 1972;82:253–262.
69. Frisbie DD, Lu Y, Colhoun H, Kawcak C, Binette F, McIlwrath CW. In vivo evaluation of a one step autologous cartilage resurfacing technique in a long term equine model. Transactions of the Orthopaedic Research Society; 2005; Poster 1355, Washington, DC.
70. Bertone A, Orban J, Grande D, et al. Articular cartilage and subchondral bone repair using a biodegradable polymer matrix and instrumentation system. Transactions of the Orthopaedic Research Society; 2005; Poster 1803, Washington, DC.
71. Mensch JS, Amstutz HC. Knee morphology as a guide to knee replacement. Clin Orthop 1975;112:231–241.
72. Potter HG, Linklater JM, Allen A, Hannafin J, Haas S. Magnetic resonance imaging of articular cartilage in the knee: an evaluation with use of fast-spin-echo imaging. J Bone Joint Surg 1998;80(A):1276–1284.

10

Autologous Chondrocyte Implantation

Deryk G. Jones, MD, and Lars Peterson, MD, PhD

Summary

Currently, autologous chondrocyte implantation (ACI) is ideally indicated for symptomatic ICRS grade III–IV lesions greater than 2 cm^2 along the femoral condyle or trochlear regions. High-demand patients between the ages of 15 to 55 years of age with excellent motivation and compliance potential should be chosen. Lars Peterson assessed his first 101 patients at intermediate to long-term follow-up. Good to excellent clinical results were seen in 92% of the isolated femoral condylar lesions, while these results decreased to 67% in patients with multiple lesions. Osteochondritis dissecans lesions demostrated 89% good-to-excellent results, and in contrast to the initial series patellar lesions did relatively well with 65% good-to-excellent results. Histologic analysis of the matrix in 37 biopsy specimens assessing for type II collagen showed a correlation between hyaline-like repair tissue and good-to-excellent clinical results. Scott Gillogly evaluated 112 patients with 139 defects treated with the ACI procedure over a 5-year period of time. Average size of the defect was 5.7 cm^2 with over 60% of patients having failed at least one prior procedure. According to the clinician evaluation portion of the Modified Cincinnati Scale 93% demonstrated good-to-excellent outcomes, while the patient evaluation portion demonstrated 89% good-to-excellent outcomes. This chapter will describe the technique of ACI first reported by the senior author (LP) in 1994, as well as additional methods to deal with the various complex problems that can arise during these demanding procedures. A further review of the current literature supporting this techique as well as those studies that compare ACI to other accepted treatment options will be undertaken as well. In addition, we will review and discuss developing literature supporting current use of various matrices in combination with autologous chondrocytes to treat this difficult patient population.

Key Words: Articular cartilage; chondrocyte; implantation; subchondral bone; collagen; scaffold.

INTRODUCTION

Injuries to joint surfaces can result from acute high-impact or repetitive shear and torsional loads to the superficial zone of the articular cartilage architecture. Two studies using direct arthroscopic visualization have shown that the overall incidence of isolated, focal articular cartilage defects is around 5%. While retrospectively reviewing more than 31,000 arthroscopic procedures, Curl et al. demonstrated a 63% incidence of chondral lesions, with an average of 2.7 lesions per knee *(1)*. With increasing age, this percentage and the number of individuals with multiple defects gradually rose. Using the modified Outerbridge classification system, they found grade IV lesions in 20% of the patients, but only 5% of individuals in this category were younger than 40 yr. Three of four people in this younger population had solitary lesions.

Interestingly, in a prospective study undertaken by Hjelle and colleagues, chondral or osteochondral lesions were found in 61% of the patients, and focal defects were found in 19%

From: *Cartilage Repair Strategies*
Edited by: Riley J. Williams © Humana Press Inc., Totowa, NJ

of the patients; these percentages were similar to those found in the retrospective analysis (2). In this prospective assessment, the mean defect size was 2.1 cm². A single, well-defined International Cartilage Repair Society (ICRS) grade III or IV defect (at least 1 cm²) in a patient younger than 40, 45, or 50 yr old accounted for 5.3, 6.1, and 7.1% of all arthroscopies, respectively. The incidence of articular lesions secondary to work-related and sporting activities has been reported to be as high as 22–50% in other studies (3,4). Such injuries alone or in combination with ligamentous instability, meniscal pathology, or mechanical malalignment can be quite debilitating for patients.

Although it is difficult to predict the long-term effects of cartilage defects in the multiply injured knee, it is certain that pain, loss of motion, effusions, and eventual joint degeneration can result from untreated cartilage injuries. Several recent studies have demonstrated that symptomatic, isolated traumatic articular defects benefit from surgical intervention (5–8). The most appropriate technique to treat these lesions has been controversial, but increasing clinical experience backed by critical outcome measures has demonstrated that implantation of autologous chondrocytes with or without a scaffold is an effective means to correct the underlying pathology by creating a hyalinelike repair tissue.

This chapter describes the technique of autologous chondrocyte implantation (ACI) first reported by the senior author in 1994 and reviews the current literature supporting this technique as well as those studies that compare ACI to other accepted treatment options (9). Furthermore, we review and discuss developing literature supporting current use of various matrices used in combination with autologous chondrocytes to treat this difficult patient population.

CLINICAL PROBLEM

Articular cartilage is an avascular, aneural tissue that protects the subchondral bone from compressive axial and shear forces. In particular, the limited vascularity in comparison to other mesenchymal tissues creates a poor environment for spontaneous repair in response to injuries to the cartilage surface. Chondrocytes also have limited migratory ability, and as a result the surrounding normal cartilage cells do not fill the defect.

Henry Mankin reported on a transient but insufficient response to injury demonstrated by the chondrocyte (10). These cells will increase mitotic activity as well as glycosaminoglycan and collagen production but only for a short period of time and to a limited degree. Normal articular cartilage also has relatively low cell numbers existing in isolated cell lacunae within the extracellular matrix, further decreasing the healing potential following injury. These factors in combination with the continued use of the extremity by the individual produce repetitive compressive and shear forces, creating an extremely poor environment for spontaneous repair.

When trauma extends through the subchondral bone, creating active bleeding, there is exposure to multipotential mesenchymal stem cells, leading to fibrocartilage formation; unfortunately, this tissue lacks the biomechanical properties required to protect the underlying subchondral bone plate, especially in the high-demand patient (11,12). In addition, as the size of the defect increases, the surrounding normal articular cartilage no longer protects the subchondral bone at the base of the lesion (Fig. 1). Exposure of the subchondral bone to repetitive axial and shear forces leads to progressive pain and disability, especially in a high-demand patient.

As a result of the clinical problem, several techniques have been used to improve the repair potential by implanting other cell or tissue phenotypes that have chondrogenic potential

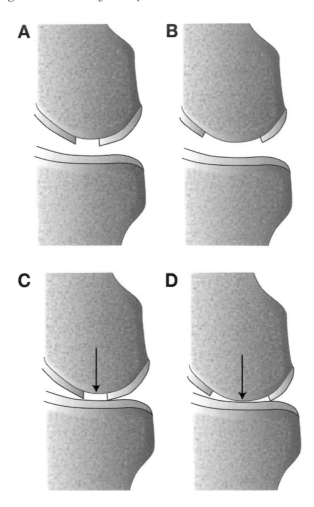

Fig. 1. Schematic representation: loading of focal femoral condyle defects. Small lesions (depicted on the left) are well contained and protect the tibial surface during activity and movement of the joint. Larger lesions, as depicted on the right, expose the subchondral bone and margins of the lesion to the tibial articular surface. Increased cartilage wear rates result along with mechanical symptoms and pain *(68)*.

(13–19). Using a rabbit model, Grande et al. first reported the successful repair of full-thickness cartilage defects through the implantation of cultured articular chondrocytes *(20)*. Based on these promising results, the technique was first used on humans in 1987 and was termed *autologous chondrocyte transplantation*. Currently, in the United States and most of Europe it is referred to as the autologous chondrocyte implantation (ACI) procedure.

Indications

Currently, ACI is ideally indicated for symptomatic ICRS grade III-IV lesions along the femoral condyle or trochlear regions *(21,22)*. High-demand patients between the ages of 15 and 55 yr with excellent motivation and compliance potential should be chosen. Failure of a previous biologic reconstructive procedure such as mosaicplasty or microfracture in a high-demand patient is not an uncommon scenario. In lesions less than 2 cm^2, it is appropriate to use the aforementioned biological procedures as a first-line option. However, in the symptomatic patient with a lesion size greater than 2 cm^2 and up to 12 cm^2, ACI is a viable option. Bone involvement is not a contraindication, but with bony involvement deeper than 6–8 mm, staged or concomitant autologous bone grafting should be undertaken.

Although the senior author (L. P.) has extensive experience and success with ACI in some high-demand patients with reciprocal or "kissing" lesions, this is currently a contraindication for the technique (23,24). However, when no other treatment options are possible in young, high-demand patients, ACI could be tried as a salvage procedure. Surgeons are increasingly using the ACI procedure to repair patellar lesions. Although the initial results in this region were not as successful, the concomitant use of tibial tubercle osteotomy and anteromedialization has significantly improved patient outcomes (9,25).

Preoperative Assessment

In identifying appropriate candidates for the ACI procedure, all factors that could compromise successful healing of the implant should be recognized and corrected in a staged or concomitant manner. Key factors to consider in evaluating patients are physiological age, desired postoperative activity level, etiology, postoperative compliance potential, and social factors such as worker's compensation claims, postoperative work conditions, and allowed time off from work.

Physical examination should focus on gait status, knee alignment, and body mass index (BMI). Weight reduction should be an integral component of the preoperative program, thus limiting postoperative stress to the healing lesion. Knee range of motion is documented and compared to the opposite side; losses of extension or flexion greater than 2–3° in comparison to the opposite side must be addressed. Any preoperative deficits should be corrected with a combination of physical therapy, dynamic splinting, and arthroscopic debridement with manipulation. Medial and lateral femoral chondral, trochlear groove, and patellar facets are palpated for tenderness and correlated with patient complaints.

While performing the arthroscopic biopsy and during chondrocyte implantation, the surgeon should keep this preoperative evaluation in mind as it is not uncommon to have isolated regions of ICRS grade II change along the articular surface; if asymptomatic or nontender during the initial evaluation, these regions should be ignored. Patellofemoral crepitus should be assessed for location and quality (i.e., coarse or fine); further, provocative maneuvers such as the patellar grind test should be performed and correlated again with symptoms. Associated ligamentous disruption and meniscal pathology should be recognized and addressed in staged or concomitant fashion as well.

Radiographic Assessment

The initial radiographic workup should include a postero-anterior (PA) weight-bearing view (Rosenberg) to assess for medial or lateral compartment narrowing, particularly in the post-menisectomized knee (26). Bilateral Merchant views to assess for medial and lateral facet wear as well as patellar subluxation and tilt are important (27). When patella alta or baja is suspected, bilateral supine lateral views at 30° flexion should be obtained and appropriate measurements made. Finally, bilateral long-leg standing films (hip to ankle) should be obtained to determine the mechanical axis and potential sites of increased load to the repair site (28).

A direct side-to-side comparison should be performed on all views. This will delineate subtle narrowing in comparison to the opposite side; demonstrated asymmetries should not be ignored but addressed to unload the affected compartment and create an optimal environment for the short- and long-term survival of the repair tissue produced by the sensitive chondrocytes that are implanted.

Magnetic Resonance Imaging

Magnetic resonance imaging (MRI) has quickly proven its worth as a reliable, noninvasive method of diagnosing osteochondral injuries. Controversy remains regarding the sensitivity and the specificity of MRI in detecting isolated chondral injuries. In 1998, Potter et al. used cartilage-sensitive pulse sequencing in detecting defects in the articular surface and reported high sensitivity and specificity for chondral pathology with minimal interobserver variability *(29)*. They concluded that MRI was an accurate and reproducible imaging modality for the diagnosis of chondral lesions in the knee.

Friemert et al. reported a sensitivity of 33–53% and specificity of 98–99% in detecting advanced articular cartilage lesions by MRI when compared directly with diagnostic arthroscopy *(30)*. Palosaari et al. found an even higher sensitivity of 80–96% when diagnosing cartilaginous lesions by MRI *(31)*. Again, findings should be correlated with clinical symptoms.

Arthroscopic Assessment and Biopsy

Arthroscopic assessment should be performed with the above workup in mind. Areas of ICRS grade III–IV change are noted and sized and the reciprocal surface visualized for degree of damage as well. If the patient is deemed an appropriate candidate for chondrocyte implantation, then a biopsy should be obtained. A preoperative discussion with the patient about the ACI procedure and the typical postoperative course is extremely helpful in determining whether a biopsy should be taken. We warn against taking unnecessary biopsies or taking cartilage immediately following other biologic reconstructive procedures, such as microfracture. These other reconstructive procedures typically need 6–12 mo to demonstrate clinical efficacy. A premature biopsy can place an unnecessary burden on the patient-surgeon relationship, forcing surgery before the procedure has had a chance to work. In addition, unused biopsies place an additional burden on the extensive resources required to process the specimen.

Biopsies are ideally taken from the superomedial edge of the femoral trochlea, but if pathology extends into this region or if there is concern about the patellofemoral articulation, the superolateral trochlear edge can be used. An additional site for biopsy is the lateral aspect of the intercondylar notch, the area of typical notchplasty used during anterior cruciate ligament surgery (Fig. 2A–C). The typical biopsy specimen is 200–300 mg total weight and should include the entire cartilage surface along with a small portion of the underlying subchondral bone. This amount of cartilage should contain approx 200,000–300,000 cells and will fill the bottom portion of the specimen container.

Studies of cartilage obtained from femoral osteophytes and debrided cartilage have demonstrated continued type II collagen production and molecular activity associated with normal articular chondrocyte phenotype *(32,33)*. Despite these findings, current recommendations are that these "abnormal" sources of cartilage should not be used to obtain the cells needed for implantation. This also applies to patients with osteochondritis dissecans (OCD) lesions. The surgeon should resist the temptation to use cartilage from the discarded OCD fragment.

Once the biopsy has been performed, cells are maintained at 4°C until processing occurs, as demonstrated in Fig. 3. Isolated defects up to 3 cm^2 can be treated with one vial allowing full coverage of the defect base with a confluent cell population. With multiple lesions and areas approaching greater than 6 cm^2, more than one vial will be required; lesion size should be taken into account when ordering cells prior to implantation.

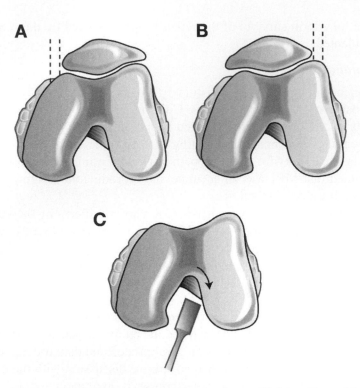

Fig. 2. Appropriate cartilage biopsy sites: (**A**) superior medial trochlear ridge; (**B**) uncovered lateral superior ridge; (**C**) lateral intercondylar notch. All sites should be sharply incised prior to harvest to avoid gouge slippage *(24)*.

SURGICAL TECHNIQUE

Exposure

Typically, a midline skin incision is utilized to facilitate exposure during any future operative interventions. However, previous surgical incisions should be taken into consideration as well as lesion location. When possible, based on defect size and location relative to the knee flexion zone, implantation can be performed through a medially or laterally based miniarthrotomy, sparing quadriceps weakness and intra-articular adhesions postoperatively. Alternatively, a sub-vastus approach can be used, particularly for medial femoral condyle lesions, as the exposure allows the surgeon to subluxate the patella laterally during knee flexion. Anterior dissection along the tibial plateau surface should be performed carefully, avoiding damage to the anterior horns and central body of the menisci. When treating tibial plateau lesions, it is necessary to reflect the meniscus through a takedown of the intermensical ligament and anterior meniscal horn of the involved compartment as described in ref. *24*. When performing a concomitant tibial tubercle osteotomy, slight lateral placement of the incision can avoid injury to the infrapatellar branch of the lesser saphenous nerve. Other concomitant procedures as well as planned periosteal graft harvest sites should also be considered prior to incision. The arthrotomy should, however, always be adjusted to allow an optimal surgical approach to the defect.

Defect Preparation

Once visualized, the lesion should be carefully debrided back to normal vertical articular cartilage margins (Fig. 4A–C). All fibrillated and partially delaminated cartilage should be

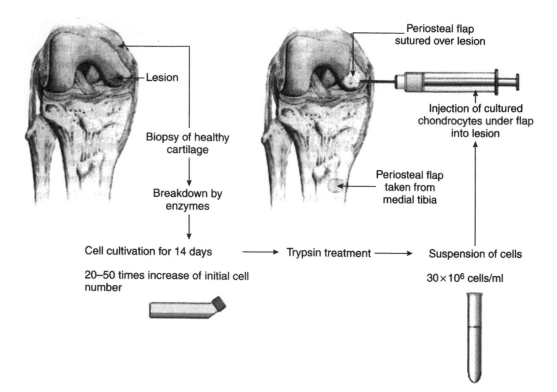

Fig. 3. Schematic drawing of cartilage biopsy preparation and autologous chondrocyte implantation (From ref. *69.* By permission of Oxford University Press).

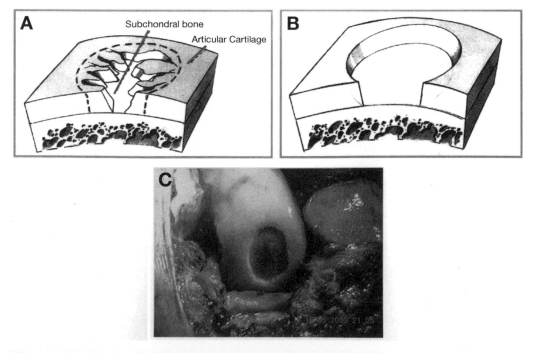

Fig. 4. Schematic drawing of defect preparation: (**A**) fibrillated cartilage lesion; (**B**) debridement to healthy cartilage margins with smooth vertical borders created on completion; (**C**) isolated cartilage lesion following debridement.

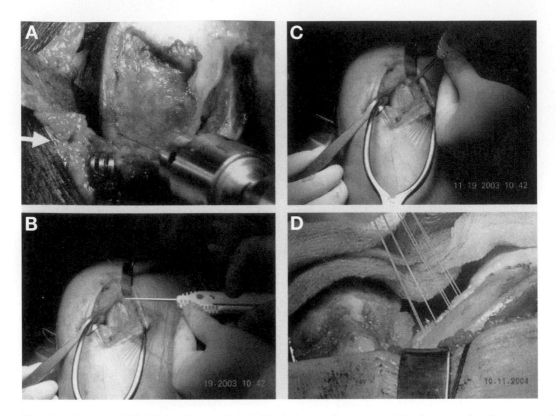

Fig. 5. (**A**) A no. 5 Keith needle used as drill bit in poorly contained lesion creating bony tunnel for later suture placement. (**B**) Microfix anchor (Mitek Inc., Raynham, MA). (**C**) Following use of the Microfix drill bit and replacement of the nonabsorbable suture with 5-0 vicryl suture, the anchor is implanted. (**D**) Application of several anchors along poorly contained border of lesion.

removed. The margins of the lesion are first demarcated with a no. 15 blade, and the damaged cartilage is then removed, typically with a ring-shaped curette, avoiding breakage through the subchondral bone plate. This prevents intraoperative bleeding into the defect, limiting exposure to the different cellular phenotypes present in human blood.

Minimally chondromalacic areas (i.e., ICRS grade I and early grade II) along the border of the lesion are left alone when appropriate suture fixation is possible. When debridement necessitates extension into poorly contained regions, the bone edge should be prepared for later suture fixation of the periosteal graft. This can be performed with the use of a no. 5 Keith needle acting as a drill bit to create a bone tunnel for later suture placement (Fig. 5A). Alternatively, small suture anchors have become commercially available (Microfix, Mitek Inc., Raynham, MA). Prior to placement, the anchors must be reloaded with a 5-0 or 6-0 vicryl suture. These anchors are ideal for poorly contained regions such as the intercondylar notch or peripheral aspect of the femoral condyle or areas such as the posterior edge of a lesion located in the 70–90° flexion zone, where it is difficult to place sutures appropriately (Fig. 5B,C). With extension into the intercondylar notch, interrupted and running suture techniques can be utilized to supplement graft fixation. As in all areas of orthopedic surgery, strong fixation of the periosteal graft to the defect is critical to prevent future graft delamination and to allow early motion of the joint.

In many instances, intralesional osteophytes or sclerotic bone regions are encountered following removal of the calcified cartilage layer or fibrocartilage. Smaller intralesional osteophytes could carefully be tapped down or curetted down to the subchondral bone level. Although it is ideal to avoid exposure to the cancellous bone, a high-speed burr should be used to remove the protuberant bone region and sclerotic bone layer. If carefully performed, a thin layer of subchondral bone should remain to serve as an appropriate viable bed for chondrocyte attachment.

Following debridement, the tourniquet, if used, should be deflated, and in those areas where bone bleeding is visualized, adequate hemostasis should be obtained. First attempts at hemostasis should involve the use of neuropatties soaked in a 1:1000 epinephrine-normal saline mixture. The patty is applied, and pressure is maintained during periosteal graft harvest. For continued bleeding, thrombin spray has been helpful. An alternative method that also works involves placing a drop of fibrin glue (Tiseel, Baxter Healthcare Corp., Glendale, CA) over the bleeding spot and compressing for a minute with a fingertip. Finally, if sites of excessive bleeding are experienced, particularly when previous bone procedures such as microfracture have been performed, a needle-tip bovie cautery unit on a low setting (20–25 coagulation setting) should be used judiciously.

As mentioned, in cases of bone deficiency deeper than 6–8 mm such as osteochondral fracture, OCD, or failed osteochondral grafting procedures, concomitant or staged bone grafting should be performed *(24)*. If performed in a staged manner, bone grafting should be performed up to the level of the subchondral bone plate. Prior to bone grafting, it is important to remove all sclerotic bone; in OCD cases in particular, drilling through the bed following debridement allows appropriate blood flow into the defect, ensuring subsequent bone graft incorporation (Fig. 6A–D). Fibrin glue, sutures, or resorbable membranes such the Restore® patch (Depuy, Raynham, MA) can be used to maintain the bone graft in place. Continuous passive motion is used postoperatively with touch-down to 25% partial weight bearing for 4 wk. Patients are then allowed to resume full weight bearing, but chondrocyte implantation is not undertaken until 6–9 mo following bone grafting to allow for appropriate reconstitution of a subchondral bone plate (Fig. 7A,B).

Alternatively, the sandwich technique as described in ref. *34* can be used. Using a high-speed burr, the sclerotic bone bed is removed down to bleeding cancellous bone, and the base is drilled as previously described. Following bone grafting to the level of the subchondral bone plate, a periosteal flap the size of the bony defect is harvested and anchored in place with the cambium layer facing up to the defect and the fibrous layer facing the bone graft. Leaving a small ridge of healthy subchondral bone can help in stabilizing this initial periosteal flap. We have successfully used Microfix anchors to help in anchori144ng the first periosteal flap (Fig. 8A–G). Fibrin glue should be injected between the periosteal flap and the bone graft to richly fill the interval. After the fibrin glue is injected for 3 min, the bone graft and periosteal cover should be compressed with a dry sponge to help fixation of the flap to the bone graft as well stabilize the bleeding. A second periosteal flap is then applied as later described in Graft Fixation following.

Periosteal Graft Harvest

Defect size should be measured with a sterile ruler to determine appropriate graft size. Alternatively, a paper template of the defect site can be created by placing it directly over the site and using a typical skin marker, tracing the defect on the paper with sequential dots. One additional technique is to use a sterile knife blade package as an aluminum template to press directly into the defect, creating an imprint of the lesion. The paper or aluminum template is created by cutting around the edge of the dots or imprint. The template should be 2 mm larger

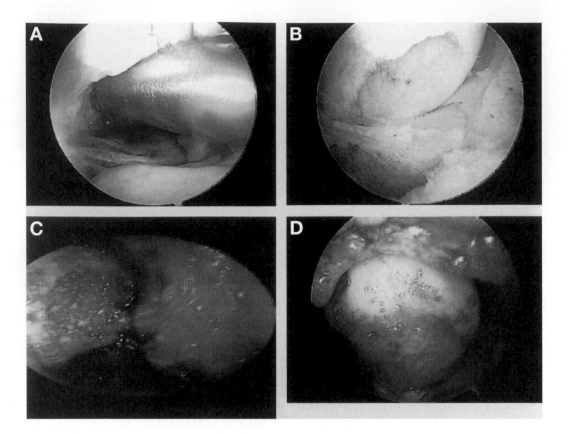

Fig. 6. (A) Debridement of osteochondritis dissecans lesion to bleeding healthy bone. **(B)** Drilled base of lesion to create bleeding. **(C)** Autologous bone graft applied arthroscopically to defect. **(D)** Fibrin glue applied over defect to maintain bone graft in place and avoid extravasation into surrounding tissues.

than the actual defect when treating the femoral condyle or tibial plateau surfaces. When grafting the trochlear groove or patellar surfaces, a template 3 mm larger than the actual lesion should be created to take into account the concave and convex surfaces, respectively *(24)*.

Several sites are available for periosteal graft harvest. The first option for harvest should be the proximal medial tibial diaphysis distal to the pes anserinus insertion or below the semitendinosis tendon insertion point. This site typically has robust but thin enough periosteum, making it ideal for implantation. Normal periosteum is a thin membrane several cell layers thick and consisting of an outer fibrogenic layer and an inner osteogenic cambium layer. In the proximal tibia, an incision is made through the subcutaneous fat and the thin fascial layer. Care should be taken to remove all overlying fascial and fatty layers prior to removal from the bone surface. This is typically best performed using sharp scissor dissection to reveal an underlying white, shiny periosteum. Attempts at periosteal debridement following harvest can cause "buttonholing" through the graft surface with resultant sites of cell leakage on implantation. No electrocautery device should be used around the periosteum prior to harvest. This will injure the periosteum and could kill the sensitive cells in the cambium layer.

Secondary sites of graft harvest include the femoral metaphyseal-diaphyseal region. During large arthrotomies, this portion of the femur is easily visualized with appropriate

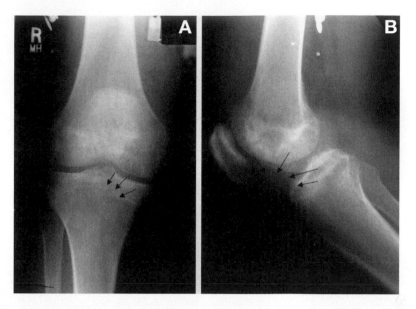

Fig. 7. (A) Postoperative anterior-posterior view 4 mo following bone graft application to defect. Notice reconstitution of subchondral bone contour following continuous passive motion machine treatment and non-weight-bearing status for 4 wk. **(B)** Lateral view demonstrating normal subchondral contour.

retraction of the quadriceps musculature. Periosteal graft harvest from this location requires carefully incision of the overlying synovium to expose the underlying periosteum. The synovium should be placed back into its normal anatomic location following graft harvest from the femur to prevent postoperative scarring. The femoral periosteum is typically thicker. This may theoretically inhibit synovial fluid diffusion and cell nutrition during the initial growth phase. Thicker periosteum may also predispose to increased rates of periosteal overgrowth. Finally, the required soft tissue dissection in the suprapatellar region can lead to bleeding and an increased incidence of postoperative intra-articular adhesions. Because of these factors, femoral periosteum should be used only as a second-line, not primary, source of periosteal graft during ACI. All periosteum should be maintained in a moist environment and, in cases of multiple lesions, labeled to prevent any confusion during graft implantation.

Resorbable membrane substitutes have become commercially available. Two examples are Chondrogide® (Geistlich Biomaterials, Wolhusen, Switzerland) and Restore® (Depuy, Raynham, MA). Haddo et al. reported on 31 patients in whom chondrogide was used in place of periosteum *(35)*. Assessment included arthroscopic second looks at 1 yr and clinical outcome evaluations at 1 and 2 yr after the second stage of the procedure. They reported no evidence of periosteal graft hypertrophy and satisfactory clinical outcomes at 2 yr. One of us (D. G. J.) has used the Restore patch as a substitute for periosteum in 30 cases as well as in cases requiring autologous bone grafting. At short-term follow-up (1–2 yr), there have been no adverse events or effects on clinical outcome (unpublished data, June 2005). Bartlett et al. reported similar results *(36)*.

When there is limited periosteum, for example because of scarring, damage from graft harvesting, poor tissue quality because of age or disuse atrophy, and in revision cases or cases with

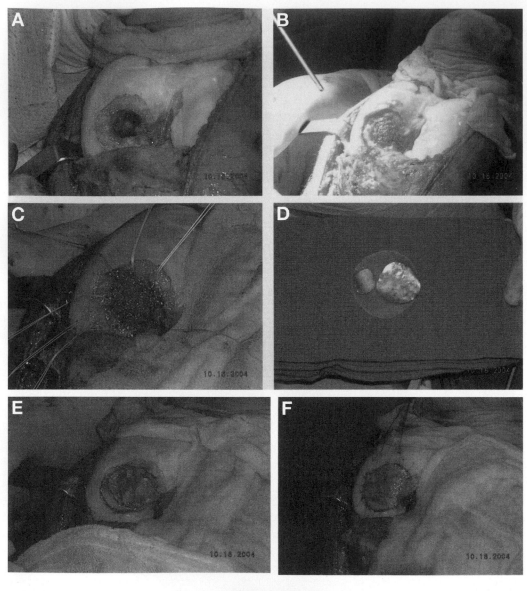

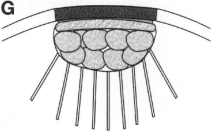

Fig. 8. (A) Bone lesion following debridement of sclerotic bone and drilling of base of lesion. Notice shelf of normal subchondral bone around bony defect. **(B)** Bone graft application up to but not over subchondral bone height. **(C)** Application of Microfix anchors around bone defect periphery. **(D)** Restore patch (Depuy Orthopaedics Inc., Warsaw, IN) with aluminum templates over graft prior to preparation

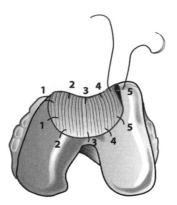

Fig. 9. Trochlear defect: It is important to create the normal trochlear configuration. The template must be oversize by approx 3 mm. The periosteal patch is then sutured sequentially from medial to lateral as denoted by numbers 1–5, taking care to re-create the normal convex surface, thus avoiding postoperative overload to the repair site *(24)*.

large surface areas, these membranes can provide an alternate source of membrane. The use of resorbable membranes as a defect cover to replace the traditional autologous periosteum has been termed the collagen-associated autologous chondrocyte implantation (CACI) procedure. Published results from the CACI procedure are discussed in more detail later in the chapter *(37)*.

Graft Fixation

The periosteal graft is fixed with 6-0 vicryl suture using a P-1 cutting needle. Ideally, the suture should be dyed to ease visualization when sewing against the normal white articular cartilage surface. Sterile mineral oil should coat the suture prior to passage through the periosteum, particularly to prevent binding between the suture-periosteal interface. The needle is first passed through the superficial surface of the periosteum approx 2 mm from the graft edge and then into the cartilage margin, entering the vertical border perpendicular to the inside wall of the defect. The needle should enter the cartilage approx 2 mm from the surface and extend peripherally, exiting the defect 4 mm from the edge of the defect (Fig. 6).

A simple instrument tying technique is used, with each throw placed parallel to the defect wall edge. This localizes the knot over the periosteum rather than placing the knot on the articular surface, where it could be exposed to shear forces, damaging fixation. During initial suture placement, all four quadrants of the graft should be tied first to stabilize the graft and then further sutures placed at 3-mm increments around the lesion to produce a water-tight seal. An exception to this method of suture placement (four quadrants first) is during trochlear ACI. In this case, sutures are first placed along the medial margin and sequentially placed from medial to lateral, producing a convex surface to allow for appropriate patellar tracking (Fig. 9). Similarly, contour of the graft should be considered with patellar ACI,

---

Fig. 8. *(Continued)*   for suture fixation. (**E**) Suture fixation of Restore patch to bone defect. (**F**) Final suture fixation of larger Restore patch and application of cells using the "sandwich" technique. (**G**) Schematic of sandwich technique; drilling base of lesion, application of bone graft, placement of bottom periosteal patch (cambium layer facing up), followed by cells and then top periosteal patch (cambium layer facing down).

especially in the centrally based patellar lesion; the normal convexity of the patella should be considered as well as height of graft placement along the defect. The significant shear forces in this area can lead to catching at the leading and trailing edges of the defect with knee motion *(24)*.

It is important to leave one region along the lesion open to allow for cell implantation. However, to prevent cell extrusion after implantation, place the sutures in the standard fashion but do not tie them immediately. Once cells are implanted simply instrument tie the sutures at that time. In large, particularly long defects, the contour of the femur may not allow placement of the angiocatheter utilized in cell implantation far enough into the defect. This can limit the ability to create an even cell suspension at the base of the lesion. In these cases, leaving a more posterior, distal second site of cell implantation is helpful. Cells are implanted in this site first and sutures tied. Cells are then implanted into the more anterior proximal site secondarily.

Prior to cell implantation, the repair should be assessed to determine whether a watertight seal has been created. Normal saline without antibiotics should be placed into the planned area of cell implantation with a 1.5-in. 18-gage angiocatheter and tuberculin syringe. The intra-articular portion of the knee is dried, and sites of leakage are noted. Further sutures are placed into the site, and testing is performed again. Only after a watertight seal has been verified should the wound edges be further sealed with fibrin glue.

Autologous fibrin glue is formed by taking the cryoprecipitate from 1 unit of the patient's whole blood and combining it with a mixture of bovine thrombin and calcium chloride. An excellent alternative to this cumbersome technique is to use the commercially available fibrin glue called Tisseel. It is important to limit the amount of Tisseel or fibrin glue placed into the joint as this has the potential to increase postoperative fibrous adhesions. Further, the senior author, using an in vivo rabbit model, demonstrated the potential deleterious effects of Tisseel on chondrocyte migration and healing potential *(38)*. As a result, care should be taken to limit the amount of Tisseel applied and to avoid its exposure to the chondrocytes.

Chondrocyte Implantation

Once a watertight seal has been created, cell implantation is undertaken. Cells, provided by Genzyme Biosurgery Corporation (Cambridge, MA), arrive in a small vial and should be maintained at 4°C until implantation. The typical concentration is 12 million cells/0.4 mL medium. One vial should cover a lesion of approx 6 cm^2. Cells are gently placed into suspension using the angiocatheter previously described and then injected into the defect. Sutures are tied, and fibrin glue or Tisseel is applied to the site of implantation.

POSTOPERATIVE REHABILITATION

Cartilage maturation occurs through several phases (Table 1). This process must be considered during the critical rehabilitation process following surgery. The first phase in cartilage metabolism, termed the *proliferative phase*, occurs during the first 6 wk when initial partial weight bearing is allowed (15–20 kg or 30–40 pounds). During the immediate postoperative period, cells are allowed to adhere to the subchondral bone plate, avoiding motion for at least 6–12 h. Continuous passive motion is initiated at this time to provide a chondrogenic stimulus as demonstrated by O'Driscoll and Salter *(14)*. Typically, this is performed during the first 4 wk for approx 6–8 h/d.

Table 1
ACI Time-Course Healing

Stage	Time	Tissue
Proliferation	0–6 wk	Soft, primitive repair tissue
Transition	7 wk–6 mo	Expansion of matrix puttylike consistency
Remodeling	6–18 mo (changes can occur for up to 3 yr)	Matrix remodeling, tissue stiffens to normal hardness

A soft, primitive repair tissue forms during this initial phase. The second phase, termed the *transition phase*, occurs during the ensuing 4–5 mo, usually ending at approx 6 mo postoperatively. This phase is characterized by expansion of the matrix released by the chondrocytes into a puttylike consistency. Weight bearing is continued progressively, increasing to full weight bearing within 12 wk after surgery. Important factors to consider at this time are the size and location of the lesion. Well-contained lesions have some degree of protection from the surrounding native cartilage, and load bearing can be initiated as early as 4 wk postoperatively (Fig. 10A,B). Conversely, poorly contained lesions require longer periods of protection. Full weight bearing in these large lesions should not occur until after about 8–14 wk (Fig. 10C,D). Patients with multiple lesions should progress more slowly as well. If there is subtle varus or valgus malalignment in the medial- or lateral-based lesions, respectively, then an unloader brace should be considered on initiation of weight bearing. Significant malalignment issues should be addressed with a concomitant or staged osteotomy as stated.

Isolated patellofemoral lesions can be protected during weight bearing if the knee is maintained in full extension during gait. A postoperative hinged immobilizer locked in extension during ambulation can achieve this goal, allowing weight bearing during the initial 6 wk. Patellofemoral lesions are susceptible to the high shear forces that occur across the implantation site; as a result, open-chain exercises should be avoided during the first 4–6 mo. The continuous passive motion machine is initiated at the same time, but progression to greater than 90° flexion should occur more slowly than with a femoral chondral lesion.

The final phase in maturation, termed the *matrix remodeling phase*, is characterized by progressive hardening of the cartilage tissue to the hard, firm quality of adjacent native cartilage. This process begins at approx 6 mo and occurs over the ensuing 6–12 mo. Although patients are allowed to resume regular activities at this time, further graft maturation can continue for up to 3 yr following implantation. Factors that affect this process are size, location, physiological age, and final activity level. Patients will have some continued symptoms along the implant site as the activity level is increased during this critical period. However, as graft maturation occurs, allowing greater protection of the subchondral bone, preoperative symptoms should resolve slowly. Preoperative patient education of this biologic process, particularly the expected length of time to recovery, is critical. This prevents the patient from exposing the graft to potentially traumatic forces during the initial phases of cartilage maturation.

POSTOPERATIVE IMAGING/EVALUATION

As our ability to assess articular cartilage, repair tissue quality, and degree of fill of defects by MRI improves, this tool becomes an increasingly important source of information that can

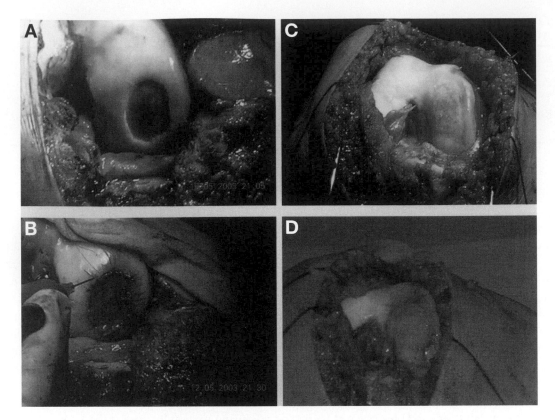

Fig. 10. (A) Well-contained lesion with normal articular cartilage borders. **(B)** Following implantation, the repair site is protected from damage, and a more aggressive rehabilitation program can be initiated. **(C)** Poorly contained lesion with limited normal articular cartilage margins. **(D)** Following implantation, the repair site is not well protected by the surrounding cartilage, and a slower rehabilitation program should be initiated with full weight bearing after 8–10 wk.

be used by the surgeon to help progress patients following biologic reconstructive procedures *(39,40)*. Henderson et al. reviewed the 2-yr treatment outcome of ACI in 53 patients (72 lesions) through clinical evaluation, MRI, second-look arthroscopy, and concomitant biopsy. MRI studies demonstrated 75.3% of defects with at least 50% defect fill, 46.3% with near-normal signal, 68.1% with mild to no effusion, and 66.7% with mild to no underlying bone marrow edema at 3 mo *(39)*. These values improved to 94.2, 86.9, 91.3, and 88.4% at 12 mo, respectively. At 24 mo, further improvements to 97, 97, 95.6, and 92.6%, respectively, were observed. Improvement in clinical outcome correlated well with information obtained from second-look arthroscopy and core biopsies as compared with MRI findings at 12 mo *(41)*.

Watrin-Pinzano et al. evaluated the ability of T_2 mapping on an 8.5-T imager to characterize morphologically and quantitatively spontaneous repair of rat patellar cartilage defects *(42)*. T_2 mapping was able morphologically to identify three types of repair tissue observed macroscopically and histologically: total, partial, and hypertrophic. Total and partial repair tissues were characterized by global T_2 values almost similar to controls, whereas hypertrophic repair tissues were characterized by T_2 global values higher than controls. They concluded that T_2 mapping with MRI was a noninvasive technique that could be used in clinical longitudinal studies of articular cartilage repair.

Brown et al. evaluated 180 MRI examinations in 112 patients who had cartilage-resurfacing procedures, including 86 microfractures and 35 ACI, at a mean of 15 and 13 mo after surgery, respectively *(43)*. ACI-treated defects showed consistently better fill at all times compared with microfracture, but there was graft hypertrophy in 63% of ACI surgeries. By contrast, the repair cartilage over the microfracture was depressed with respect to native cartilage and had a propensity for bone development and loss of adjacent cartilage with progressive follow-up.

Stefan Marlovits and colleagues used a surface phased array coil over the knee on a 1-T MRI scanner to obtain high-resolution images in 45 patients treated with three different techniques for cartilage repair (microfracture, autologous osteochondral transplantation, and ACI) *(44)*. Patients were analyzed 6 and 12 mo after the procedure, and pertinent variables were defined to describe the repair tissue. Nine pertinent variables were described: the degree of filling of the defect, the integration to the border zone, the description of the surface and structure, the signal intensity, the status of the subchondral lamina and subchondral bone, the appearance of adhesions, and the presence of synovitis.

It becomes clear that MRI is a useful tool to assess cartilage repair, and as our imaging techniques improve and our grading systems based on these images are refined, this will become an important clinical tool to evaluate the repair tissue, which will help in determining postoperative rehabilitation and the appropriate time for the patient to return to higher impact activities.

Schneider et al., as part of a prospective clinical pilot study, evaluated 17 patients at 6 wk as well as 3, 6, and 12 mo after ACI. A synovial analysis was performed, and molecular markers for bone and cartilage metabolism were determined. A number of parameters, including deoxypyridinolin, matrix metalloproteinase 1 and 3, as well as proteoglycan levels were analyzed. The levels were referenced to the total protein concentration of the synovial fluid, and analyses were compared with clinical parameters (Larson score) and MRI examinations. The most notable marker was deoxypyridinolin, which increased continuously between surgery and wk 12 and then disappeared after the repair process was complete 1 yr after surgery. All molecular markers for cartilage degradation increased initially after surgery and dropped off below the original levels 3–6 mo later *(45)*. This is a potential adjunct to MRI that is minimally invasive and less expensive. Further studies to define the appropriate markers that correlate with clinical outcome are required prior to recommending widespread use of this method.

Arthroscopic assessment remains the gold standard for postoperative evaluation as it allows direct visualization of the repair site; in conjunction with histomorphologic biopsy assessment and probe analysis, this method provides the most thorough postoperative information *(46)*. Arthroscopic probe indentation stiffness testing is increasingly used to evaluate clinical outcomes *(47)*. Vasara et al. arthroscopically evaluated 30 patients following ACI, and indentation stiffness was measured and clinical evaluations performed. Stiffness of the repair tissue improved to 62% (mean 2.04 ± 0.83 N, mean ± standard deviation) of adjacent cartilage (3.58 ± 1.04 N). In 6 patients, the normalized stiffness was at least 80%, suggesting hyalinelike repair; indentation stiffness of the OCD lesion repairs (1.45 ± 0.46 N; $n = 7$) was less than that of the non-OCD lesion repair sites (2.37 ± 0.72 N; $n = 19$). Gadolinium-enhanced MRI of the cartilage during follow-up of 4 patients suggested proteoglycan replenishment. The authors concluded that low stiffness values may indicate incomplete maturation or predominantly fibrous repair; increasing stiffness in comparison to the adjacent cartilage correlated with improved clinical outcomes.

LITERATURE REVIEW/CLINICAL OUTCOMES

In a landmark article, the senior author (L. P.) published his initial experience with ACI in 1994 *(9)*. Twenty-three patients were treated in this initial series, with 14 of 16 patients who were implanted along the distal femur obtaining good-to-excellent results. Only 2 of 7 patients who were implanted in the patellar region obtained promising results. Second-look biopsies were obtained, and hyalinelike cartilage was demonstrated in 11 of 15 distal femoral lesions; only 1 of 7 patellar lesions demonstrated hyalinelike repair tissue. Biopsy results correlated well with clinical outcome, demonstrating a direct correlation between hyalinelike repair tissue and good-to-excellent function 2 yr following the surgery.

This same experience was further evaluated during the intermediate- to long-term period (2–9 yr), and this initial trend continued, as well as a clear demonstration of a significant learning curve that occurs as the surgeon gains experience with the procedure (25). In this study, graft failure occurred in 7 patients, with 4 occurring in the first 23 patients but only 3 occurring in the next 78 patients. Clinical, arthroscopic, and histologic results from the first 101 patients treated using this technique were reported in this study. Patient- and physician-derived clinical rating scales were used as well as arthroscopic assessment of cartilage fill, integration, and surface hardness. Biopsies were obtained, and standard histochemical techniques were utilized in the assessment. Ninety-four patients of this initial group underwent reevaluation. Good-to-excellent clinical results were seen in 92% of the isolated femoral condylar lesions; these results decreased to 67% in patients with multiple lesions. OCD lesions also did well (89% good-to-excellent results). In contrast to the initial series, patellar lesions did relatively well, with 65% good-to-excellent results. Strict attention to patellofemoral tracking and malalignment issues were important; concomitant tibial tubercle advancement and trochleoplasty procedures protected the patellofemoral implant during postoperative rehabilitation, accounting for the improved clinical results in this area in comparison to the initial series. Patients who underwent femoral condylar implantation with concomitant anterior cruciate ligament reconstruction demonstrated 75% good-to-excellent results. Periosteal overgrowth, as demonstrated by arthroscopy, was identified in 26 patients, but only 7 were symptomatic and resolved after arthroscopic trimming. Histologic analysis of the matrix in 37 biopsy specimens assessing for type II collagen showed a correlation between hyalinelike repair tissue and good-to-excellent clinical results.

Using this same group of patients, arthroscopic evaluation was performed on a subset of patients treated for isolated cartilage defects on the femoral condyle or the patella (46). Sixty-one patients with a mean follow-up of 7.4 yr (range 5–11) were assessed for durability by comparing the clinical status at long-term follow-up with that found 2 yr after transplantation. Of 61 patients, 50 had good or excellent clinical results at 2 yr, increasing to 51 of 61 good or excellent results at 5–11 yr. Hyalinelike repair tissue was demonstrated in 8 of 12 biopsies as characterized by Safranin O staining and homogeneous appearance under polarized light. Three fibrous and eight hyaline biopsy specimens stained positive to aggrecan and to cartilage oligomeric matrix protein. Hyalinelike specimens stained positive for type II collagen; fibrous specimens stained positive for type I collagen.

An electromechanical indentation probe was used to assess the grafted areas from 11 patients during a second-look arthroscopy procedure (mean follow-up 54.3 mo; range 33–84 mo); 8 patients demonstrated stiffness measurements that were 90% or more in comparison to normal cartilage measurements. The mean stiffness of grafted areas with hyalinelike repair tissue, as determined by histologic assessment, was 3.0 ± 1.1 N. By contrast, the mean stiffness of grafted areas with fibrous tissue was 1.5 ± 0.35 N. Again, good or excellent clinical outcomes were directly correlated with the demonstration of a hyalinelike repair tissue at the implanted site; fibrous fill correlated with poorer clinical outcomes. More important, durability of the repair tissue was clearly demonstrated with results at 9 yr that were equal to or better than the initial 2-yr results.

Genzyme Tissue Repair (Cambridge, MA) initiated an international registry assessing the clinical effectiveness of the ACI procedure. Data from this registry were used to evaluate the first 50 patients treated in the United States *(22)*. Mean age was 36 yr, and mean defect size was 4.2 cm^2, with minimum 3-yr follow-up. Seventy-eight percent had undergone previous articular cartilage repair procedures on the affected knee during the previous 5 yr. Failed marrow stimulation technique had occurred in 18% of the patients. Outcome was measured with the modified Cincinnati Knee Rating system, with graft failure defined as replacement or removal of the graft because of mechanical symptoms or pain. Statistically significant median improvement in the clinician-based portion of the evaluation was 4; the patient-based portion of the evaluation increased by 5 points ($p < 0.001$). Previous treatment with marrow stimulation techniques or the size of defect did not have an impact on the results with ACI. Three patients had graft failure, and Kaplan-Meier-estimated freedom from graft failure was 94% at 36 mo postoperatively (95% CI = 88–100%).

Using this same registry, the first 76 patients treated in the United States were evaluated 6 yr following implantation *(48)*. Mean age remained at 36 yr, with 57 patients having single lesions with a mean size of 4.4 cm^2. Nineteen patients had multiple lesions with a mean total surface area of 10.8 cm^2. Nine treatment failures occurred, with 7 occurring within the first 24 mo following the procedure. Including these failed patients, overall condition scores improved from 3.1 preoperatively to 6.0 at 6-yr follow-up ($p < 0.001$). Pain and swelling scores improved 2.7 and 2.6 points from baseline to follow-up, respectively.

Scott Gillogly evaluated 112 patients with 139 defects treated with the ACI procedure over a 5-yr period of time *(49–51)*. Average size of the defect was 5.7 cm^2, with over 60% of patients having failed at least one prior procedure. Of the patients, 22 had multiple defects. Forty-two patients had patellofemoral lesions (27 trochlea, 15 patella). Outcomes were measured using the Modified Cincinnati Rating Scale, Sports Score, and Knee Society Rating Scale. There were three clinical failures, and three patients were lost to follow-up. Average follow-up was 43 mo, with a range from 24 to 65 mo. Using the clinician evaluation portion of the Modified Cincinnati scale, 93% demonstrated good-to-excellent outcomes; the patient evaluation portion demonstrated 89% good-to-excellent outcomes. Importantly, no deterioration in outcomes occurred during the 2- to 5-yr follow-up period. Worker's compensation claims had no effect on clinical outcomes.

Two other studies have assessed ACI in the worker's compensation sector. Seidner and Zaslav assessed direct medical and nonmedical costs as well as return-to-work status in patients undergoing ACI who used the same claims system for a single worker's compensation insurer *(52)*. In comparison to a matched control group, 24 patients treated with ACI (mean age 35 yr) were followed to claim closure. Occupations ranged from light- to heavy-demand work status. In the ACI group, total medical costs averaged $90,235 per patient, and average indemnity costs were $64,704; overall, 71% returned to work. By comparison, the control group had total medical costs averaging $80,407 ($p < 0.001$) and indemnity costs averaging $89,226 ($p < 0.001$); overall, 83% returned to work in this group, which was not statistically different from the ACI group ($p = 0.24$). They concluded that ACI results in similar return to work at an average cost savings of $15,000/patient in comparison to the controls.

James Yates performed a prospective longitudinal study in 24 worker's compensation patients with lesions greater than 2 cm^2 (mean lesion size was 4.7 cm^2, range 2–10 cm^2) *(8)*. Five lesions were on the patella; the remaining 19 lesions were on the distal femur. The

Modified Cincinnati Knee Rating scale was used with clinician and patient evaluations. Overall clinical scores improved from a mean of 3.2 at baseline to 6.8 at 1 yr after the operation. Good-to-excellent results were demonstrated in 78% of the patients. In patients with greater than 1-yr follow-up, 63% returned to unrestricted work status at a mean of 7 mo, with an additional 22% returning to modified work status.

Minas evaluated the health economics of the ACI procedure *(53)*. He prospectively examined the efficacy of treatment and quality of life in 44 patients undergoing the procedure and calculated the average cost per additional quality-adjusted life year. At 12-mo follow-up, ACI treatment showed improvement in patient function as measured by both the Knee Society score (114.02–140.67, $p < 0.001$) and the Western Ontario and McMaster Universities Osteoarthritis Index (35.30–23.82, $p < 0.05$). Quality of life was measured by the Short Form-36 Physical Component Summary and improved from 33.32 prior to biopsy to 41.48 ($p < 0.05$) 12 mo after implantation. Improvement on all three outcomes measures occurred during the following 12–24 mo. As a result of these findings, an estimated cost per additional quality-adjusted life year was $6791. He concluded that ACI improved quality of life in patients and was a cost-effective treatment for cartilage lesions.

Comparative Assessments

Several comparative studies have been reported assessing ACI directly with other biologic reconstructive procedures. Horas et al. compared ACI to osteochondral cylinder transplantation (OCT) in a prospective, single-center study investigating 2-yr outcomes in 40 patients *(6)*. Mean lesion size was 3.86 cm^2, and mean age was 31.4 yr in the ACI group. Mean lesion size was 3.63 cm^2, and mean age was 35.4 yr in the OCT group. Of 20 patients in the ACI group, 7 had undergone previous abrasion arthroplasty. In the OCT group, 2 patients had undergone abrasion arthroplasty, and 2 had undergone microfracture.

Recovery after ACI was slower than with OCT at 6 mo as assessed by Lysholm score; both groups demonstrated substantial improvement at 2 yr as assessed by the Meyers score and Tegner activity score. The one treatment failure in the study occurred in the ACI group but represented the only patellofemoral patient in either group. This patient had a large (5.6 cm^2) patellofemoral lesion, and failure was considered a result of poor rehabilitation. Histomorphologic assessment was performed on 7 biopsies in 6 ACI patients, with 2 biopsies coming from the patellofemoral patient; 5 biopsies were obtained from the OCT group.

In all ACI cases except for the one failure, gross evaluation demonstrated a complete, mechanically stable resurfacing of the defect. Biopsies from the ACI group demonstrated predominant areas of fibrocartilage with localized areas of hyalinelike regenerative tissue close to the subchondral bone. In the OCT group, all biopsies demonstrated hyaline articular cartilage that was histomorphologically similar to the surrounding cartilage. All OCT specimens demonstrated a persistent interface between the transplant and the surrounding cartilage, however.

One significant limitation of the study is the small number of patients in each treatment group, raising questions regarding the effect of the learning curve associated with the ACI procedure in particular. This study also had relatively short-term follow-up. With longer follow-up, the durability of the repair in both groups would be better delineated. Further, the one treatment failure in the ACI group was in the trochlear groove, with a surface area much larger than the other defects treated, placing this patient at higher risk for delamination or poor clinical outcome.

In a similar prospective, randomized study of ACI and mosaicplasty, Bentley et al. assessed 100 consecutive patients (mean age 31.3 yr and defect size 4.66 cm^2) *(5)*. Mean duration of symptoms prior to operative repair was 7.2 yr, and mean number of previous operative procedures, excluding arthroscopy, was 1.5 yr. Mean follow-up was 19 mo. Fifty-eight patients underwent ACI; 42 patients underwent microfracture. Using modified Cincinnati and Stanmore functional rating systems as well as objective clinical assessment, excellent or good results were seen in 88% of the ACI patients compared to 69% after mosaicplasty. Lesions were assessed based on the ICRS grading system using arthroscopic evaluation at 1 yr. Grade I–II appearance was demonstrated in 31 of 37 ACI patients (84%) compared with only 8 of 23 patients treated with microfracture (35%). They noted that 50% of the ACI patients demonstrated a soft consistency on probe assessment at 1 yr. Biopsies were obtained for 19 ACI patients at 1 yr, 3 from patellar lesions and 16 from femoral condylar lesions. Seven patients' biopsies demonstrated hyalinelike cartilage as assessed by Safranin O staining, polarized light, and S100 protein immunostaining. Seven patients demonstrated a mix of hyalinelike and fibrocartilaginous regions; 5 patients' biopsies demonstrated a fibrocartilagenous appearance that was well bonded to the subchondral bone. One patient biopsy had a mixed appearance; the patient was rebiopsied at 2 yr, and the lesions had converted to hyalinelike cartilage consistent with the maturation process. There were 7 poor results in the mosaicplasty group, demonstrating poor graft incorporation in the interface in 4, graft disintegration in 3, and exposed subchondral bone at the margin in 1.

Two studies have assessed ACI in comparison to the Steadman microfracture technique *(54)*. In a prospective, concurrently controlled study, Anderson et al. compared the two techniques with 23 patients in each group *(55)*. Defects less than 2 cm^2 as well as patellar and tibial lesions were excluded. No differences were noted in overall defect area, body mass index, number of prior procedures, or baseline scores. A worker's compensation claim was filed in 39% of the ACI group as opposed to 14% of the microfracture group. Mean improvements in overall condition score from baseline was 3.1 in the ACI group as opposed to 1.3 in the microfracture group. Two ACI and 6 microfracture patients met the study criteria for treatment failure. When treatment failures were excluded from each group, ACI patients had a mean improvement of 4.7 in overall condition score, and microfracture patients improved by 2.8. This difference was statistically significant ($p = 0.023$).

In a separate study, Knutsen et al. evaluated 80 patients, each with a single symptomatic cartilage defect of the femoral condyle, who were treated with either ACI or microfracture (40 per group) *(56)*. ICRS, Lysholm, Short Form-36 (SF-36), and Tegner standardized scoring systems were used to evaluate patients, with an independent observer performing follow-up assessments at 12 and 24 mo. Arthroscopic biopsy was performed 2 yr postoperatively; histological evaluation was performed by a pathologist and a clinical scientist, with both evaluators blinded to each patient's operative treatment. At 2 yr, both groups had significant clinical improvement. However, by SF-36 physical component score, improvements in the microfracture group were significantly better than in the ACI group ($p = 0.004$). Two failures occurred in the ACI group; one occurred in the microfracture group. Eighty-four percent of patients underwent arthroscopic biopsy. Hyalinelike tissue was seen in 72% of specimens evaluated in the ACI group; 25% demonstrated a mixed hyaline-fibrocartilage appearance. Only 3% demonstrated true fibrocartilage in the ACI group. In the microfracture group, 40% demonstrated hyalinelike tissue, and 29% demonstrated a mixed hyaline-fibrocartilage appearance. Fibrocartilage was demonstrated in 31% of specimens from the microfracture group. No correlation between histologic appearance and clinical outcome was demonstrated in this study.

One important question following a critical review of this study *(56)* is whether the ACI procedure would have been used as a first-line treatment in many of these patients. Baseline

Table 2
Lesion Size and Operative Treatment Recommended

Recommended treatment	Lesion size
Microfracture	$1–2.5$ cm^2
	Well-shouldered, protected edges
Osteochondral autograft	$1–2.5$ cm^2
	Grafts need to be perpendicular and flush to surface
Autologous chondrocyte	>2 cm^2
	Background factors need to be addressed; compliant with rehab
Osteochondral allografts	>4 cm^2
	Large lesion uncontained involving significant bony loss

scores in the ACI group were higher than baseline scores in the microfracture group. Currently, the ACI procedure necessitates a concomitant arthrotomy with associated morbidity as opposed to the microfracture technique. Based on the reported sizes of the defects, many of these patients might have been more appropriately treated with a less-invasive option. At this time, for isolated lesions less than 2 cm^2, most surgeons would probably consider use of the microfracture or the mosaicplasty procedure first and use the ACI procedure for treatment failures after at least 1 yr has been allowed for healing *(57,58)* (Table 2).

Further, the multicenter nature of the study raises concerns about the learning curve associated with the ACI procedure and how this may have affected treatment outcomes in the ACI group. Critical biostatistical assessment using comparative study designs suggests that a minimum of 120 patients would be needed in each study arm to determine clear superiority of one technique over the other. Thus, as the authors concluded *(56)*, each technique demonstrated clinical efficacy with statistically significant improvements in function at short-term follow-up in both groups. As there were demonstrated histologic differences in appearance between the two techniques, it will be interesting to see the clinical results with return to normal activities at the intermediate and long-term follow-up time-points.

Matrix-Supported Autologous Chondrocyte Implantation

With the introduction of the ACI procedure, the significant regenerative potential of cultured chondrocytes was recognized. Simultaneously, interest in possible carriers and matrices that would potentially expedite the maturation process arose. In 1994, Hendrickson et al. used fibrin as a vehicle for the implantation of articular chondrocytes into 12-mm full-thickness defects in horses *(59)*. The chondrocytes, isolated from a 9-d-old foal, were mixed 1:1 with fibrinogen and thrombin and injected into 12-mm circular defects on the lateral trochlea of the distal femur of eight normal horses. Similar defects created in the contralateral knee were left empty and served as the controls. Statistically significant ($p < 0.05$) increases in type II collagen (61.2% grafted, 25.1% control) as well as aggrecan levels (58.8 μg/mg grafted, 27.4 μg/mg control; $p < 0.05$) were noted in the grafted tissue at 8 mo.

Lee et al. isolated chondrocytes from adult canine knees; cells were expanded in number in monolayer for 3 wk, seeded into porous type II collagen scaffolds, and cultured for an additional 4 wk in vitro *(60)*. The populated scaffolds were then implanted into chondral defects in the trochlear groove of the opposite knee joint. The reparative tissue filled $88 \pm 6\%$ (mean $\pm$ standard error of the mean; range 70–100%) of the cross-sectional area of the original defect, with hyaline cartilage accounting for $42 \pm 10\%$ (range 7–67%) of defect area. These values were greater than those reported previously for untreated defects and defects implanted with a type II collagen scaffold seeded with autologous chondrocytes within 12 h prior to implantation *(61)*.

Based on these preliminary studies and the promise of decreased surgical time and morbidity, Hyalograft® C (Fidia Biopolymers Inc; Abano Terme, Italy) was introduced. This innovative tissue-engineering approach uses a three-dimensional hyaluronan-based scaffold entirely made of HYAFF 11, a benzyl ester of hyaluronic acid with 20-μm fibers. Autologous chondrocytes are grown under laboratory conditions on the scaffold prior to implantation into knee cartilage defects. Pavesio et al. reported on a cohort of 67 patients treated with Hyalograft C with a mean follow-up of 17.5 mo following implantation. Patients were evaluated arthroscopically and histologically. Subjective evaluation of patients' knee conditions demonstrated 97% improvement; quality-of-life assessment demonstrated 94% improvement. Surgeons' knee functional testing produced best scores in 87% of the patients; arthroscopic evaluation of cartilage repair revealed 96.7% biologically acceptable results, and histological assessment of the grafted site demonstrated hyalinelike tissue in a majority of specimens.

Marcacci et al. reported on a retrospective cohort, multicenter study investigating the subjective symptomatic, functional, and health-related quality-of-life outcomes of patients treated with Hyalograft C. A cohort of 141 patients with follow-up assessments ranging from 2 to 5 yr (average 38 mo) demonstrated that 91.5% of patients improved according to the International Knee Documentation Committee (IKDC) subjective evaluation, 76% had no pain as assessed by a visual analog scale, and 88% of patients had no mobility problems based on quality-of-life assessment. Surgeon evaluations revealed 95.7% of the patients had normal or nearly normal findings in the treated knee; Arthroscopic assessment of the cartilage repair demonstrated normal or nearly normal findings in 96.4% of the knees evaluated. Histological assessment of 21 second-look biopsies demonstrated hyalinelike tissue in 12 specimens, mixed hyaline and fibrocartilaginous findings were demonstrated in 5 specimens, and 4 cases demonstrated fibrocartilaginous findings. Interestingly, no fixation was used in 57.4% of cases, with the other cases using sutures or fibrin glue. A limited number of complications were recorded as well, with the authors concluding that Hyalograft C is a potentially safe and effective therapeutic option for the treatment of articular cartilage lesions. At the 2004 International Cartilage Repair Society, Marcacci reported on 88 patients treated arthroscopically with the Hyalograft C implant using no fixation. Computed tomographic and MRI evaluations were performed on all patients at 6, 12, and 24 mo, with no complications reported. Average preoperative IKDC scores were 41 and increased to 76 at 24-mo follow-up *(62)*.

Marlovits and coworkers reported on 16 patients with full-thickness, weight-bearing chondral defects of the femoral condyle *(63)*. All patients were treated with a three-dimensional collagen type I–III membrane seeded with cultured autologous chondrocytes (Fig. 11A,B). Fibrin glue was used with no periosteal cover or further surgical fixation. All patients were prospectively assessed using high-resolution MRI to determine the early postoperative attachment rate (range 22–47 d) after scaffold implantation. Implants were completely attached in 14 of 16 patients (87.5%), and full coverage was demonstrated in these patients as well. One patient had a partial detachment, and a patient had a complete detachment of the graft. At 24-mo

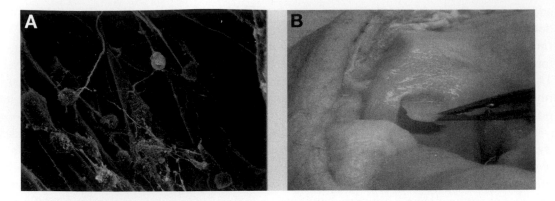

Fig. 11. (A) Electron microscopy of type I/III collagen scaffold seeded with articular chondrocytes. **(B)** Matrix on implantation into cartilage defect.

follow-up, significant improvements in IKDC, knee injury and osteoarthritis outcome, Lysholm, and modified Cincinnati scores were demonstrated in a majority of patients as well.

The term matrix-induced autologous chondrocyte implantation (MACI) has been used to describe procedures that specifically use a scaffold in addition to the autologous chondrocytes. Bartlett et al. performed a prospective, randomized study comparing the CACI procedure using a porcine-derived type I/III collagen cover to the MACI procedure using a bilayer of type I/III collagen *(37)*. Symptomatic chondral defects of the knee were evaluated in 91 patients, with 44 patients receiving the CACI procedure and 47 patients receiving the MACI procedure. Mean modified Cincinnati knee score at 1 yr increased by 17.6 in the CACI group and 19.6 in the MACI group ($p = 0.32$); good-to-excellent ICRS scores were demonstrated in 79.2% of CACI patients, and 66.6% of MACI patients had good-to-excellent results. Hyalinelike cartilage or hyalinelike cartilage with fibrocartilagenous regions were found in the biopsies of 43.9% of the CACI and 36.4% of the MACI grafts after 1 yr. Minimal graft hypertrophy and reoperation rates were noted in both groups. The authors concluded that the MACI procedure was technically attractive, but further long-term studies would be required before the technique is widely adopted.

CONCLUSIONS

The numerous matrices available in Europe and initial clinical reports associated with these devices are encouraging. The MACI procedure offers the benefit of sutureless fixation, minimally invasive or arthroscopic implantation, and fewer postoperative adhesions. The framework for future tissue engineering advances has clearly been laid. Several studies have demonstrated that articular chondrocytes, mesenchymal cells, and other cell phenotypes can be modulated by a variety of means to create hyalinelike articular cartilage.

Smith et al. exposed high-density primary cultures of bovine chondrocytes to hydrostatic pressure applied intermittently at 1 Hz or constantly for 4 h in serum-free medium or in medium containing 1% fetal bovine serum *(64)*. In serum-free medium, intermittent pressure increased aggrecan messenger ribonucleic acid (mRNA) signal by 14%, and constant pressure decreased type II collagen mRNA signal by 16% ($p < 0.05$). In the presence of 1% fetal bovine serum, intermittent pressure increased aggrecan and type II collagen mRNA signals by 31% ($p < 0.01$) and 36% ($p < 0.001$), respectively, whereas constant pressure had no effect on either mRNA. Intermittent and constant pressure stimulated glycosaminoglycan synthesis 65% ($p < 0.001$) and 32% ($p < 0.05$), respectively. These results were reproduced using human articular chondrocytes, simultaneously demonstrating that the duration and magnitude of applied IHP differentially altered chondrocyte matrix protein expression and anabolism *(65)*.

Nawata et al. used muscle-derived mesenchymal cells from postcoital rat embryos that were then propagated in vitro in monolayer culture for 10 d and packed within diffusion chambers together with type I collagen (CI) and 0, 1, or 10 µg rHuBMP-2; cells were implanted into abdominal subfascial pockets of adult rats *(66)*. Tissue pellets generated in the chamber 5 wk after implantation were transplanted into a full-thickness cartilage defect made in the patellar groove of the same strain of adult rat. In the presence of 10 µg recombinant bone morphogenic protein-2 (rHuBMP-2), muscle-derived mesenchymal cells expressed type II collagen (CII) messenger RNA at 4 d after transplantation, and a mature cartilage mass was formed 5 wk after transplantation in the diffusion chamber. Cartilage was not formed in the presence of 1 µg rHuBMP-2 or in the absence of rHuBMP-2. Defects receiving cartilage engineered with 10 µg rHuBMP-2 were repaired and restored to normal morphologic condition within 6 mo after transplantation.

Zhou et al. used bone marrow-derived stromal cells (BMSCs) in a porcine knee joint model to test this cell phenotype's ability to repair articular osteochondral defects in a minimal weight-bearing area of porcine knee joints *(67)*. BMSCs were cultured, in vitro expanded, and induced with dexamethasone (group A) or with dexamethasone and transforming growth factor-β1 (TGF-β1) (group B). Cells were seeded on a construct of polyglycolic acid (PGA) and polylactic acid (PLA) and co-cultured for 1 wk before implantation. Four osteochondral defects (8-mm diameter, 5 mm deep) were created in each animal on both sides. The defects were repaired with dexamethasone-induced BMSC-PGA/PLA construct in group A, with dexamethasone and TGF-β1-induced BMSC-PGA/PLA construct in group B, with PGA/PLA construct alone (group C), or left untreated (group D) as controls.

Stronger expression of type II collagen and aggrecan were observed in BMSCs induced with both dexamethasone and TGF-β1 *(67)*. At 3- and 6-mo time-points, gross observation and histologic evaluation showed that a majority of defects in group A were repaired by fibro-cartilage and cancellous bone with an irregular surface. However, most of group B defects were completely repaired by engineered hyaline cartilage and cancellous bone. No repair tissue or fibrous tissue was observed in groups C and D. The compressive moduli of repaired cartilage in groups A and B reached 30.37 and 43.82% of normal values at 3 mo and 62.69 and 80.27% at 6 mo, respectively; further, high levels of GAG contents in engineered cartilage of group A (78.03% of normal contents) and group B (no statistical difference from normal contents) were noted. Confocal microscopy revealed the presence of green fluorescent protein-labeled cells in engineered cartilage lacuna and repair of underlying cancellous bone. The authors concluded that implanted BMSCs can differentiate into either chondrocytes or osteoblasts at different local environments and repair a complex articular defect with both engineered cartilage and bone. TGF-β1 and dexamethasone in vitro induction promoted chondrogenic differentiation of BMSCs and improved the results of repairing articular defects.

The above studies demonstrate that cells of variable phenotypes can be modulated, and under appropriate conditions mature hyalinelike or normal articular cartilage is regenerated. Certainly, in light of the results with the MACI procedure, the in vitro manipulation and subsequent implantation of maturing cartilage constructs will be attempted.

Our experience with the traditional ACI technique using autologous chondrocytes with an autologous periosteal patch has been quite promising as well. In a majority of these patients, prior operative interventions had failed, or the total surface area of involvement was too extensive for less-versatile techniques. At this time, when the lesion size is less than 2 cm^2, minimally invasive procedures such as the microfracture or mosaicplasty techniques should be considered. However, for lesions greater than or equal to 2 cm^2 or when there are multiple lesions, the surgeon should consider the ACI procedure (Table 2). Critical evaluation of the biologic repair process has clearly demonstrated a reproducible sequence of events that occur as the tissue matures. If preoperative attention is given to those potential factors that could delay or prevent this process, failures can be avoided and the desired outcomes achieved.

Potential long-term benefits of the ACI procedure include durable repair tissue that can function in a manner similar to normal hyaline cartilage, withstanding the high shear and compressive loads applied during daily and sporting activities. The senior author has clearly demonstrated results in patients up to 11 yr following the ACI procedure that are equal to or better than those demonstrated at the initial 2-yr time-point. Further, as delineated in this chapter in the review of literature, second-look biopsies that demonstrated hyalinelike or mixed hyaline-fibrocartilaginous tissue reacted to indentation probe assessment in a manner similar to the adjacent host cartilage, suggesting a more normal response to physiologic loads; in line with these findings, a direct correlation between hyalinelike biopsies and better clinical results has been demonstrated in several studies as well.

The future of biologic regeneration and tissue engineering of articular cartilage to heal defects looks promising, and with further modifications in the techniques, arthroscopic or minimally invasive repair of these defects will be obtained, and successful return of patients to normal activity will be achieved on a regular basis.

REFERENCES

1. Curl WW, Krome J, Gordon ES, Rushing J, Smith BP, Poehling GG. Cartilage injuries: a review of 31,516 knee arthroscopies. Arthroscopy 1997;13:456–460.
2. Hjelle K, Solheim E, Strand T, Muri R, Brittberg M. Articular cartilage defects in 1000 knee arthroscopies. Arthroscopy 2002;18:730–734.
3. Piasecki DP, Spindler KP, Warren TA, Andrish JT, Parker RD. Intraarticular injuries associated with anterior cruciate ligament tear: findings at ligament reconstruction in high school and recreational athletes. An analysis of sex-based differences. Am J Sports Med 2003;31: 601–605.
4. Shelbourne KD, Jari S, Gray T. Outcome of untreated traumatic articular cartilage defects of the knee: a natural history study. J Bone Joint Surg Am 2003;85-A(suppl 2):8–16.
5. Bentley G, Biant LC, Carrington RW, et al. A prospective, randomised comparison of autologous chondrocyte implantation vs mosaicplasty for osteochondral defects in the knee. J Bone Joint Surg Br 2003;85:223–230.
6. Horas U, Pelinkovic D, Herr G, Aigner T, Schnettler R. Autologous chondrocyte implantation and osteochondral cylinder transplantation in cartilage repair of the knee joint. A prospective, comparative trial. J Bone Joint Surg Am 2003;85-A:185–192.
7. Wada Y, Watanabe A, Yamashita T, Isobe T, Moriya H. Evaluation of articular cartilage with 3D-SPGR MRI after autologous chondrocyte implantation. J Orthop Sci 2003;8:514–517.
8. Yates JW Jr. The effectiveness of autologous chondrocyte implantation for treatment of full-thickness articular cartilage lesions in workers' compensation patients. Orthopedics 2003;26: 295–300.
9. Brittberg M, Lindahl A, Nilsson A, Ohlsson C, Isaksson O, Peterson L. Treatment of deep cartilage defects in the knee with autologous chondrocyte transplantation. N Engl J Med 1994; 331:889–895.

10. Mankin HJ. The response of articular cartilage to mechanical injury. J Bone Joint Surg Am 1982;64:460–466.

11. Robinson D, Nevo Z. Articular cartilage chondrocytes are more advantageous for generating hyaline-like cartilage than mesenchymal cells isolated from microfracture repairs. Cell Tissue Bank 2001;2:23–30.

12. Nehrer S, Spector M, Minas T. Histologic analysis of tissue after failed cartilage repair procedures. Clin Orthop Relat Res 1999;365:149–162.

13. O'Driscoll SW, Keeley FW, Salter RB. The chondrogenic potential of free autogenous periosteal grafts for biological resurfacing of major full-thickness defects in joint surfaces under the influence of continuous passive motion. An experimental investigation in the rabbit. J Bone Joint Surg Am 1986;68:1017–1035.

14. O'Driscoll SW, Salter RB. The repair of major osteochondral defects in joint surfaces by neochondrogenesis with autogenous osteoperiosteal grafts stimulated by continuous passive motion. An experimental investigation in the rabbit. Clin Orthop Relat Res 1986;208:131–140.

15. Homminga GN, Bulstra SK, Bouwmeester PS, van der Linden AJ. Perichondral grafting for cartilage lesions of the knee. J Bone Joint Surg Br 1990;72:1003–1007.

16. Bulstra SK, Homminga GN, Buurman WA, Terwindt-Rouwenhorst E, van der Linden AJ. The potential of adult human perichondrium to form hyaline cartilage in vitro. J Orthop Res 1990;8:328–335.

17. Nakahara H, Dennis JE, Bruder SP, Haynesworth SE, Lennon DP, Caplan AI. In vitro differentiation of bone and hypertrophic cartilage from periosteal-derived cells. Exp Cell Res 1991;195: 492–503.

18. Nakahara H, Goldberg VM, Caplan AI. Culture-expanded human periosteal-derived cells exhibit osteochondral potential in vivo. J Orthop Res 1991;9:465–476.

19. Caplan AI, Elyaderani M, Mochizuki Y, Wakitani S, Goldberg VM. Principles of cartilage repair and regeneration. Clin Orthop Relat Res 1997;254:254–269.

20. Grande DA, Pitman MI, Peterson L, Menche D, Klein M. The repair of experimentally produced defects in rabbit articular cartilage by autologous chondrocyte transplantation. J Orthop Res 1989;7:208–218.

21. King PJ, Bryant T, Minas T. Autologous chondrocyte implantation for chondral defects of the knee: indications and technique. J Knee Surg 2002;15:177–184.

22. Micheli LJ, Browne JE, Erggelet C, et al. Autologous chondrocyte implantation of the knee: multicenter experience and minimum 3-yr follow-up. Clin J Sport Med 2001;11:223–228.

23. Minas T. Autologous chondrocyte implantation in the arthritic knee. Orthopedics 2003;26: 945–947.

24. Minas T, Peterson L. Advanced techniques in autologous chondrocyte transplantation. Clin Sports Med 1999;18:13–44.

25. Peterson L, Minas T, Brittberg M, Nilsson A, Sjogren-Jansson E, Lindahl A. Two- to 9-yr outcome after autologous chondrocyte transplantation of the knee. Clin Orthop Relat Res May 2000; 374:212–234.

26. Rosenberg TD, Paulos LE, Parker RD, Coward DB, Scott SM. The 45° posteroanterior flexion weight-bearing radiograph of the knee. J Bone Joint Surg Am 1988;70:1479–1483.

27. Insall JN. Patella pain syndromes and chondromalacia patellae. Instr Course Lect 1981;30: 342–56.

28. Petersen TD, Rohr W Jr. Improved assessment of lower extremity alignment using new roentgenographic techniques. Clin Orthop Relat Res 1987;219:112–119.

29. Potter HG, Linklater JM, Allen AA, Hannafin JA, Haas SB. Magnetic resonance imaging of articular cartilage in the knee. An evaluation with use of fast-spin-echo imaging. J Bone Joint Surg Am 1998;80:1276–1284.

30. Friemert B, Oberlander Y, Schwarz W, et al. Diagnosis of chondral lesions of the knee joint: can MRI replace arthroscopy? A prospective study. Knee Surg Sports Traumatol Arthrosc 2004;12: 58–64.

31. Palosaari K, Ojala R, Blanco-Sequeiros R, Tervonen O. Fat suppression gradient-echo magnetic resonance imaging of experimental articular cartilage lesions: comparison between phase-contrast method at 0.23T and chemical shift selective method at 1.5 T. J Magn Reson Imaging 2003;18:225–231.

32. Alonge TO, Rooney P, Oni OO. Osteophytes—an alternative source of chondrocytes for transplantation? West Afr J Med 2004;23:224–227.

33. Chaipinyo K, Oakes BW, Van Damme MP. The use of debrided human articular cartilage for autologous chondrocyte implantation: maintenance of chondrocyte differentiation and proliferation in type I collagen gels. J Orthop Res 2004;22:446–455.

34. Peterson L, Minas T, Brittberg M, Lindahl A. Treatment of osteochondritis dissecans of the knee with autologous chondrocyte transplantation: results at 2 to 10 yr. J Bone Joint Surg Am 2003; 85-A(suppl 2):17–24.

35. Haddo O, Mahroof S, Higgs D, et al. The use of chondrogide membrane in autologous chondrocyte implantation. Knee 2004;11:51–55.

36. Bartlett W, Gooding CR, Carrington RW, Skinner JA, Briggs TW, Bentley G. Autologous chondrocyte implantation at the knee using a bilayer collagen membrane with bone graft. A preliminary report. J Bone Joint Surg Br 2005;87:330–332.

37. Bartlett W, Skinner JA, Gooding CR, et al. Autologous chondrocyte implantation vs matrix-induced autologous chondrocyte implantation for osteochondral defects of the knee: a prospective, randomised study. J Bone Joint Surg Br 2005;87:640–645.

38. Brittberg M, Sjogren-Jansson E, Lindahl A, Peterson L. Influence of fibrin sealant (Tisseel) on osteochondral defect repair in the rabbit knee. Biomaterials 1997;18:235–242.

39. Henderson I, Francisco R, Oakes B, Cameron J. Autologous chondrocyte implantation for treatment of focal chondral defects of the knee—a clinical, arthroscopic, MRI and histologic evaluation at 2 years. Knee 2005;12:209–216.

40. Polster J, Recht M. Postoperative MR evaluation of chondral repair in the knee. Eur J Radiol 2005;54:206–213.

41. Henderson IJ, Tuy B, Connell D, Oakes B, Hettwer WH. Prospective clinical study of autologous chondrocyte implantation and correlation with MRI at 3 and 12 months. J Bone Joint Surg Br 2003;85:1060–1066.

42. Watrin-Pinzano A, Ruaud JP, Cheli Y, et al. T_2 mapping: an efficient MR quantitative technique to evaluate spontaneous cartilage repair in rat patella. Osteoarthritis Cartilage 2004;12: 191–200.

43. Brown WE, Potter HG, Marx RG, Wickiewicz TL, Warren RF. Magnetic resonance imaging appearance of cartilage repair in the knee. Clin Orthop Relat Res May 2004;422:214–223.

44. Marlovits S, Striessnig G, Resinger CT, et al. Definition of pertinent parameters for the evaluation of articular cartilage repair tissue with high-resolution magnetic resonance imaging. Eur J Radiol 2004;52:310–319.

45. Schneider U, Schlegel U, Bauer S, Siebert CH. Molecular markers in the evaluation of autologous chondrocyte implantation. Arthroscopy 2003;19:397–403.

46. Peterson L, Brittberg M, Kiviranta I, Akerlund EL, Lindahl A. Autologous chondrocyte transplantation. Biomechanics and long-term durability. Am J Sports Med 2002;30:2–12.

47. Vasara AI, Nieminen MT, Jurvelin JS, Peterson L, Lindahl A, Kiviranta I. Indentation stiffness of repair tissue after autologous chondrocyte transplantation. Clin Orthop Relat Res 2005;433: 233–242.

48. Moseley JB, Micheli L, Erggelet C, et al. 6-Year patient outcomes with autologous chondrocyte implantation. Read at the annual meeting of the American Academy of Orthopaedic Surgeons, Feb 2003, New Orleans.

49. Gillogly SD. Autologous chondrocyte implantation: complex defects and concomitant procedures. Operative Tech Sports Med 2002;10:120–128.

50. Gillogly SD. Treatment of large full-thickness chondral defects of the knee with autologous chondrocyte implantation. Arthroscopy 2003;19(suppl 1):147–153.

51. Gillogly SD. Clinical results of autologous chondrocyte implantation for large full-thickness chondral defects of the knee: 5-yr experience with 112 consecutive patients. Read at the annual meeting of the American Society for Sports Medicine, June 2001, Keystone, CO.

52. Seidner AL, Zaslav K. Articular cartilage lesions of the knee in patients receiving worker's compensation: effect of autologous chondrocyte implantation on costs and return to work status. Poster presented at the annual meeting of the American Academy of Orthopaedic Surgeons, Feb 2001, San Francisco, CA.

53. Minas T. Chondrocyte implantation in the repair of chondral lesions of the knee: economics and quality of life. Am J Orthop 1998;27:739–744.

54. Steadman JR, Briggs KK, Rodrigo JJ, Kocher MS, Gill TJ, Rodkey WG. Outcomes of microfracture for traumatic chondral defects of the knee: average 11-yr follow-up. Arthroscopy 2003;19: 477–484.

55. Anderson AF, Fu F, Mandelbaum B, et al. A controlled study of autologous chondrocyte implantation vs microfracture for articular cartilage lesions of the femur. Read at the annual meeting of the American Academy of Orthopaedic Surgeons, Feb 2002, Dallas, TX.

56. Knutsen G, Engebretsen L, Ludvigsen TC, et al. Autologous chondrocyte implantation compared with microfracture in the knee. A randomized trial. J Bone Joint Surg Am 2004;86-A:455–464.

57. Sgaglione NA, Miniaci A, Gillogly SD, Carter TR. Update on advanced surgical techniques in the treatment of traumatic focal articular cartilage lesions in the knee. Arthroscopy 2002;18(2 suppl 1):9–32.

58. Farr J, Lewis P, Cole BJ. Patient evaluation and surgical decision making. J Knee Surg 2004;17: 219–228.

59. Hendrickson DA, Nixon AJ, Grande DA, et al. Chondrocyte-fibrin matrix transplants for resurfacing extensive articular cartilage defects. J Orthop Res 1994;12:485–497.

60. Lee CR, Grodzinsky AJ, Hsu HP, Spector M. Effects of a cultured autologous chondrocyte-seeded type II collagen scaffold on the healing of a chondral defect in a canine model. J Orthop Res 2003;21:272–281.

61. Nehrer S, Breinan HA, Ramappa A, et al. Chondrocyte-seeded collagen matrices implanted in a chondral defect in a canine model. Biomaterials 1998;19:2313–2328.

62. Marcacci M, Kon E, Zaffagnini S, Marchesini L, Iacono F, Neri MP. Arthroscopic autologous chondrocyte transplantation. prospective study results at 1 and 2 yr follow-up. Read at the 5th Symposium of the International Cartilage Repair Society, Ghent, Belgium, 2004.

63. Marlovits S, Striessnig G, Kutscha-Lissberg F, et al. Early postoperative adherence of matrix-induced autologous chondrocyte implantation for the treatment of full-thickness cartilage defects of the femoral condyle. Knee Surg Sports Traumatol Arthrosc 2005 Sep;13(6):451–457.

64. Smith RL, Rusk SF, Ellison BE, et al. In vitro stimulation of articular chondrocyte mRNA and extracellular matrix synthesis by hydrostatic pressure. J Orthop Res 1996;14:53–60.

65. Ikenoue T, Trindade MC, Lee MS, et al. Mechanoregulation of human articular chondrocyte aggrecan and type II collagen expression by intermittent hydrostatic pressure in vitro. J Orthop Res 2003;21:110–116.

66. Nawata M, Wakitani S, Nakaya H, et al. Use of bone morphogenetic protein 2 and diffusion chambers to engineer cartilage tissue for the repair of defects in articular cartilage. Arthritis Rheum 2005;52:155–163.

67. Zhou GD, Wang XY, Miao CL, et al. Repairing porcine knee joint osteochondral defects at non-weight bearing area by autologous BMSC. Zhonghua Yi Xue Za Zhi 2004;84:925–931.

68. Minas T, Nehrer S. Current concepts in treatment of articular cartilage defects. Orthopedics 1997;20:525–538.

69. Brittberg M, Peterson L. Autologous chondrocyte transplantation can effectively treat most articular cartilage lesions of the knee? In: Williams R, Johnson D (ed) Controversies in Knee Surgery, New York: Oxford University Press Inc., 2004, p. 439–454.

11

Osteochondral Allograft Transplantation

Joseph Yu, MD, and William D. Bugbee, MD

Summary

Fresh osteochondral allografting is a reconstructive technique with a long clinical history. In fresh allografting, diseased or damaged articular cartilage is replaced with living mature hyaline cartilage from a suitable donor. The bony portion of the allograft serves as an attachment vehicle or to reconstruct associated osseous defects. Fresh allografts can be used for a wide spectrum of pathology, ranging from focal chondral lesions to posttraumatic arthrosis. The surgical technique involves fashioning the allograft to fit into a prepared recipient site. Outcomes of fresh allografting for focal femoral condyle lesions are 75–90% successful while results in salvage situations range from 50–75% successful at follow-up intervals from 2 to 15 years. Many unique clinical issues associated with fresh osteochondral allografting require further investigation, but clinical success supports the use of fresh allografts as a cartilage repair technique.

Key Words: Allograft; cartilage injury; cartilage repair; cartilage transplant; osteochondral allograft.

HISTORICAL BACKGROUND

Initial experimentation with fresh joint transplantation started with Erich Lexer in the early 1900s *(1)*; however, in the modern era, fresh small-fragment osteochondral allografting for the treatment of articular cartilage injury and disease began in the 1970s. This clinical experience, along with basic scientific investigation, has provided an understanding of the rationale and support for the use of fresh osteochondral allografts.

Currently, fresh osteochondral allografts are utilized to treat a broad spectrum of articular cartilage pathology, from focal chondral defects *(2,3)* to joints with established osteoarthrosis *(4)*. Most commonly, allografts have successfully treated osteochondritis dissecans (OCD) lesions *(5)*, osteonecrosis *(6)*, and posttraumatic cartilage defects of the knee *(7,8)*. Allografts also have been successfully utilized in the treatment of osteochondral lesions of the ankle and hip joints *(9–11)*.

RATIONALE

The fundamental concept governing fresh osteochondral allografting is the transplantation of architecturally mature hyaline cartilage with living chondrocytes. It is the notion that these living chondrocytes survive transplantation and are thus capable of supporting the cartilage matrix indefinitely following implantation into the host knee. Hyaline cartilage possesses characteristics that make it attractive for transplantation. It is an avascular tissue and therefore does not require a blood supply, meeting its metabolic needs through diffusion

From: *Cartilage Repair Strategies*
Edited by: Riley J. Williams © Humana Press Inc., Totowa, NJ

from synovial fluid. It is an aneural structure as well and does not require innervation for function. Third, articular cartilage is relatively immunoprivileged *(12)* as the chondrocytes are embedded within the articular cartilage matrix and are relatively protected from host immune surveillance.

The second component of the osteochondral allograft is the osseous portion. The bony portion of the fresh osteochondral allograft is dead (void of cells) and functions as a support for the living articular cartilage layer and as a vehicle that facilitates attachment and fixation of the graft to the host. The osseous portion of the graft is quite different from the hyaline portion because it is a vascularized tissue, and cells are not thought to survive transplantation; rather, the osseous structure functions as a scaffold for healing to the host by creeping substitution (similar to other types of bone graft). Generally, the osseous portion of the graft should be limited to a few millimeters; however, depending on the clinical situation, the allograft may contain more extensive amounts of bone, as might be required to restore injured or absent subchondral tissue. Large osteochondral lesions such as those associated with OCD, osteonecrosis, or posttraumatic reconstruction may require the transplantation of a large bony component.

In light of the aforementioned concepts, it is helpful to consider a fresh osteochondral allograft as a composite graft of both bone and cartilage, with a living mature hyaline cartilage portion and a nonliving subchondral bone portion. It is also helpful to understand the allografting procedure in the context of a tissue or organ transplantation. The graft essentially is transplanted as an intact structural and functional unit replacing a diseased or absent component in the recipient joint. The transplantation of mature hyaline cartilage obviates the need to rely on techniques, which are central to other restorative procedures, that induce cells to form cartilage tissue; however, the allograft has its own set of clinic issues, including the following:

1. Complexities of acquisition, processing, and storage of the donor tissue.
2. Safety concerns with respect to disease transmission from donor tissue to host.
3. Immunological behavior of the allograft.
4. The allograft–host bone interaction.

DONOR TISSUE

Graft Acquisition

The cornerstone of an allografting procedure is the availability of fresh osteochondral tissue. It is important to note that currently, in fresh osteochondral allografting, the small-fragment allografts are not human lymphocyte antigen- (HLA) or blood type-matched and are utilized fresh rather than frozen or processed, such as is used in other bulk allografting or tumor-reconstructive procedures. The rationale for fresh tissue use in this application is predicated on the concept of maximizing the quality of the articular cartilage in the graft. This is in distinction to cases of large osseous reconstructions, for which restoration of the osseous defect is the primary goal and for which frozen tissue may be more appropriate.

Despite numerous efforts at cryopreservation and other freezing protocols that might maintain chondrocyte viability, it has been demonstrated that the cryopreservation freezing process kills chondrocytes *(13)*, and that this effectively eliminates more than 95% of viable chondrocytes in the articular cartilage portion of osteochondral grafts. Furthermore, clinical experience has shown that the articular matrix in transplanted frozen allografts deteriorates over time; this phenomenon presumably occurs because there are no cells within the implanted matrix to maintain tissue structure *(14)*. Conversely, with fresh osteo-chondral allografts, it has been demonstrated, primarily through retrieval studies *(15,16)*, that viable chondrocytes and relatively preserved cartilage matrix are present many years after transplantation. These experiences have generally supported the use of fresh vs frozen tissue for small osteochondral allografts in the setting of reconstruction of chondral and osteochondral defects.

Allograft Testing and Safety

Understanding the process of tissue procurement, testing, and storage is important in the allografting procedure. Historically, the obstacles presented by these fundamental components have led to the development of fresh allograft programs only at specialized centers that not only have a close association with an experienced tissue bank but also have put significant investment of resources into setting up specific protocols for safe and effective transplantation of fresh osteochondral tissue.

Fresh osteochondral grafts have become commercially available and thus more accessible to the orthopedic surgical community. Procurement, processing, and testing of donor tissue follow guidelines established by the American Association of Tissue Banks (AATB) *(17)*. The screening process is extensive and includes inquiry into the donor's medical, social, and sexual history. Current guidelines include serologic testing for HIV 1/2 antibody, human T-lymphotropic virus (HTLV 1/HTLV 2) antibody, hepatitis B surface antigen (HBsAg), hepatitis C virus, syphilis, and hepatitis B core antibody. The age criterion for the donor pool for fresh grafts is generally between 15 and 40 yr. The joint surface must also pass a visual inspection for cartilage quality. These criteria ensure, but do not guarantee, acceptable tissue for transplantation.

Experienced allograft surgeons often will discuss particular donor characteristics with tissue bank personnel. It is extremely important to acknowledge that fresh human tissue is unique, and no two donors have the same characteristics. Therefore, strict adherence to tissue-banking standards and adherence to protocols and processes in quality control are paramount. Furthermore, an essential part of the informed consent process is a discussion of the risk of bacterial or viral disease transmission.

As with any transplantation of allogeneic organs or tissue, there exists the risk of transmission of infectious disease despite donor screening and testing. Advances in serological testing has improved safety, but a measurable risk does remain; both the surgeon and the patient considering the allografting procedure should be well aware of the risk for transmission of infectious disease. Unfortunately, this risk is difficult to quantify. With more than 5 million allograft transplants performed over the past decade, there are very few documented incidents of disease transmission, especially for fresh osteochondral allografts *(18)*. There has been one reported death from transmission of *Clostridium sordelli* by a fresh osteochondral allograft.

In our institution's 20-yr experience involving more than 450 fresh allografts, there have been no documented cases of transmission of disease from donor to recipient. We feel that strict adherence to the guidelines set forth by the AATB and knowledge of the individual tissue banks that provide transplanted tissue can minimize the documented risks of disease transmission. Overall, inherent safety of the graft is based on good tissue recovery and processing practices, including donor screening and physical examination and serological and bacterological testing.

Allograft Storage

The storage of fresh osteochondral allografts prior to transplantation has recently become a more important issue. Historically, fresh grafts were transplanted within 5 d of donor death, obviating the need for prolonged tissue storage. The majority of the basic science and clinical studies reflect the situation by which the grafts were recovered, stored in lactated Ringer's solution, and transplanted within 5 d. Current tissue bank protocols, however, call for storage of fresh osteochondral allografts while tests for bacterial and viral contamination are carried out. Because some anaerobic organisms require 14 d to grow in ideal solution, the tissue currently recovered today is usually transplanted no sooner than 14 d and sometimes as long as 40 d after recovery from the donor. Recent studies of allograft storage have shown significant deterioration in cell viability, cell density, and metabolic activity with prolonged storage of fresh osteochondral allografts *(19,20)*. Small, but statistically significant, changes are first detected after storage for 14 d; these changes are pronounced after storage for 28 d *(21)*. Conversely, the hyaline matrix appears to be relatively preserved at 28 d. The clinical consequences of these storage-induced graft changes have yet to be determined.

Immunology

The immunology of fresh osteochondral allografts is another important consideration. Although it appears that hyaline cartilage is relatively immunoprivileged *(12)*, it is also evident that fresh unmatched osteochondral allografts do elicit a variable immune response. In a canine study comparing the immune response to fresh and frozen leukocyte antigen-matched and -mismatched allografts, Stevenson demonstrated that fresh mismatched osteochondral allografts generated the largest immune response *(22)*. Conversely, in humans, allograft retrieval studies *(14,23)* have consistently shown little or no histologic evidence of immune-mediated pathology; however, in another study of fresh osteochondral allografts, 50% of individuals generated serum anti-HLA antibodies *(24)*. The presence of the anti-HLA antibodies correlated with inferior appearance of the graft–host interface on magnetic resonance imaging (MRI) studies. This suggests that humoral immunity may play a role in the outcome of fresh allografting. Current clinical practice does not include either HLA or blood-type matching of donor and recipient; however, preliminary evidence suggests that blood typing may be important to clinical outcomes *(25)*. It is clearly an area in which more knowledge is necessary.

INDICATIONS

Knee

Fresh osteochondral allografts possess the ability to restore a wide spectrum of articular and osteoarticular pathology. As a result, the clinical indications cover a broad range of pathology. As is true for other restorative procedures, the careful assessment of the entire joint is important in addition to evaluating the articular lesion. Many proposed treatment algorithms suggest the use of allografts for large lesions (>2–3 cm^2) or for salvage in difficult reconstructive situations. In our experience, allografts can be considered as a primary treatment option for osteochondral lesions greater than 2 cm in diameter, as is typically seen in OCD and osteonecrosis.

In addition, allografts often are used primarily for salvage reconstruction of posttraumatic defects of the tibial plateau or the femoral condyle *(7,8)*. Allografts also have been utilized in the treatment of epiphyseal tumors, for which a significant amount of joint surface

Table 1
Indications for Fresh Osteochondral Allografting

Knee	Ankle	Hip
Osteonecrosis	Osteonecrosis	Osteonecrosis
Osteochondritis dissecans	Osteochondritis dissecans	Osteochondral fracture
Posttraumatic reconstruction (tibial plateau fracture, femoral condyle fracture)	Posttraumatic arthrosis	
Chondral lesions (traumatic, degenerative)	Hemophilic arthropathy	
Salvage of previous cartilage procedure		
Patellofemoral chondrosis or arthrosis		
Unicompartmental arthrosis		

requires reconstruction. Other indications for allografting in the knee include treatment of patellofemoral chondrosis or arthrosis *(26)* and select cases of unicompartmental tibiofemoral arthrosis *(6)*. Plus, allografts are useful as a salvage procedure when other cartilage-restorative procedures, such as microfracture, osteochondral autograft transfer system (OATS), or autologous chondrocyte implantation, have been unsuccessful.

Ankle

In the ankle joint, fresh allografts are indicated in posttraumatic reconstruction, including resurfacing of the tibiotalar joint with posttraumatic arthrosis, osteonecrosis of the talus, and OCD lesions not amenable to OATS or other restorative procedures *(9,10)*. The use of fresh allografts for bipolar resurfacing of the tibiotalar joint is unique to the ankle as total joint resurfacing has not been proven successful in the knee; the use of bipolar joint resurfacing in the ankle also reflects the limited options for the younger individual with end-stage arthrosis of the tibiotalar joint.

Hip

In the hip, osteochondral allografts have been utilized with mixed results in the treatment of osteonecrosis of the femoral head *(11)*. Current indications are evolving and include symptomatic Ficat stage II or III lesions with limited head involvement (Steinberg classification B) that have not responded to other treatments. Fresh osteochondral allografts also may be useful in posttraumatic reconstruction of femoral head fractures or treatment of large chondral lesions, although clinical experience is limited, and no published data are available (Table 1).

CONTRAINDICATIONS

Relative contraindications to the allografting procedure include uncorrected joint instability or uncorrected malalignment of the limb. An allograft may be considered in combination or as part of a staged procedure in these settings. In the knee, allografting should not be considered an alternative to prosthetic arthroplasty in an individual with symptoms and acceptable age and activity level for prosthetic replacement. In the younger individual, bipolar and multicompartment allografting have been modestly successful; however, advanced multicompartment arthrosis, even in the younger individual, is a relative contraindication to the allografting procedure.

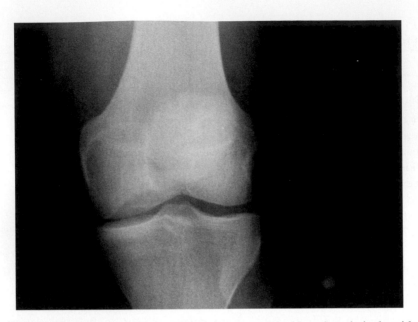

Fig. 1. Osteochondritis dissecans of the medial femoral condyle. Note the relatively wide, flat contour of the condyle.

The presence of inflammatory disease or crystal-induced arthropathy is considered a relative contraindication as well, as is any unexplained synovitis. The use of fresh osteochondral allografts in individuals with altered bone metabolism, such as is seen in chronic steroid use, smoking, or even use of nonsteroidal anti-inflammatory agents, has not been studied extensively. Results in the knee and in the hip have demonstrated mixed results in the treatment of steroid-induced avascular necrosis, but this may represent the extent of disease rather than the effect of steroid usage.

TECHNIQUE OF OSTEOCHONDRAL ALLOGRAFTING

The surgical technique for fresh osteochondral allografting depends on the joint and surface to be grafted. Common to all fresh allografting procedures is matching the donor with recipient. This is done on the basis of size. In the knee, an anteroposterior (AP) radiograph with a magnification marker is used, and a measurement of the medial-lateral dimension of the tibia, just below the joint surface, is made. This corrected measurement is utilized, and the tissue bank makes a direct measurement on the donor tibial plateau. Alternatively, a measurement of the affected condyle can be performed.

A match is considered acceptable when the graft dimensions fall within 2 mm of that of the host bone; however, it should be noted that there is a significant variability in anatomy not reflected in size measurements. In particular, in treating OCD, the pathological condyle typically is larger, wider, and flatter; therefore, a larger donor generally should be used (Fig. 1). In the ankle, a similar measurement is made of the medial-lateral dimension of the talus from an AP or mortise view; and a direct measurement is made on the talus at the time of tissue processing. Similarly, the diameter of the femoral head is measured from the radiograph and is correlated to a direct measurement on the donor.

Most femoral condyle lesions can be treated utilizing dowel-type grafts. Commercially available instruments (Arthrex, Naples, FL) simplify the preparation, harvesting, and insertion of these grafts, which may be up to 35 mm in size.

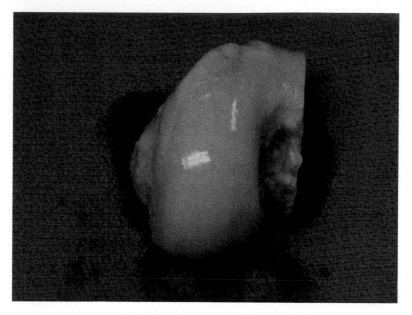

Fig. 2. Medial femoral condyle allograft.

Surgical Technique

Femoral Condyle

For most femoral condyle lesions, allografting can be performed through a miniarthrotomy. In most situations, a diagnostic arthroscopy has been performed recently and is not a necessary component of the allografting procedure; however, if there are any unanswered questions regarding meniscal status or the status of the other compartments, then a diagnostic arthroscopy can be performed prior to the allografting procedure.

The patient is positioned supine, with a tourniquet on the thigh. A leg holder is valuable in this procedure for positioning the leg in between 70 and 100° of flexion to access the lesion. Prior to incision, the fresh graft, which should be placed in chilled saline, is inspected to confirm the adequacy of the size match and quality of the tissue (Fig. 2).

A standard midline incision is made from the center of the patella to the tip of the tibial tubercle. Depending on the location of the lesion (either medial or lateral), a retinacular incision is then made beginning from the superior aspect of the patella. Great care is taken to enter the joint and incise the fat pad without disrupting the anterior horn of the meniscus. In some cases when the lesion is posterior or very large, the meniscus must be taken down; generally, this can be done safely, leaving a small cuff of tissue adjacent to the anterior attachment of the meniscus for later repair.

Once the joint capsule and synovium have been incised and the joint has been entered, retractors are placed medially and laterally to expose the condyle (Fig. 3). Care is taken for the positioning of the retractor within the notch to protect the cruciate ligaments and articular cartilage. The knee is then flexed and extended until the proper degree of flexion is noted that presents the lesion into the arthrotomy site. Excessive degrees of flexion limit the ability to mobilize the patella. The lesion then is inspected and palpated with a probe to determine the extent, margins, and maximum size. A guidewire is driven into the center of the lesion perpendicular to the curvature of the articular surface.

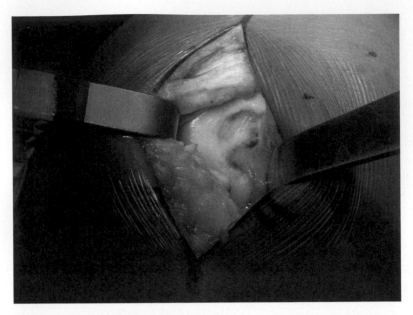

Fig. 3. Exposure of the osteochondritis dissecans lesion in the medial femoral condyle.

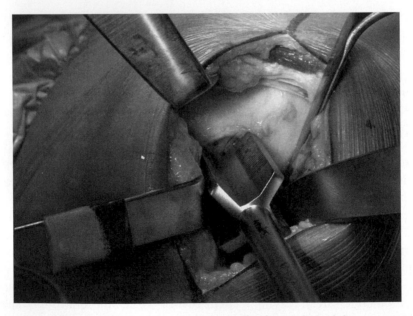

Fig. 4. Reaming the diseased medial femoral condyle.

The size of the proposed graft is determined by utilizing sizing dowels; a special reamer is used to remove the remaining articular cartilage and 3–4 mm of subchondral bone (Fig. 4). In deeper lesions, the pathologic bone is removed until there is healthy, bleeding bone. Generally, the preparation does not exceed 6–10 mm, and usually bone grafting is performed to fill any deeper or more extensive osseous defects. After removal of the guide pin, depth measurements are made in the four quadrants of the prepared recipient site.

The corresponding anatomic location of the recipient site then is identified on the graft. The graft is placed into a graft holder (or alternately, held with bone-holding forceps). A saw

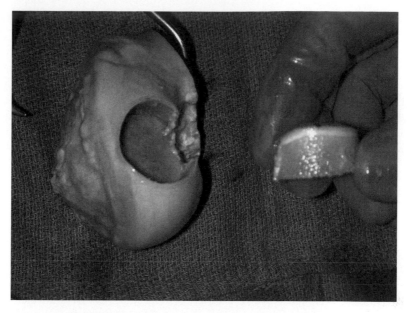

Fig. 5. Allograft is cut from the femoral condyle.

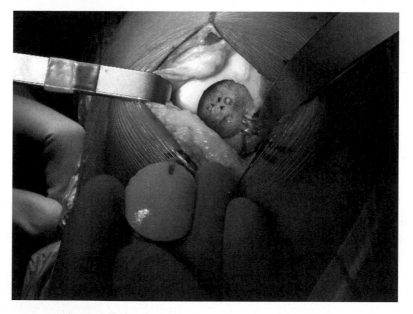

Fig. 6. Allograft trimmed and ready for implantation.

guide then is placed in the appropriate position, again perpendicular to the articular surface; and the appropriate size tube saw is used to core out the graft (Fig. 5). Once the graft is removed, depth measurements, which were taken from the recipient, are transferred to the graft; this graft is cut with an oscillating saw and then trimmed with a rasp to the appropriate thickness in all four quadrants. Often, trimming must be done multiple times to ensure precise thickness, matching the prepared defect in the patient (Fig. 6).

The graft should be irrigated copiously with a high-pressure lavage to remove all marrow elements.

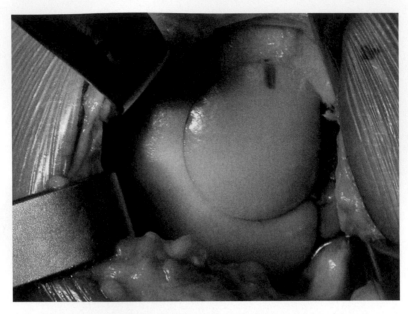

Fig. 7. Graft is inserted in place.

The graft is then inserted by hand in the appropriate rotation and is gently tamped in place until it is flush (Fig. 7). If the graft does not fit, then the recipient site can be dilated, or the recipient site or the graft itself is refashioned carefully.

Once the graft is seated, a determination is made whether additional fixation is required. Typically, absorbable pins are utilized, particularly if the graft is large or has an exposed edge. Often, the graft needs to be trimmed in the notch region to prevent impingement. The knee is then brought through a complete range of motion to confirm that the graft is stable and that there is no mechanical blockage or soft-tissue obstruction (Fig. 8).

Trochlear Allografts

Lesions of the trochlea are approached in a similar manner; however, these are much more technically challenging as the anatomy of the trochlea is much more complex, leading to technical issues in creating symmetric matching recipient sites and donor grafts. In this setting, extensive care must be taken to match the anatomic location and the angle of approach as most larger grafts will end up elliptical because of the anatomy of the trochlear groove. Cases of patellofemoral arthrosis, in which the entire trochlea is removed, are performed similar to arthroplasty, with resection of the anterior femur. The graft is resected similarly and is fixed in place with interfragmentary screws both medially and laterally. Great care must be taken not to thin the graft in the central portion of the trochlea, which can lead to fracture.

Patellar Allografts

The patella is often entirely resurfaced when using an osteochondral allograft. In this setting, a technique similar to that used in arthroplasty resurfacing is utilized. Patellar thickness is first measured, and resection of the articular surfaces is performed, maintaining at least 12–15 mm of residual patellar bone. The graft is then resected freehand in a similar fashion, ensuring minimal thickness in the medial and lateral facets. This generally leads to a maximal thickness of 10–12 mm. The graft is seated in appropriate position and rotation, and tracking

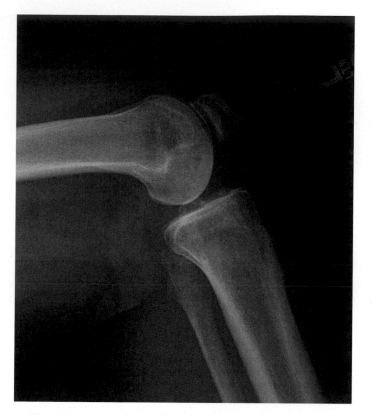

Fig. 8. Postoperative radiograph of the allograft at 3 mo.

is noted. The patellar graft can be moved a few millimeters on the recipient surface to optimize patellar tracking. Fixation typically is performed with interfragmentary screw fixation from the anterior surface of the patella into the median ridge of the graft, which has adequate bone for small screw purchase. An extensive lateral release is routinely performed. Proximal or distal patellar realignment is optional. Smaller patellar lesions can be treated with dowel-type grafts, with a technique similar to that for the femoral condyle.

Tibial Plateau Allografts

The surgical technique of tibial plateau allografting utilizes principles similar to those in unicompartmental arthroplasty (Figs. 9 and 10). The tibial plateau graft typically can be performed through an arthrotomy that does not require patellar eversion. Great care, however, must be taken to protect cruciate ligament attachments, as well as meniscal attachments, when the meniscus is preserved. Fluoroscopy is utilized extensively in this procedure. Two guidewires are placed in the tibial metaphyseal bone parallel to the desired slope and depth of resection of the diseased tibial surface. The more central pin also acts as a guide for the level of vertical resection of the tibia and the AP direction of the cut.

After placement of the pins is confirmed, a freehand cut is made, resecting a minimal amount of subchondral bone. After removal of all diseased or damaged tissue, particularly in the back of the joint, the knee is brought out into appropriate alignment, and the width of the resected surface is measured, as is the joint space gap from the femoral condyle to the resected surface. This measurement allows estimation of the required allograft thickness. The tibial

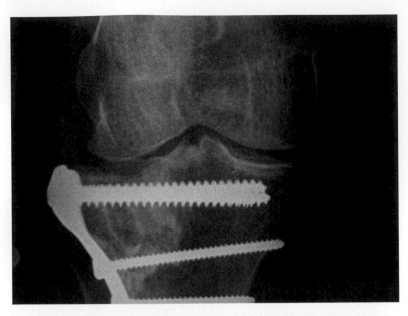

Fig. 9. Radiograph of posttraumatic arthritis after a lateral tibial plateau fracture.

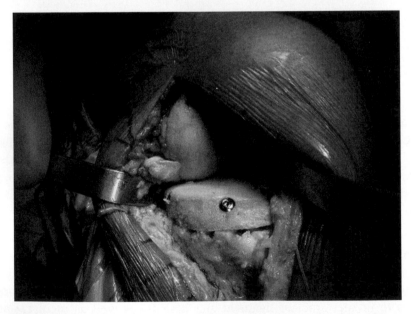

Fig. 10. Lateral tibial plateau allograft restoring the height of the plateau.

allograft then is placed in the graft holder, and the desired thickness is measured and marked on the graft. Typically, grafts are at least 12 mm thick, with a minimum of 10 mm. A reciprocating saw cut is then made. If meniscal transplantation is performed, this includes the meniscal attachments. An oscillating saw cut then is made, utilizing the guide marks placed on the graft margins. At this point, the graft is measured for appropriate width and length and often needs to be thinned in the medial-lateral direction. Trimming is then performed as necessary.

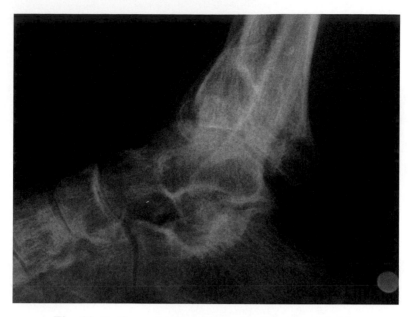

Fig. 11. Radiograph of posttraumatic tibiotalar arthritis.

When the graft size is confirmed for the recipient site, the graft is then lavaged; the knee is brought into flexion; and unloading stress of the compartment is performed. The graft is gently placed under the femoral condyle, taking care not to entrap the native meniscus and to ensure that the associated allograft meniscus is seated under the condyle. Once this is done, the knee is brought through range of motion, and the graft is visualized, both clinically and under fluoroscopy, for appropriate position, restoration of joint line, slope, and the proper orientation of the femur relative to the tibial surface. Revisions are made as necessary; and grafts are fixed with interfragmentary screw fixation from the submeniscal articular margin at the midcoronal and anterior positions. The meniscus then is repaired, or in the case of associated meniscal allograft, suturing is performed in the standard fashion. It should be noted that it is vitally important to ensure stability of the tibial graft and to prevent mechanical overloading of the graft either by overstuffing the compartment or underfilling the compartment, creating an angular deformity and stress on the grafted side.

Ankle Allografts

The surgical procedure for allografting the ankle depends on the surfaces to be grafted. Focal lesions of the talus are amenable to either anterior arthrotomy or, in some cases, a medial malleolar or fibular osteotomy to access more posterior medial or lateral talar lesions. These lesions generally can be treated with small dowel-type allografts, as described in treating the femoral condyle lesions. In cases of extensive talar involvement, such as large necrotic segments from osteonecrosis or large OCD lesions, half or the entire talar articular surface is replaced (Fig. 11). An anterior arthrotomy is performed, and the talar dome is resected, under fluoroscopic guidance, from the articular margin anteriorly to posteriorly. The talar graft then is resected freehand in a similar manner, again using the landmarks of the anterior articular margin to the posterior articular margin. This generally creates a maximum graft thickness at the center of the talar dome of between 9 mm and 11 mm. Bringing the foot into maximum plantar flexion aids in inserting the graft under the tibial

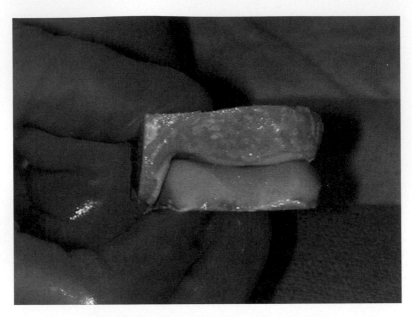

Fig. 12. Harvested tibia and talus allograft.

plafond. In many cases, an external fixator for distraction is useful to aid in allografting of the talus.

Bipolar allografting of the tibiotalar joint represents perhaps the most complex of the fresh allografting procedures. The procedure essentially parallels that utilized for prosthetic replacement of the ankle *(10)*. Initially, an external fixator is placed on the medial side of the ankle, and the ankle is distracted. An extensile anterior arthrotomy is performed, and the joint is entered. Under fluoroscopic guidance, the Agility Ankle Jig (DePuy, Warsaw, IN) with the appropriate size cutting block is placed on the ankle. Using the guide, matched resections of the tibial and talar surface are performed, with the joint in neutral position and the ankle distracted 6–10 mm. Great care is taken to avoid overresection of the medial malleolus or injury to neurovascular structures. The resected diseased surfaces then are removed, and the graft is measured.

The tibia and talar grafts are prepared separately. Utilizing the next larger size cutting jig (i.e., recipient cut with size 2, donor with size 3), this is placed onto the tibial graft in appropriate position and rotation under fluoroscopic guidance. Great care is taken to match rotation, slope, and position as the precise fitting of this graft is critical. The talus then is resected freehand, again utilizing the anterior and posterior articular margins, with a goal of 9–11 mm maximum thickness. Once these grafts are prepared, the composite thickness is measured and compared to the resection gap of the recipient (Fig. 12).

The grafts are irrigated, and trial fittings are performed. Commonly, the medial malleolus requires trimming. The external fixator is removed, and the ankle is brought through range of motion to help center the grafts. Fluoroscopy is used to ensure that the tibial and talar grafts are centered appropriately, and a check for AP impingement is performed. The grafts are then fixed with small fragment screws or pins (Fig. 13).

Hip Allografts

Allografting of the hip is performed generally through an anterior or anterolateral approach, with gentle anterior dislocation of the femoral head. As most lesions typically

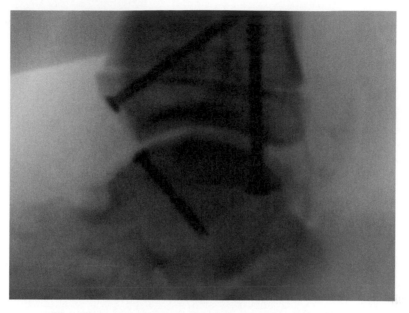

Fig. 13. Postoperative radiograph of ankle allografting.

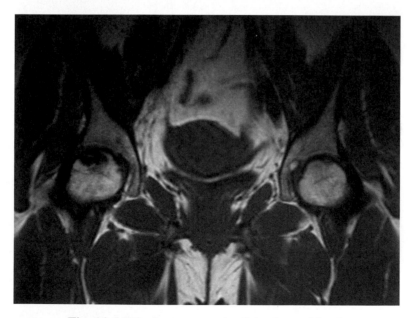

Fig. 14. MRI of osteonecrosis of the femoral head.

are anterior-superior (Fig. 14), this approach facilitates visualization and exposure. Debridement of the lesion is performed, and the graft is fashioned, either utilizing instruments to create a dowel-type graft or performed freehand utilizing small power burrs and cutting instruments. Fixation of these grafts is typically with pins or screws through the articular surface (Figs. 15, 16).

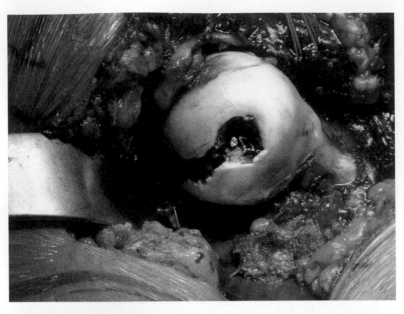

Fig. 15. Exposure of the osteonecrosis lesion in the femoral head.

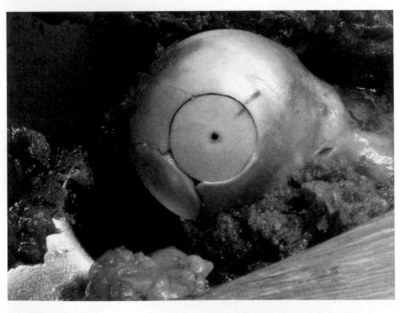

Fig. 16. After placement of the allograft into the femoral head.

POSTOPERATIVE MANAGEMENT AND REHABILITATION

In the knee, early postoperative management includes attention to control of pain, swelling, and restoration of limb control and range of motion. Patients generally are maintained on touch-down weight bearing for a minimum of 6 wk and typically closer to 8–12 wk, depending on the size of the graft and stability of fixation. Patients with patellofemoral grafts are allowed weight bearing as tolerated in extension and generally are limited to 45° of flexion for the first 4 wk, utilizing an immobilizer or range-of-motion brace. Tibial or bipolar grafts, and those with an associated osteotomy, are fitted with a range-of-motion brace to control varus/valgus stress. Tibial grafts associated with meniscal allografting are often limited to 90° of flexion for the initial 6 wk. Weight bearing progresses slowly between the second and fourth months, with full weight bearing utilizing a cane or crutch. Full weight bearing and normal gait pattern are generally tolerated between the third and fourth months. Recreation and sports are not reintroduced until joint rehabilitation is complete and radiographic healing has been demonstrated, which generally occurs no earlier than 6 mo postoperatively.

The rehabilitation protocol is straightforward, assuming confidence with graft fixation. Continuous passive motion use is considered optional and often is used only in the hospital setting. Restoration of range of motion and quadriceps/hamstring function with isometrics and avoidance of open-chain exercises are principal. Stationary cycling is begun at 4–6 wk, and pool therapy can be utilized at this time as well.

Clinical follow-up includes radiographs at 4–6 wk, 3 mo, 6 mo, and yearly thereafter. Careful radiographic assessment of the graft–host interface is important. Any concern of delayed healing should lead to a more cautious approach to weight bearing and other high-stress activities.

Postoperative protocol for ankle allografting includes the use of a bulky splint to control swelling and to allow wound healing for the first 1–2 wk. A fracture brace or removable cast is then employed, and a nonweight-bearing status is maintained for up to 3 mo for large and bipolar allografts. Gentle range-of-motion exercises are performed three to four times a day, with great care in avoiding forcing extreme ranges of motion, which may lead to excessive forces on the graft–host interface. At 6 wk, attention is given to increasing range of motion, particularly in dorsiflexion and Achilles stretching. Progressive weight bearing, first in the fracture brace at 3 mo and then out of the brace at 4 mo, is performed. A cane is often utilized at this time. Unprotected weight bearing is begun between 4 and 6 mo if radiographic confirmation of interface healing is demonstrated.

Typically, patients undergoing the allografting procedure will demonstrate continued incremental improvement over the first postoperative year. A plateau in recovery typically can be expected at 1 yr, although often patients demonstrate continued functional improvement between years 1 and 2. Often, this depends on patient motivation, desired activities, and persistence with the rehabilitation program.

COMPLICATIONS OF FRESH OSTEOCHONDRAL ALLOGRAFTING

Complications of the allografting procedure can be divided as early or late.

Early Complications

Early complications unique to the allografting procedure are few. There does not appear to be any increased risk of surgical site infection with the use of allografts compared with other procedures. The use of a miniarthrotomy in the knee decreases the risk of postoperative stiffness. Occasionally, one sees a persistent effusion, which is typically a sign of overuse, but may indicate an immune-mediated synovitis. Delayed union or nonunion of the fresh allograft is the most common early finding, evidenced by persistent discomfort or visible graft–host interface on serial radiographic evaluation.

Delayed union or nonunion is more common in larger grafts, such as those used in the tibial plateau, or in the setting of compromised bone, such as in the treatment of osteonecrosis. In this setting, patience is essential, as complete healing and recovery may take an extended period. Decreasing activities, the institution of weight-bearing precautions or use of braces, and possible use of external bone stimulators may be helpful in the early management of delayed healing. In this setting, careful evaluation of serial radiographs can provide insight into the healing process; MRI scans are rarely helpful, particularly prior to 6 mo postoperative, as they typically show extensive signal abnormality that is difficult to interpret. It should be noted that, with adequate attention to postoperative weight-bearing restrictions and adequate graft fixation, delayed or nonunion requiring repeat surgical intervention within the first year is extremely uncommon.

The natural history of the graft that fails to osteointegrate is unpredictable. Clinical symptoms may be minimal, or there may be progressive clinical deterioration and radiographic evidence of fragmentation, fracture, or collapse. This is most commonly seen in grafts of the tibial plateau or ankle joint. Typical symptoms of this type of graft failure include sudden onset of increased pain, often associated with minor trauma. Effusion, crepitus, or focal pain are commonly seen. Careful evaluation of serial radiographs typically will demonstrate collapse, subsidence, fracture, or fragmentation. MRI or computed tomography scanning also can be utilized to assess graft failure.

Treatment of this type of graft failure generally requires either allograft revision or, in cases where the allograft was used as a salvage, conversion to arthroplasty or arthrodesis.

Late Complications

As noted, the requisite event for a successful fresh allograft procedure is healing of the host–graft bony interface and integration of the host bone into the osseous portion of the allograft. This process of so-called creeping substitution is well described in the paradigm of bone-graft healing. Revascularization of the allograft bone by the host may take many years and may not be complete *(23)*. The amount of bone within the allograft may be important in this process, and it is likely that thinner grafts will have more complete revascularization than thicker grafts. Retrieval studies *(14–16,23)* of failed fresh osteochondral allografts have provided tremendous insight into the allograft healing process and have led to the understanding that fresh osteochondral allografts rarely fail because of the cartilage portion of the graft; rather, most failures originate within the osseous portion of the graft or from progression of the host joint disease process (i.e., osteoarthrosis). It is likely that late allograft failure, which has been seen between 2 and 17 yr, is the result of graft subsidence collapse or fragmentation caused by fatigue failure, very much like that seen with bulk allografts placed under repetitive loading situations. This clinical finding underscores the need to pay close attention to joint alignment and stability in the initial treatment of the patient.

Clinically, the patient will present with new pain or mechanical symptoms, of either insidious or acute onset. Radiographs will show cysts or sclerosis or perhaps subchondral collapse, typically in the center of the graft, which may be most distant from the revascularization process or an area that has been under higher load because of activity of the patient or malalignment. Again, careful review of serial radiographs is important. MRI also may be useful and generally is obtained to confirm the allograft pathology and to rule out other sources of pain or sites of pathology in the knee joint. It is important to note that the allografted joint may suffer from the same pathology that is present in any other joint, such as meniscus or ligamentous injury. It should also be noted that radiographic and MRI abnormalities are

Table 2
Results of Fresh Osteochondral Allografting

Reference	*Site*	*Diagnosis*	*Number*	*Mean follow-up (yr)*	*Successful outcome*
Ghazavi et al. *(7)*	Knee	Trauma	126	7.5	85% survivorship
Meyers et al. *(2)*	Knee	Multiple	31	3.5	77%
Chu et al. *(3)*	Knee	Multiple	55	6.2	84% good or excellent
Bugbee *(6)*	Knee	Arthrosis	41	4.5	54% good or excellent
Görtz and Bugbee *(29)*	Knee	Trauma	78	5.5	79% good or excellent
Park and Bugbee *(31)*	Knee	Arthrosis	34	2.6	74% good or excellent
Aubin et al. *(8)*	Femoral condyle	Trauma	60	10.0	85% survivorship
Garrett et al. *(5)*	Femoral condyle	OCD	17	2–9	16/17 good or excellent
Bugbee et al. *(28)*	Femoral condyle	OCD	69	5.2	80% good or excellent
Jamili and Bugbee *(32)*	Femoral condyle	AVN	18	5.3	100% survivorship
Jamali et al. *(26)*	Patellofemoral	Multiple	29	4.5	52% good or excellent
Gross et al. *(9)*	Talus	OCD	9	12.0	6/9 survivorship
Kim et al. *(10)*	Ankle	Arthrosis	7	10.0	4/7 good or excellent
Meehan et al. *(33)*	Ankle	Multiple	11	2.8	72% good or excellent

commonly noted even in well-functioning allografts *(24)*, and great care must be taken in interpreting and correlating the imaging studies with clinical findings.

Treatment options for failed allografts include observation if the patient is minimally symptomatic and the joint is thought to be at low risk for further progression of disease. Arthroscopic evaluation and debridement also may be utilized *(6,7)*. In many cases, revision allografting is performed and generally has led to a success rate equivalent to primary allografting. This appears to be one of the particular advantages to fresh osteochondral allografting in that fresh allografting does not preclude a revision allograft as a salvage procedure for failure of the initial allograft. In cases of more extensive joint disease, particularly in older individuals, conversion to prosthetic arthroplasty is appropriate.

RESULTS

Results of fresh osteochondral allografting are shown in Table 2.

Knee Allografts

In the knee, fresh allografts are effective as primary treatment for small chondral femoral condyle lesions, but in our experience they are often used as salvage after other grafting procedures, such as microfracture, osteochondral autografting, or autologous chondrocyte implantation, have failed. Fresh allografts also have been utilized in the treatment of osteonecrosis *(2,27)*.

The experience at University of California, San Diego extends over two decades. To date, 365 fresh osteochondral allograft procedures have been performed in the knee alone. Of these procedures, 29% were performed for salvage involving complex reconstruction of traumatic or degenerative conditions, 27% for OCD of the femoral condyle, 22% for isolated focal chondral lesions secondary to traumatic and degenerative conditions, 14% for patellofemoral disease, and 8% for osteonecrosis (Table 3). Of the 365 operations in the knee, 35% were on the medial femoral condyle, 17% on the lateral femoral condyle, 4% on the trochlea, 4% on the patella, 5%

Table 3
Indications for Allograft Procedures to the Knee (Total Procedures = 365)

Indication	Percentage of procedures
Salvage or complex reconstruction of trauma or degenerative conditions	29
Osteochondritis dissecans of the femoral condyle	27
Focal chondral lesions (traumatic and degenerative conditions)	22
Patellofemoral disease	14
Osteonecrosis	8

Table 4
Sites of Knee Allografts Performed (Total Procedures = 365)

Sites	Percentage of allografts
Medial femoral condyle	35
Lateral femoral condyle	17
Trochlea	4
Patella	4
Patella and trochlea	5
Lateral tibial plateau	4
Medial tibial plateau	1
Multiple sites	30

Table 5
Reoperations in Knee Allografts (Total Reoperation Rate = 20%)

Reason for reoperation	Percentage of allografts
Arthroscopy	6
Revision allograft	5
Total vs unicompartmental arthroplasty	5
Removal of metal fixation	2
Other	2

on the patella and trochlea combined, 4% on the lateral tibial plateau, 1% on the medial tibial plateau, and 30% on multiple sites (Table 4). The total reoperation rate has been 20%; among these, 6% were arthroscopic procedures, 5% were revision allografts, 5% were total knee or unicompartmental arthroplasties, and 2% involved removal of metal fixation (Table 5).

Osteochondritis Dissecans of the Femoral Condyle

Fresh osteochondral allografts are most commonly utilized in the treatment of OCD of the femoral condyle. These lesions typically are large and involve defects in subchondral bone, characteristics that make allografting attractive because the graft can address both the osseous and the chondral components of the lesion.

Garrett *(5)* first reported on 17 patients treated with fresh osteochondral allografts for OCD of the lateral femoral condyle. All patients had failed previous surgery, and in a 2- to 9-yr follow-up period, 16 of 17 patients were reported as asymptomatic.

We reviewed our experience in the treatment of OCD of the medial and lateral femoral condyle *(28)*. Sixty-nine knees in 66 patients were evaluated at a mean of 5.2 yr postoperatively. All allografts were implanted within 5 d of procurement. Patients were prospectively evaluated using an 18-point modified D'Aubigne and Postel scale; subjective assessment was performed with a patient questionnaire. In this group, there were 49 males and 17 females, with a mean age of 28 yr (range 15–54 yr). Forty lesions involved the medial femoral condyle and 29 the lateral femoral condyle. An average of 1.6 surgeries had been performed on the knee prior to the allograft procedure. Allograft size was highly variable, with a range from 1 to 13 cm^2. The average allograft size was 7.4 cm^2. Two knees were lost to follow-up.

Overall, 53 out of 67 (79%) knees were rated good or excellent, scoring 15 or above on the 18-point scale; 10 out of 67 (15%) were rated fair, and 6 of 67 (9%) were rated poor. The average clinical score improved from 13 preoperatively to 15.8 postoperatively ($p > 0.01$). Six patients had reoperations on the allograft; 1 was converted to total knee arthroplasty, and 6 underwent revision allografting at 1, 2, 5, 7, and 8 yr after the initial allograft. Of 66 patients, 49 completed questionnaires: 96% reported satisfaction with their treatment; 86% reported less pain. Subjective knee function improved from a mean of 3.5 to 7.9 on a 10-point scale.

Posttraumatic Tibiofemoral Lesions

Fresh osteochondral allografts have a particularly valuable role in the treatment of posttraumatic knee reconstruction, after periarticular fractures of the tibial plateau or femoral condyle, in individuals considered too young for prosthetic arthroplasty. The Toronto group has long-term experience with allografts for posttraumatic reconstruction. Ghazavi et al. *(7)* reviewed 126 knees in 123 patients with osteochondral defects primarily secondary to trauma. The average age of these individuals was 35 yr (range 15–64 yr). There were 81 males and 42 females. In this group, 63 lesions involved the tibial plateau, 50 involved the femoral condyle, and 7 were bipolar lesions. In 47 cases, the meniscus was included with the transplant, and 68 knees underwent osteotomy to correct alignment. Patients were evaluated both clinically and radiographically. Survivorship analysis demonstrated 95% survivorship at 5 yr, 71% survivorship at 10 yr, and 66% survivorship at 20 yr. Among 18 failures, 1 underwent arthrodesis, 8 underwent total knee arthroplasty, 1 graft was removed, and 8 failed because of low clinical score but still retained their grafts.

At our institution, we reviewed 82 knees (81 patients) from a patient database of traumatic chondral and osteochondral lesions of the femoral condyle *(29)*. Clinical evaluation was performed with a modified D'Aubigne and Postel (18-point) scale. The mean age was 35 yr (range 14–67 yr), with a mean follow-up of 5.5 yr (range 1–14 yr). In this group, 52 lesions involved the medial femoral condyle, and 32 involved the lateral femoral condyle. Six patients were lost to follow-up. Of the 78 patients, 62 (79%) had a successful outcome. Nine patients had repeat surgeries, with two revision allografts, two unicompartmental arthroplasties, and five total knee arthroplasties; four patients who had poor scores had no further surgery.

Tibiofemoral Arthrosis

Fresh osteochondral allografts also have been utilized for salvage of advanced tibiofemoral arthrosis in carefully selected cases *(4,30)*. Forty-one knees were reviewed at a mean of 4.5-yr follow-up. Of these knees, 12 underwent unipolar or single-surface grafting, 26 underwent bipolar femoral and tibial grafting, and 3 underwent multisurface grafting. Fifteen of the tibial grafts had associated meniscal transplantation. In this group, 54% of grafts were considered successful, and 47% were considered unsuccessful. Seven patients were revised to total knee arthroplasty, 5 underwent revision allografting, and 5 failed because of low clinical scores. It is important to note that, in this group, unipolar grafts performed far better than bipolar grafts (70 vs 48% successful).

The second author *(30)* identified 40 patients who had knee allografts performed for osteoarthritis. Clinical evaluation was performed with an 18-point modified D'Aubigne and Postel scale and an International Knee Documentation Committee evaluation. There were 26 males and 14 females; mean age was 41 yr. Contact was lost in 6 patients. The mean follow-up was 31.4 mo. Twenty allografts were unipolar (16 femoral condyle, 3 tibial plateau, 1 trochlea); 10 were bipolar (femoral-tibial, trochlea-patella surfaces); and 4 involved multiple surfaces. The mean allograft area was 10.2 cm^2. Of the surgeries, 74% were considered successful (good or excellent on an 18-point scale), and 26% were unsuccessful, with 3 converted to knee arthroplasties, 2 with repeat allografting, and 4 with fair or poor scores with no further surgery. Subjective International Knee Documentation Committee scores improved from 31.7 to 60.2 ($p < 0.01$), with 18 of 34 (53%) extremely satisfied, 33 of 34 (97%) were at least satisfied, and 1 of 34 (3%) somewhat satisfied.

Patellofemoral Lesions

In the patellofemoral joint, allografts have been used for treating patellar or trochlear chondral lesions, avascular necrosis, and patellofemoral arthrosis caused by chronic malalignment *(26)*. In this group, 29 knees have been evaluated at a mean of 4.5-yr follow-up. Twenty-two underwent complete patellar resurfacing, 1 underwent trochlear resurfacing, and 7 underwent combined patellar and trochlear grafting. In this difficult group, 57% were considered as having good or excellent results, and 40% of results were considered fair, poor, or requiring reoperation. The reoperations included 4 revision allografts, 3 total knee arthroplasties, and 1 arthrodesis for sepsis. Four required no further surgery but failed because of a low clinical score.

Other Results

Chu et al. *(3)* reported on 55 consecutive knees undergoing osteochondral allografting. This group included patients with diagnoses such as traumatic chondral injury, avascular necrosis, OCD, and patellofemoral disease. The mean age of this group was 35.6 yr, with follow-up averaging 75 mo (range 11–147 mo). Of the 55 knees, 43 were unipolar allografts, and 12 were bipolar allografts. On an 18-point scale, grafting for 42 of 55 (76%) of these knees was rated good to excellent, and 3 of 55 grafts were rated fair, for an overall success rate of 82%. It is important to note that 84% of the knees that underwent unipolar femoral grafts were rated good to excellent, and only 50% of the knees with bipolar grafts achieved good or excellent status.

Aubin et al. *(8)* reported on the Toronto experience with fresh osteochondral allografts of the femoral condyle. Sixty knees were reviewed, with a mean follow-up of 10 yr (range 5 to 23 yr). The etiology of the osteochondral lesion was trauma in 36, osteochondritis in 17, osteonecrosis in 6, and arthrosis in 1. Realignment osteotomy was performed in 41 patients and meniscal transplantation in 17. Twelve knees required graft removal or conversion to total knee arthroplasty. The remaining 48 patients averaged a Hospital for Special Surgery score of 83 points. The authors reported 85% graft survivorship at 10 yr.

Ankle Allografts

There are limited published data on ankle allografts. Gross et al. *(9)* reported on nine patients treated for osteochondral lesions of the talus caused by OCD or fracture. Six of nine grafts remained *in situ* at mean follow-up of 12 yr (range 4–20 yr). Three ankles required arthrodesis.

Kim et al. *(10)* reported on bipolar tibiotalar allografting for posttraumatic arthrosis in seven patients. At mean 10-yr follow-up, four of seven patients' results were rated good/excellent, one did not improve, and two underwent arthrodesis.

Since 1998, there have been 82 fresh osteochondral allograft procedures performed at University of California, San Diego: 84% bipolar tibia and talus allografts, 11% partial talar dome allografts, 3% entire talar dome allografts, and 2% entire tibial plafond allografts. The overall revision rate was 15%. There was only one ankle that was converted to a total ankle arthroplasty. No arthrodesis was performed.

FUTURE DIRECTIONS

Clinical experience with fresh, small-fragment osteochondral allograft transplantation extends nearly three decades. The value of this procedure in reconstructing large or difficult chondral and osteochondral lesions is reflected in the increasing utilization of allografts in cartilage and joint reconstructive procedures. Despite the extensive clinical experience and basic scientific investigation, there are large gaps in our understanding of fresh osteochondral allografts. As with other cartilage restorative procedures, the indications for the use of fresh osteochondral allografts are still evolving regarding the use of allografts in the treatment of focal femoral condyle lesions as well as the use of allografts in more extensive disease states that typify the arthritic joint.

One can envision applying allografting techniques to other anatomic locations in special circumstances. The technical aspects of the procedure are evolving rapidly as well, and it is anticipated that improved surgical instrumentation, techniques, and innovations will allow more reproducible results and will decrease the number of technical-related early failures.

With respect to the fresh grafts, we can anticipate further improvements in tissue-banking techniques; not only to improve safety, but also to enhance the graft quality; perhaps innovation in storage of allografts will prolong the storage life of fresh allografts, allowing more widespread access to this procedure. Further understanding of the immunological behavior of fresh allografts is clearly needed. Modulating the immunologic response, either by donor–recipient matching or other therapies, may lead to breakthroughs in short- and long-term success of allograft procedures.

Advancements in tissue engineering of cartilage could profoundly change the management of articular lesions. Chondrocytes cultured in scaffolds are approaching the mechanical and biochemical properties of hyaline cartilage. Osteochondral constructs could be made from a chondral layer integrated onto a trabecular subchondral bony layer, with the hypothesis that the bone layer would provide a suitable interface for in vivo bony ingrowth. Integration of these constructs into the damaged articular surface could be fixed with the same method as a fresh osteochondral allograft. With tissue-engineered allografts, surgeons could order prefabricated osteochondral allografts based on radiographic dimensions of the patient's bone. Alternatively, a patient with a complex osteochondral lesion could have a custom allograft created based on preoperative imaging. Other future benefits of such technology include the elimination of immunological reaction and disease transmission, more accurate shape and size matching of the cartilage lesion, and increased availability.

The rapidly emerging field of growth factors and other bioactive substances could provide new methods that would serve to enhance bone healing and may improve the integration of the allograft bone to the recipient, which is currently the most important event for clinically successful allografting. Processing or manipulation of the osseous portion of the allograft with the addition of growth factors may allow the allograft bone to act more like an autograft and to enhance or facilitate the osseointegration so vital to the success of the allograft. We may also envision the application of growth factors or other substances to the hyaline cartilage portion of the graft to improve matrix properties or cellular function, effect integrative cartilage repair of allograft to host, and to limit the detrimental effect of storage on the allografts. In summary, fresh osteochondral allografts have enjoyed a long and successful clinical history, particularly considering their application in difficult clinical situations for which few other options exist. Rapid advancement in our understanding of the biology and technical aspects should further expand indications and utility of osteochondral transplantation.

REFERENCES

1. Lexer E. Joint transplantations and arthroplasty. Surg Gynecol Obstet 1925;40:782–809.
2. Meyers MH, Akeson WA, Convery FR. Resurfacing of the knee with fresh osteochondral allograft. J Bone Joint Surg Am 1989;71A:704–713.
3. Chu CR, Convery FR, Akeson WA, et al. Articular cartilage transplantation: clinical results in the knee. Clin Orthop Relat Res 1999;36:159–168.
4. Bugbee WD, Jamali A, Rabbani R. Fresh osteochondral allografting in the treatment of tibiofemoral arthrosis. Proceedings of the 69th meeting AAOS; February 2002; Dallas, TX.
5. Garrett JC. Fresh osteochondral allografts for treatment of articular defects in osteochondritis dissecans of the lateral femoral condyle in adults. Clin Orthop Relat Res 1994;303:33–37.
6. Bugbee WD. Fresh osteochondral allografts. Semin Arthroplasty 2000;11:1–7.
7. Ghazavi MT, Pritzker RP, Davis AM, et al. Fresh osteochondral allografts for post-traumatic osteochondral defects of the knee. J Bone Joint Surg Br 1997;79B:1008–1013.
8. Aubin PP, Cheah HK, Davis AM, Gross AE. Long term follow-up of fresh femoral osteochondral allografts for post-traumatic knee defects. Clin Orthop Relat Res suppl Articular Cartilage Repair 2001; 391-S:318–327.
9. Gross AE, Agnidis A, Hutchison CR. Osteochondral defects of the talus treated with fresh osteochondral allograft transplantation. Foot Ankle Int 2001;22:385–391.
10. Kim CW, Tontz WL, Jamali A, Convery FR, Brage ME, Bugbee WD. Treatment of post-traumatic ankle arthrosis with bipolar tibiotalar osteochondral shell allografts. Foot Ankle Int 2002; 23:1091–1102.
11. Meyers MH. Resurfacing of the femoral head with fresh osteochondral allografts: long-term results. Clin Orthop Relat Res 1985;197:111–114.
12. Langer F, Gross AE. Immunogenicity of allograft articular cartilage. J Bone Joint Surg Am 1974;56A:297–304.
13. Ohlendorf C, Tomford WM, Mankin HJ. Chondrocyte survival in cryopreserved osteochondral articular cartilage. J Orthop Res 1996;14:413–416.
14. Enneking WF, Campanacci DA. Retrieved human allografts: a clinicopathological study. J Bone Joint Surg Am 2001;83:971–986.
15. Czitrom AA, Keating S, Gross AE. The viability of articular cartilage in fresh osteochondral allografts after clinical transplantation. J Bone Joint Surg Am 1990;72:574–581.
16. Convery FR, Akeson WH, Meyers MH. The operative technique of fresh osteochondral allografting of the knee. Operative Tech Orthop October 1997;340–344.
17. American Association of Tissue Banks. Standards for Tissue Banking. Arlington, VA: American Association of Tissue Banks; 1987.

18. Centers for Disease Control. allograft associated bacterial infections. MMWR Morb Mortal Wkly Rep 2002;51:207–210.
19. Ball S, Chen AC, Tontz WL, Jr, et al. Preservation of fresh human osteochondral allografts: effects of storage conditions on biological, biochemical, and biomechanical properties. Trans Orthop Res Soc 2002;27:441.
20. Williams SK, Amiel D, Ball ST, et al. Fresh osteochondral allografts: time-dependent storage effects. Session 57: Podium Presentation 6 at: International Cartilage Repair Society Annual Meeting; June 2002; Toronto, Canada.
21. Williams SK, Amiel D, Ball ST, et al. Prolonged storage effects of articular cartilage of fresh human osteochondral allografts. J Bone Joint Surg Am 2003;85:2111–2120.
22. Stevenson S. The immune response to osteochondral allografts in dogs. J Bone Joint Surg Am 1987;69:573–582.
23. Oakeshott RD, Farine I, Pritzker KP, et al. A clinical and histologic analysis of failed fresh osteochondral allografts. Clin Orthop Relat Res 1988;233:283–294.
24. Sirlin CB, Brossman J, Boutin RD, et al. Shell osteochondral allografts of the knee: comparison of MR imaging findings and immunologic responses. Radiology 2001;219:35–43.
25. Bugbee WD, Kwak C, Lebeck L, Brage M. The effect of ABO blood type on outcome of fresh osteochondral allograft transplantation. Paper 110 presented at: AAOS 71st Annual Meeting; February, 2004, San Francisco, CA.
26. Jamali A, Bugbee WD, Chu C, Convery FR. Fresh osteochondral allografting of the patellofemoral joint. Paper 177 presented at: AAOS 68th Annual Meeting; February 2001; San Francisco, CA.
27. Gross AE, McKee NH, Pritzker KP. Reconstruction of skeletal deficits of the knee: a comprehensive osteochondral transplant program. Clin Orthop Relat Res 1983;174:96–106.
28. Bugbee WD, Emmerson BC, Jamali A. Fresh osteochondral allografting in the treatment of osteochondritis dissecans of the femoral condyle. Paper 054 presented at: AAOS 70th Annual Meeting; February 2003; New Orleans, CA.
29. Görtz S, Ho A, Bugbee W. Fresh osteochondral allograft transplantation for cartilage lesions in the knee. Presentation at the 73rd Annual Meeting of the American Academy of Orthopaedic Surgeons; March 2006, Chicago, IL.
30. Gross AE, Silverstein EA, Falk J. The allotransplantation of partial joints in the treatment of osteoarthritis of the knee. Clin Orthop Relat Res 1975;108:7–14.
31. Park DY, Bugbee WD. Clinical outcomes of fresh osteochondral allografts for younger, active individuals with established osteoarthritis of the knee. Unpublished manuscript.
32. Jamili A, Bugbee WD. Fresh osteochondral allografting in the treatment of osteonecrosis of the knee. Paper 108 presented at: AAOS 71st Annual Meeting; February 2004; San Francisco, CA.
33. Meehan RE, Tonz W, McFarlin S, Bugbee WD, Brage ME. Fresh ankle osteochondral allograft transplantation for tibiotalar joint arthritis. Foot Ankle Int 2005; in press.

Matrix-Induced Autologous Chondrocyte Implantation

David Wood, MBBS, MS, FRCS, FRACS
and Ming Hao Zheng, PhD, DM, FRCPath

Summary

Matrix-induced autologous chondrocyte implantation (MACI) by means of direct inoculation of chondrocytes on a type I/IV collagen membrane for surgical implantation is less invasive and obviates periosteal harvest and suturing in most cases. It allows manufacturers to deliver a standard cell density for implantation. This chapter describes the characteristics of collagen membrane and the surgical procedures of MACI. The early clinical results based on 43 implantations in 40 patients were reported. It concluded that MACI achieves a comparable functional and histological outcomes as does conventional ACI technology.

Key Words: Hyaline-like cartilage; matrix-induced autologous chondrocyte implantation; MACI; type I/IV collagen membrane; fibrin sealant; fibro cartilage.

INTRODUCTION

Conventional autologous chondrocyte implantation (ACI) was the first surgical technique to highlight the therapeutic potential of autologous cell techniques, but the use of periosteum to seal the defects has various complications *(1–5)*. The use of a type I/IV collagen membrane instead of periosteum, however, facilitates reduced postoperative tissue hypertrophy, decreased surgical invasiveness, shortened operative time, minimized donor-site morbidity, and subsequent postoperative pain *(6,7)*. Although collagen-covered ACI has exhibited commendable histological outcomes, its efficiency is impeded by the need to microsuture the membrane to the defect circumference, a tedious task that increases the length and technicality of the surgical procedure. Some concern also remains about cell delivery.

The use of a collagen membrane in place of periosteum has led to the development of matrix-induced autologous chondrocyte implantation (MACI). Instead of injection of chondrocytes under the collagen membrane into the sealed defect compartment, autologous chondrocytes can be directly inoculated on the type I/III collagen membrane and delivered as a cell-scaffold construct for implantation. The recipient bed is prepared in the same way as the periosteum technique. A thin layer of fibrin glue is applied to the base of the defect; the cell seeded membrane is cut to match the defect geometry, applied with the cells facing subchondral bone, and held in place for about 30 s to allow graft fixation. The reconstruction is then stable in most contained defects, and the wound is closed. Even application of 1 million cells/cm^2 is made to the area of the repairing lesion, and there is generally no need for sutures to fix the graft.

This simple surgical technique obviates periosteal harvest, is generally suture free, and is less invasive than traditional methods. Early mobilization of the joint is safe, and structured

From: *Cartilage Repair Strategies*
Edited by: Riley J. Williams © Humana Press Inc., Totowa, NJ

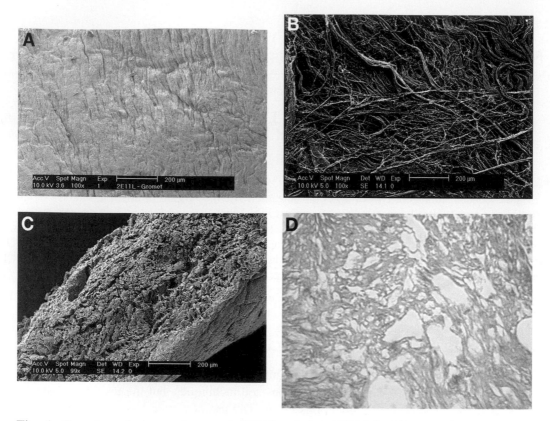

Fig. 1. Scanning electron micrograph (SEM) of the ACI-Maix bilayer collagen membrane microstructure. SEM of the cell-occlusive compact arrangement of collagen in the smooth surface **(A)**, compared to the rough surface showing loose collagen matrix **(B)** of the membrane. Cross-sectional imaging **(C)** of the membrane shows the differential organization of the collagen matrix. Surface histology **(D)** of the membrane illustrates the porous organization of membrane collagen fibers that allows chondrocyte integration (hematoxylin and eosin staining; 25×).

rehabilitation is routine. Since the MACI technique was first used in 1998, more than 3000 patients have been treated across Europe and Australia. In this chapter, we describe the characteristics of the collagen membrane and its impact on chondrocyte phenotype, review the efficacy of cartilage regeneration induced by MACI through progressive histological observation of biopsied tissue following graft implantation, and discuss the clinical outcomes of this technique.

CHARACTERIZATION OF CHONDROCYTES ON COLLAGEN MEMBRANE

The type I/III collagen membrane has been widely used for various clinical applications (e.g., dental and plastic surgery) and has undergone extensive biocompatibility evaluation testing. The current sources of type I/III collagen membrane are from Matricel GmbH (ACI-maix) and Geistish Group (Chondro-Gide). It is a class III product for use in orthopedic surgery and extensive testing has shown no evidence of an immune reaction following intra-articular implantation and subcutaneous or systemic injection. The membrane is acellular, shows no evidence of genotoxicity, and on broad-band viral testing was declared virus free.

The ACI-Maix type I/III collagen membrane for MACI is obtained from the porcine peritoneal cavity followed by several disinfection and sterilization steps during processing. The materials are sterilized with low-dose γ-irradiation before release for use. Scanning electronic microscopic examination reveals that the collagen membrane has a bilayer microstructure (Fig. 1). Cross-sectional imaging of the membrane shows compact collagen fiber arrangement on the smooth outer surface of the membrane (Fig. 1A) compared to the loose arrangement of fibers on the rough surface (Fig. 1B). The flat topology of the superficial side of the smooth surface is also illustrated by cross-sectional viewing of the membrane (Fig. 1C). The rough surface is well characterized by its loose, porous collagen fiber arrangement capable of chondrocyte integration (Fig. 1B).

The highly purified natural type I/III collagen fibers crosslinked to manufacture the membrane are well illustrated by high magnification of the rough surface. In contrast, magnification of the smooth membrane surface shows the cell-occlusive compact arrangement of collagen fibers (Fig. 1A). Fibers on the smooth surface are seen aggregating together to provide a slick surface reminiscent of superficial articular cartilage collagen fibers. Basic cross-sectional histology of the membrane also exhibits the porous organization of collagen fibers and shows no evidence of porcine cells or cell fragments (Fig. 1).

Chondrocytes cultured in monolayer dedifferentiate and cease type II collagen and gyclosaminaoglycan synthesis, presenting a fibroblasticlike phenotype after early passages *(8)*. Subsequently, chondrocytes transplanted as a cell suspension, as in conventional ACI, may not be capable of differentiating into the chondrocyte phenotype necessary to facilitate active regeneration. Direct inoculation of chondrocytes on type I/III collagen membrane seems to stabilize the phenotypic profile of chondrolineage cells. Chondrocytic integration into the ACI-Maix collagen membrane can be evidenced by immunohistochemical and electron microscopic analysis (Fig. 2).

Scanning electron microscopy of the chondrocyte-seeded membranes shows the integration and attachment of chondrocytes within the collagen matrix of the membrane and their differentiated globular appearance (Fig. 2A). Furthermore, transmission electron microscopic assessment of chondrocyte integration into the membrane illustrates the presence of cytoplasmic projections from chondrocytes into the fibers of the collagen membrane, anchoring the cells and facilitating matrix synthesis (Fig. 2B). S-100 (chondrocyte marker) staining, while also showing seeded cells to be chondrolineage cells, confirms the integration and attachment of chondrocytes within the collagen matrix of the membrane (Fig. 2C). Type II collagen staining in the seeded cells was also positive prior to implantation (Fig. 2D), demonstrating these chondrolineage cells are capable of producing type II collagen, a necessary component for hyaline cartilage matrix.

FIBRIN GLUE

The chondrocyte-seeded membrane is secured in place with a thin layer of fibrin glue applied to the base of the defect. The subchondral plate should not be penetrated during preparation of the recipient bed; however, should the bone bleed despite the application of adrenaline, a small amount of fibrin glue provides excellent hemostasis. Contained defect grafts are usually stable, but with uncontained defect grafts, judicious sutures, anchors, or resorbable pins may be required. Concern has been raised about fibrin glue and the potential to cause apoptosis among chondrolineage cells *(10)*. However, our experiments have demonstrated that fibrin glue acts as a chemoattractant to chondrocytes, and that cells from the chondrocyte lineage penetrate the fibrin glue with time (Fig. 3). Although the morphology of cells changes as it penetrates the fibrin glue, they retain the chondrocyte phenotype *(11)*.

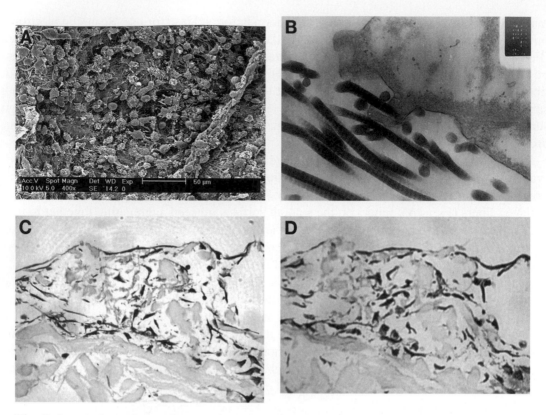

Fig. 2. Integration of chondrocytes into the ACI-Maix collagen membrane. Scanning electron micrographic (SEM) imaging of the membrane evidences the differentiated globular chondrocyte appearance and attachment to the collagen fibers of the membrane (**A**). S-100 positive staining proves that the integrated cells within the collagen matrix are chondrolineage (**C**) and illustrates their distribution throughout the membrane (25× magnification). Transmission electron micrographic (TEM) imaging of chondrocyte attachment with the membrane (**B**) showing the presence of cytoplasmic projections anchoring cells to the collagen fibers of the membrane (15,000× magnification). Staining of the chondrocyte-seeded membrane for type II collagen (**D**) is positive, indicating that the synthesis of collagenous matrix in the seeded membrane is active prior to implantation.

SURGICAL PROCEDURES AND POSTOPERATIVE CARE

Harvesting of Cartilage

Biopsy harvesting of cartilage can be performed as day surgery. Arthroscopically, a cartilage chip about 5 mm long is excised from the nonweight-bearing supracondylar region of the femoral condyles of the operative knee, placed into serum-free nutrient medium, and transported to good manufacturing practice culture laboratories. A biopsy of 50–100 mg should contain about 100,000–200,000 cells, to be expanded to approx 12 million cells over 4–6 wk of cultivation. After acceptable cell density is achieved in vitro, cells are seeded onto a type I/III collagen membrane and transported for implantation.

Surgical Technique

For contained defects, the defect site is accessed via a parapatellar arthrotomy approach in a tourniquet-controlled field. If an additional realignment of ligament reconstruction is

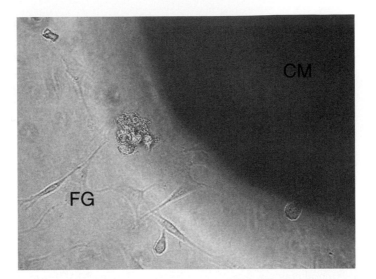

Fig. 3. Chondrocyte migration from the ACI-Maix collagen membrane (CM) into fibrin glue (FG) at 15 d in vitro.

required, then the surgical approach is modified. Access to the tibia is challenging with an open procedure, a possible arthroscopic approach has been reported *(12)*. Contained defects are thoroughly curetted to remove native fibrous tissue buildup and define vertical defect walls, ideally composed of normal native cartilage. Persistent bleeding is occasionally troublesome, but hemostasis can be achieved with a thin layer of fibrin sealant and direct pressure.

Once membranes are correctly shaped to match defect geometry, a thin layer of fibrin glue (Baxter AG, Vienna, Austria) is injected into the defect bed. Once the fibrin sealant foundations are laid, the shaped membrane is transferred to the defect. The seeded membrane is then press-fit into the defect, and the membrane–cartilage interface is sealed with minimal fibrin sealant to optimize surface continuity. The periphery of the membrane is everted to juxtapose the vertical wall of contained defects, presenting cells to the cartilage-graft interface to facilitate chondral union. Excess surface fibrin glue is meticulously excised. The joint is put through a full range of movement 5–10 times prior to closure to ensure implant stability. Should the membrane appear unstable, sutures may be used to assist fixation. Figure 4 shows the MACI graft after surgery.

The same surgical technique is used in uncontained defects, such as osteochondritis dissecans lesions. Bone graft has not been used in defects greater than 1 cm deep, but progressive growth and formation of the subchondral bone plate has been seen in such defects. Osteoarthritic patient grafts are routinely peripherally fixed with resorbable anchors. Opposing defects should not be grafted simultaneously as the two grafts tend to adhere to each other and dislodge; however, multiple nonopposing defects may be grafted at one surgery (Fig. 4).

Postoperative Care

Continuous passive motion is commenced 1 d after surgery, and the patients are gradually returned to weight-bearing activity over the ensuing months by participation in a graduated rehabilitation program designed specifically for ACI.

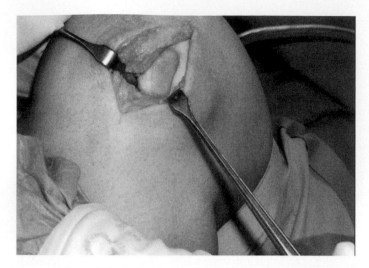

Fig. 4. Medial femoral condyle defect immediately following MACI graft implantation.

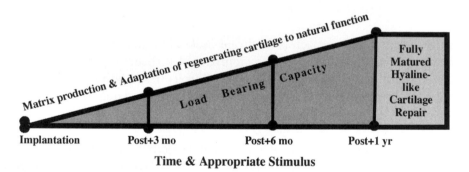
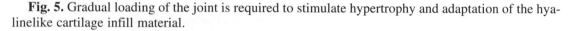

Time & Appropriate Stimulus

Fig. 5. Gradual loading of the joint is required to stimulate hypertrophy and adaptation of the hyalinelike cartilage infill material.

To prepare patients both physically and mentally for the rigors of surgery and the lengthy postoperative recovery, rehabilitation started prior to surgery. Following surgery, patients underwent an intensive specialized rehabilitation program that underpinned the chondrocyte maturation process (Fig. 5). Patients were required to protect their repair from full weight-bearing stresses and were restricted to toe-touch ambulation with two crutches for the first 6 wk postoperatively.

Over the following 6 wk, a stepwise increase in weight bearing occurred, so that by 12 wk postsurgery, patients were ready to fully bear their own weight. At the 12-wk time-point, compressive and decompressive forces provided by full weight bearing further stimulated the chondrocytes to synthesize the correct matrix molecules.

Return to work, sport, and recreational activities was carefully controlled, however, and progressed gradually. Although the cartilage defect may well have been filled with hyaline-type cartilage within the first few months, it was deemed ill advised to undertake stressful joint extension or weight-bearing activities, such as squats or running, before 9–12 mo, depending on defect characteristics.

Table 1
Patient Demographics

Mean age 38 yr (13–67 yr)
Male:female ratio 28:15
Mean height 174.14 cm (154–190 cm)
Mean weight 78.64 kg (47–108 kg)

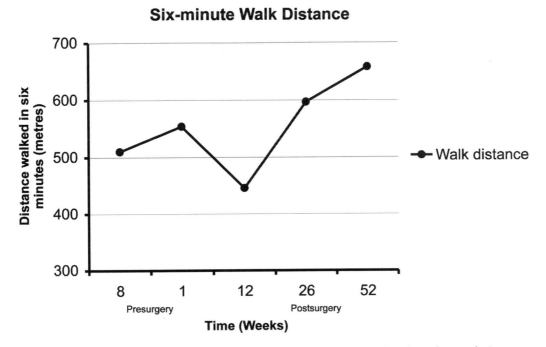

Fig. 6. Six-minute walk assessment of MACI patients ($n = 14$ at 1-yr time-point).

Clinical Assessment of MACI

A consecutive series of 43 implantations was made in 40 patients aged between 13 and 67 yr (Table 1). All patients were suffering from full-thickness chondral lesions between 1.5 and 10 cm². Those patients with established osteoarthritis were considered a separate, more complex group. All patients had an acceptable body mass index. Joint instability or malalignment was corrected at the time of implantation. Auxiliary procedures included patellar realignment, anterior cruciate ligament reconstruction, and corrective proximal tibial osteotomy.

Functional Outcome

There are many functional assessment protocols for the cartilage repair. A simple test of functional outcome has proved to be the 6-min walk test: The distance covered showed a non-significant improvement during preoperative rehabilitation, which naturally diminished around the time of surgery. Our study of 45 MACI patients showed that the distance covered rose to significantly above preoperative levels by 6 mo and continued to improve to 1 yr (Fig. 6).

In addition, other functional assessment showed that the average knee injury and osteoarthritis outcome score (KOOS) for all parameters improved significantly by 1 yr ($p < 0.05$) (Fig. 7).

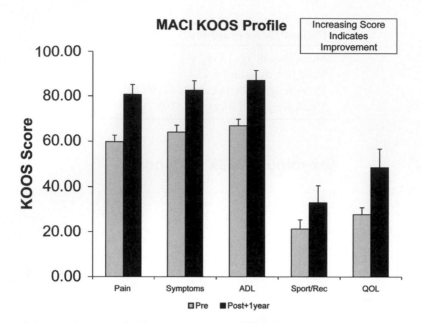

Fig. 7. Knee injury and osteoarthritis outcome score (KOOS) assessment of MACI patients ($n = 14$ at 1-yr time-point). ADL, activities of daily living; QOL, knee-related quality of life.

Arthroscopic and biopsy assessment of regenerative tissue following ACI are reliable indicators of surgical success. However, patient consent for biopsy is rare, and both are undesirable given the invasiveness of the procedure. Magnetic resonance imaging (MRI) is considered to be the best assessment option for ACI when histological assessment is not possible *(13–17)*. MRI usually assesses cartilage repair by defect fill, signal intensity of repair site compared to adjacent native cartilage, effusion, and bone marrow edema underneath the graft site. Furthermore, MRI has been shown to correlate with histology of biopsied specimens following ACI *(15–17)*. Sequential MRIs have been conducted preoperatively, then at 3 mo and 1 yr postoperatively.

Our study based on 43 patients with MACI indicated that, at postoperative MRI scans at 3 mo, there was edematous tissue at the defect sites, contrasting with the fluid-filled defects seen preoperatively. MRI scans at 1 yr show similar to full-thickness hyalinelike tissue infill in 60% of patients, partial-thickness hyalinelike tissue infill in 30% of patients, and a thin cover of hyalinelike tissue in 10% of patients assessed at the 1-yr time-point (Figs. 8 and 9).

Histological Outcome

Various other studies have reported on histological outcomes subsequent to the implantation of autologous chondrocytes in patients *(1,6,15,18)*. ACI using periosteum has consistently reported more than 65% hyalinelike cartilage regeneration (80% in Brittberg's group), with the remainder comprised of fibrocartilage or a fibro-/hyaline cartilage hybrid tissue *(1,15,18)*. Richardson et al. noted that fibrocartilage tissue outcome is always consistent with positive type II collagen results, suggesting a hyalinelike matrix production in these fibroblasticlike cells *(18)*. Briggs et al. have documented 57% good-to-excellent results with hyalinelike cartilage regeneration after ACI using collagen membrane *(6)*. Similar to the previous studies, Briggs et al. noted that all fibrocartilage outcomes were type II collagen positive and

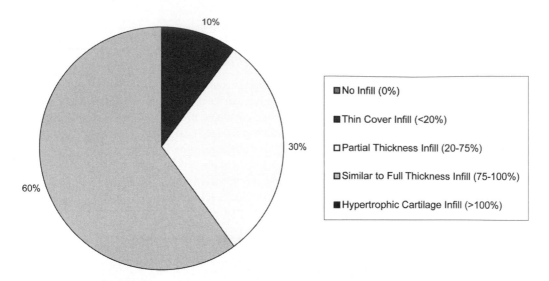

Legend:
- ■ No Infill (0%)
- ■ Thin Cover Infill (<20%)
- □ Partial Thickness Infill (20-75%)
- ■ Similar to Full Thickness Infill (75-100%)
- ■ Hypertrophic Cartilage Infill (>100%)

Fig. 8. Magnetic resonance imaging outcomes 1 yr following MACI surgery for medial femoral condyle (MFC) lesions.

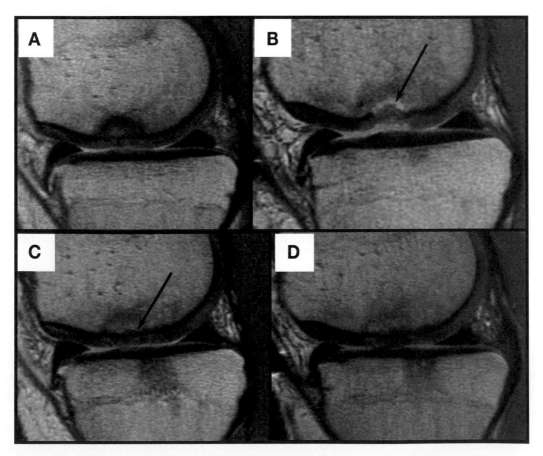

Fig. 9. Magnetic resonance imaging following MACI surgery: **(A)** preoperative; **(B)** 3 mo postsurgery; **(C)** 1 yr postsurgery; **(D)** 2 yr postsurgery.

Table 2
Histology of Patient Biopsies at Different Time-Points

Patient	Time of Biopsy	Histological Appearance
1	48 h	Chondrolineage cells mixed with fibrin glue
2	21 d	Cartilagelike matrix mixed with mesenchymal tissue
3	6 mo	Hyalinelike cartilage, high cell density, type II collagen +
4	8 mo	Hyalinelike cartilage, type II collagen +
5	12 mo I	Hyalinelike cartilage, type II collagen +
6	12 mo II	Hyalinelike cartilage, type II collagen +
7	12 mo III	Mix of hyalinelike and fibrocartilage
8	18 mo	Hyalinelike cartilage, type II collagen +

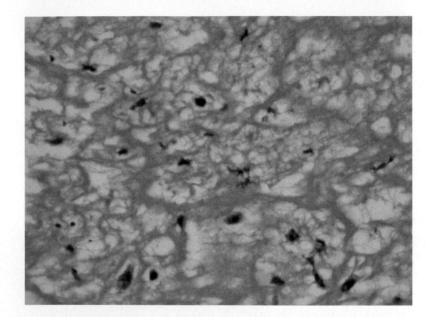

Fig. 10. Histology micrograph of regenerative tissue 48 hr postoperatively. Spherical chondrocytes and some spindle-shaped cells were seen within the transitional zone of the regenerative tissue (hematoxylin and eosin stain; 200×).

noted fibrous tissue repair in two cases. Although conventional ACI also produces hyaline-like tissue regeneration, all outcome evaluation has been conducted beyond 1 yr postoperatively, leaving questions relating to the time frame of regeneration.

Similarly, MACI has been shown to form hyalinelike repair cartilage regeneration up to 2 yr following surgery. Biopsies at 48 h, 21 d, 6, 8, 12, and 24 mo after MACI treatment in respective patients showed a steady progression of the regenerating tissue toward the formation of hyaline cartilage. Table 2 outlines the basic histological outcomes of biopsies at each time-point.

At 48 h, the repair tissue was observed to be a mix of spindle-shaped to round chondrolineage cells scattered among their fibrin glue housing, with no obvious cartilage matrix formation evidenced (Fig. 10). It appears that most chondrolineage cells have already migrated out of the collagen scaffold into the fibrin glue matrix; in some areas, chondrolineage cells are already diffusely distributed within the fibrin glue matrix.

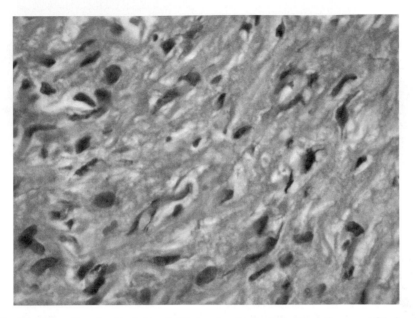

Fig. 11. The high density of cells through fibrin glue in the transitional zone at 21 d, with evidence of matrix formation at high power (hematoxylin and eosin stain; 200×).

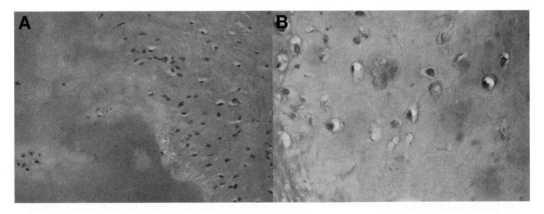

Fig. 12. Histology of hyalinelike regeneration of a patient at 6 mo postoperatively. **(A)** At the base of the defect, the regenerative tissue was seen to integrate well with the healthy tissue at the defect interface (hematoxylin and eosin stain; 100×). **(B)** Hyalinelike cartilage was seen in the intermediate zone of the regenerative tissue, with mature chondrocytes visible within their hyalinelike matrix (hematoxylin and eosin stain; 200×).

After 21 d, a heterologous mix of cartilagelike matrix within mesenchymal tissue in the biopsied defect tissue was noted (Fig. 11). Cells located within foci of cartilagelike matrix appear round and resemble chondrocytes, whereas cells within the mesenchymal tissue matrix appear more elongated and contain large nuclei characteristic of mesenchymal cells (Fig. 11).

At 6 mo, biopsies showed hyalinelike cartilage morphologic features, with chondrocytes within matured lacunae and zonal cellular organization similar to that of healthy tissue (Fig. 12). Also, chondrocytes were noted to be at very high density within collagen II-positive

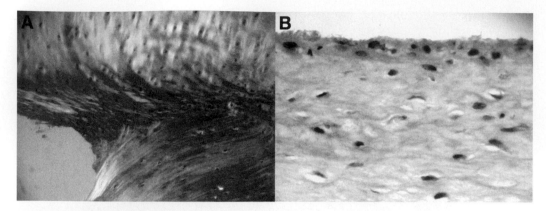

Fig. 13. Histology at 8 mo illustrates cartilage regeneration. (**A**) Polarized imaging demonstrates the integration of collagen fibers from the regenerative tissue into the subchondral bone (hematoxylin and eosin stain; 40×). (**B**) Spindle-shaped chondrocytes can be seen in the superficial layer. Collagen fibers were also observed. (Hematoxylin and eosin stain; 200×.)

matrix. Regenerative tissue integrated well with the native cartilage for the provision of stable biomechanics (Fig. 12A). Cellular morphology of chondrocytes within the matrix regions ranged from spherical to spindle shaped, and most cells were individual to their surrounding matrix rather than in clusters (Fig. 12B).

At 8 mo, hyaline to hyalinelike cartilage tissue was seen (Fig. 13). Polarized imaging demonstrated excellent integration of deep zone collagen fibers into the subchondral bone collagen matrix (Fig. 13A). Chondrocytes exhibit columnar arrangements or clusters within the matrix, arranging mainly as spindle-shaped cells in the superficial zone (Fig. 13B), and round chondrocytes within their lacunae in the deeper zones. Large amounts of collagen fibrils were still obvious in the intermediate zone, but the matrix produced by chondrocytes in the deep zone was mainly hyaline cartilage. It is noteworthy that a small amount of fibrin glue remained within the matrix of the transitional cartilage zone in this patient.

At 12 mo, one of three biopsies displayed hyalinelike cartilage with fibrocartilage, whereas the existing two cases displayed uniformly characteristic hyalinelike cartilage regeneration tissue throughout, with good tissue infiltration of the subchondral bone. Figure 14 shows the mix of hyaline-like and fibrocartilage regeneration by MACI. The superficial layer of the regenerated cartilage in both cases contained elongated chondrocytes and displayed a very smooth surface, similar to the 8-mo histology. Distribution of chondrocytes in both these cases was a mix of columnar organization and clusters. Type II collagen matrix production at 12 mo (Fig. 14B) was also similar to that of healthy hyaline articular cartilage compared to native staining. In one of three cases, residual implanted collagen was seen in the cartilage matrix, but no inflammatory response or lymphocytic infiltration was observed. In the region where fibrocartilage forms, no obvious tide mark was observed (Fig. 14C). The 18-mo histology (data not shown) and type II collagen where identical to those at 12 mo.

COMPLICATIONS

There has been one complication directly related to the surgical process: a graft detachment. This problem was successfully treated with a second procedure 3 d following the initial implantation. There were also postoperative complications in five patients: one deep vein

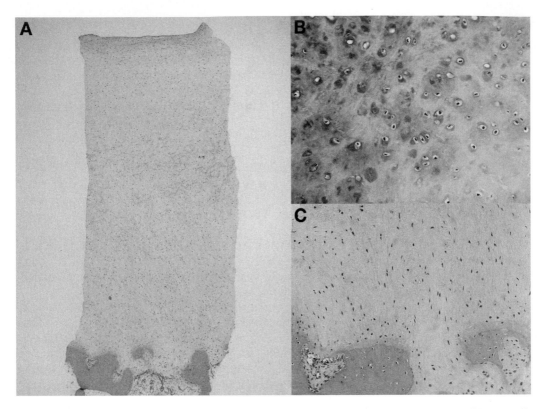

Fig. 14. Biopsy histology at 12 mo postoperatively. **(A)** Mix of hyalinelike and fibro-cartilage regenerated cartilage can be seen at low magnification (hematoxylin and eosin stain; 25×). **(B)** Moreover, higher magnification with immunohistochemistry (monoclonal antihuman type II collagen mouse immunoglobulin G) exhibits the spherical cellular morphology and positive collagen II staining of the regenerative tissue (100×). **(C)** No tide mark was observed in the fibro cartilage region. (Hematoxylin and eosin stain; 100×.)

thrombosis, a hemarthrosis, and three cases of superficial wound infection, which were successfully treated with antibiotics.

CONCLUSION

MACI is a convenient system of cell delivery, with chondrocytes seeded onto a collagen membrane in the laboratory prior to implantation. The simple surgical technique obviates periosteal harvest, is usually suture free, and is less invasive than traditional methods. Early mobilization of the joint is safe, and staged rehabilitation is routine. The indications for use of this convenient technique may be expanded to include osteoarthritis defects, although opposing areas cannot be grafted simultaneously.

ACKNOWLEDGMENTS

Unless otherwise specified, the data given in this review are based on work carried out at the University of Western Australia.

We would like to acknowledge Tim Ackland and Brett Robertson in relation to the rehabilitation section.

REFERENCES

1. Brittberg M, Lindahl A, Nilsson A, Ohlsson C, Isaksson O, Peterson L. Treatment of deep cartilage defects in the knee with autologous chondrocyte transplantation. N Engl J Med 1994;331:889–895.
2. King PJ, Bryant T, Minas T. Autologous chondrocyte implantation for chondral defects of the knee: indications and technique. J Knee Surg 2002;15:177–184.
3. Minas T, Nehrer S. Current concepts in the treatment of articular cartilage defects. Orthopedics 1997;20:525–538.
4. Driesang IM, Hunziker EB. Delamination rates of tissue flaps in articular cartilage repair. J Orthop Res 2000;18:909–911.
5. Ueno T, Kagawa T, Mizukawa N, Nakamura H, Sugahara T, Yamamoto T. Cellular origin of endochondral ossification from grafted periosteum. Anat Rec 2001;264:348–357.
6. Briggs TWR, Mahroof S, David LA, Flannelly J, Pringle J, Bayliss M. Histological evaluation of chondral defects after autologous chondrocyte implantation of the knee. J Bone Joint Surg 2003;85-B:1077–1083.
7. Cherubino P, Grassi FA, Bulgheroni P, Ronga M. Autologous chondrocyte implantation using a bilayer collagen membrane. J Orthop Surg 2003;11:10–15.
8. Zheng MH, King E, Kirilak Y, et al. Molecular characterization of chondrocytes in autologous chondrocyte implantation. Int J Mol Med 2004;13:623–628.
9. Brittberg M, Sjogren-Jansson E, Lindahl A, Peterson L. Influence of fibrin sealant (Tisseel) on osteochondral defect repair in the rabbit knee. Biomaterials 1997;18:235–242.
10. Benya PD, Shaffer JD. Dedifferentiated chondrocytes re-express the differentiated collagen phenotype when cultured in agarose gels. Cell 1982;30:215–224.
11. Kirilak Y, Pavlos NJ, Willers CR, et al. Fibrin sealant promotes migration and proliferation of human articular chondrocytes: possible involvement of thrombin and protease-activated receptors. Int J Mol Med 2006;17(4):551–558.
12. Ronga M, Grassi FA, Bulgheroni P. Arthroscopic autologous chondrocyte implantation for the treatment of a chondral defect in the tibial plateau of the knee. Arthroscopy 2004;20(1):79–84.
13. Bachmann G, Basad E, Lommel D, Steinmeyer J. MRI in the follow-up of matrix-supported autologous chondrocyte transplantation (MACI) and microfracture. Radiologe 2004;44:773–782.
14. Chung CB, Frank LR, Resnick D. Cartilage imaging techniques: current clinical applications and state of the art imaging. Clin Orthop Relat Res. 2001;(391 suppl):S370–S378.
15. Henderson IJ, Tuy B, Connell D, Oakes B, Hettwer WH. Prospective clinical study of autologous chondrocyte implantation and correlation with MRI at 3 and 12 mo. J Bone Joint Surg Br 2003;85:1060–1066.
16. Marlovits S, Striessnig G, Kutscha-Lissberg F, et al. Early postoperative adherence of matrix-induced autologous chondrocyte implantation for the treatment of full-thickness cartilage defects of the femoral condyle. Knee Surg Sports Traumatol Arthrosc, October 2004, p. 20.
17. Roberts S, McCall IW, Darby AJ, et al. Autologous chondrocyte implantation for cartilage repair: monitoring its success by magnetic resonance imaging and histology. Arthritis Res Ther 2003;5:R60–R73.
18. Richardson JB, Caterson B, Evans EH, Ashton BA, Roberts S. Repair of human articular cartilage after implantation of autologous chondrocytes. J Bone Joint Surg Br 1999;81B:1064–1068.

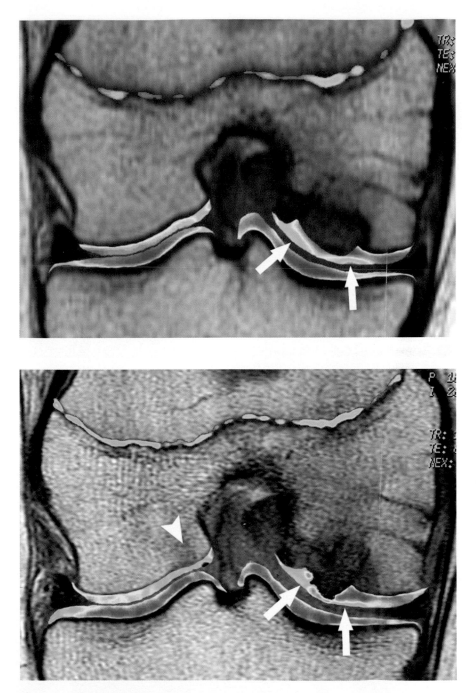

Color Plate 1 Coronal T2 relaxation time maps of the femorotibial articular cartilage of a 13-yr-old girl with osteochondritis dissecans (OCD). (Fig. 11A,B, Chapter 3; *see* complete caption on p. 31 and discussion on p. 30.)

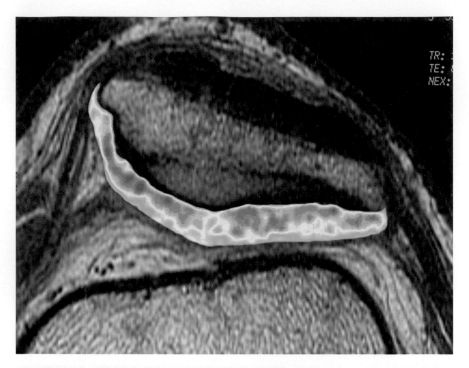

Color Plate 2 Axial T2 relaxation time map from a 27-yr-old man with chronic patellofemoral overload. (Fig. 6, Chapter 3; *see* complete caption p. 26 and discussion on p. 25.)

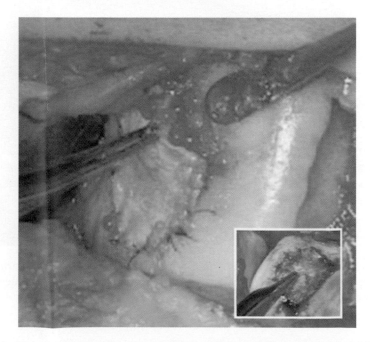

Color Plate 3 (Fig. 4, Chapter 14; *see* complete caption and discussion on p. 226.)

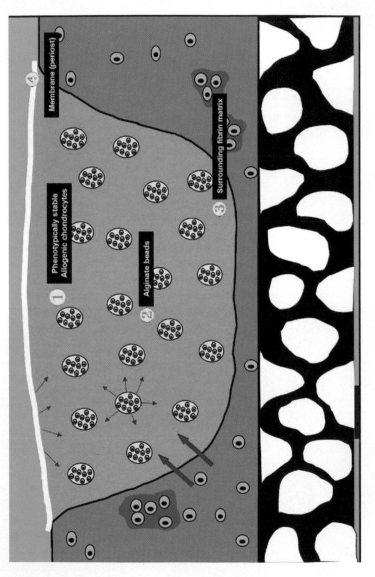

Color Plate 4 The allogeneic chondrocyte-alginate-fibrin concept. (Fig. 1, Chapter 14; *see* complete caption on p. 221 and discussion on p. 220.)

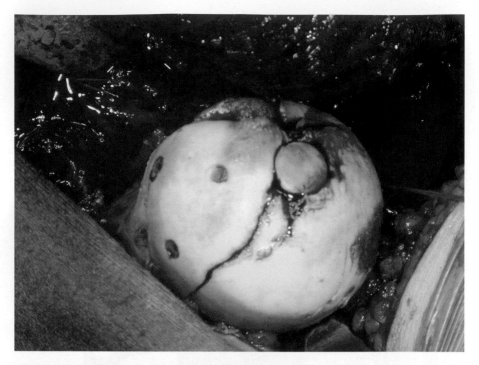

Color Plate 5 Autogenous osteochondral transfer in the hip: view of the femoral head following fixation of the major fragment and delivery of the osteochondral plug. (Fig. 5B, Chapter 19; *see* complete caption on p. 320 and discussion on p. 319.)

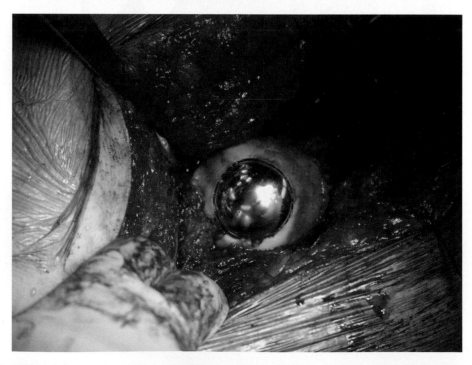

Color Plate 6 Conventional hip replacement: partial resurfacing implant. (Fig. 6B, Chapter 19; *see* complete caption and discussion on pp. 320–321.)

13

Cell-Based Cartilage Repair Using the Hyalograft Transplant

Maurilio Marcacci, MD, Elizaveta Kon, MD,
Stefano Zaffagnini, MD, Leonardo Marchesini Reggiani, MD,
Maria Pia Neri, MD, and Francesco Iacono, MD

Summary

Autologous chondrocyte implantation (ACI) is an effective means of treating symptomatic articular cartilage defects. This two-stage cartilage repair strategy relies on the cultured expansion of harvested chondrocytes; these cells are subsequently reimplanted into the host defect and covered (periosteum, collagen patch). The ACI technique has been shown by many authors to result in improved clinical outcomes by facilitating the creation of a hyaline-like cartilage repair tissue. However, it has been demonstrated that defect fill can be variable, and that the procedure itself is technically demanding. Over the past few years, so called "second generation" ACI techniques have been available for clinical use in many parts of the world. These second generation techniques rely on the combination of autologous chondrocytes with absorbable scaffolds. It is believed that the addition of a stable matrix scaffold facilitates the creation of a more hyaline-like cartilage repair tissue. We describe, herein, such a technique. The Hyalograft C implant has been used to treat symptomatic cartilage defects at our institution for many years. This implant consists of autologous chondrocytes that are seeded on a hyaluronan-based scaffold. Implantation of the Hyalograft C scaffold simplifies the method by which autologous chondrocytes may be used to repair a cartilage defect. Moreover, we believe this is the first method by which autologous chondrocytes may be implanted using minimally invasive arthroscopic techniques. The Hyalograft C implant effectively treats symptomatic cartilage defects in a manner that is less morbid, simpler, and more predictable than first-generation ACI methods.

Key Words: Arthroscopy; autologous chondrocyte implantation; cartilage; cell therapy; chondrocyte; hyaluronan, Hyalograft.

The incidence of articular cartilage lesions has grown because of a marked increase in sports participation and greater emphasis on physical activity in all age groups worldwide. The functional expectation of patients following treatment for such cartilage lesions have risen as well. Curl et al. *(1)* found a 63% incidence of chondral lesions in a survey of 31,516 knee arthroscopies. Articular cartilage lesions are difficult to treat because of the avascular structure of the cartilage matrix. In the Curl et al. series *(1)*, grade IV lesions were noted in 20% of patients, and only 35% had no accompanying meniscal or ligamentous lesions. It is therefore difficult to determine which tissue injury is responsible for a given patient's symptoms.

Options for the treatment of cartilage lesions are numerous and fall into one of two broad categories: reparative and regenerative. Reparative treatments are directed to the local recruitment

From: *Cartilage Repair Strategies*
Edited by: Riley J. Williams © Humana Press Inc., Totowa, NJ

of bone marrow cells to the cartilage lesion to facilitate the creation of repair tissue. Marrow stimulation techniques promote the migration of stem cells from the marrow cavity to the fibrin clot that is created in the defect following such procedures *(2)*. However, these treatment options, which include abrasion arthroplasty, drilling, and the microfracture technique, tend to produce a predominantly fibrocartilaginous repair tissue that is composed mostly of type I collagen, fibrocytes, and unorganized matrix *(2,3)*. Such repair tissue lacks the biomechanical and viscoelastic characteristics of normal hyaline cartilage and may be predisposed to degeneration on exposure to typical joint reactive forces over the long term *(2,4)*.

Steadman et al. *(5)* reported highly satisfactory results at 11-yr follow-up with the microfracture technique, but patients had to adjust their activity level to that of the affected knee. The authors stressed the importance of a meticulous postoperative program that included the use of continuous passive motion (CPM) and 8 wk of restricted weight bearing. The microfracture technique is simple and can be used in small lesions or in wide degenerative lesions. However, the repair tissue response can be variable and unpredictable. Nehrer et al. *(6)* frequently found soft, spongiform, fibrous tissue combined with central degeneration in the treated cartilage defect following the microfracture technique. Moreover, clinical failure was observed at an average follow-up of 21 mo.

More reconstructive surgical treatments have been developed, such as osteochondral autograft transfer as proposed by Hangody et al. *(7)* and mosaicplasty *(8)*. These procedures are technically demanding; the location of the donor site and the size of the harvested grafts play a key role in patient outcome following surgery. Complete defect coverage, the mechanical stability of the plugs, and the restoration of joint surface congruity are difficult to achieve in every case. Moreover, there is limited donor graft availability, which severely reduces the use of this procedure in the treatment of larger lesions.

The cell-based repair strategy was initially put to clinical use of with the development of the autologous chondrocyte implantation (ACI) technique and was pioneered in Sweden in 1987 *(2,9)*. The first clinical report in 1994 demonstrated highly satisfactory results, with biopsy samples showing hyalinelike cartilage. Peterson et al. *(3)* showed that the early results obtained with the ACI technique are long lasting; after 2 yr, 50 of 61 patients had good-to-excellent results. At 5- to 11-yr follow-up, 51 of 61 patients had satisfactory results. Biomechanical evaluation of the grafted area, using an indentation probe, demonstrated stiffness values that were approximatly 90% of normal cartilage measurements. These studies demonstrated that 84–91% of the patients were able to achieve good-to-excellent results and return to active lifestyles. Sgaglione et al. *(10)* suggested that ACI is a safe, effective treatment that should be considered a viable option to restore "normal cartilage" in young patients with cartilage lesions greater than 2 cm^2 and who want to resume an active lifestyle.

A study by Knutsen and colleagues *(11)* prospectively compared microfracture to ACI. This study showed that Lysholm and Visual Analog Scale pain score improved in both groups at 2 yr; Tegner score improved only in the microfracture group. Microfracture had fewer failures and reoperations than ACI. However, biopsies from patients treated with the ACI technique had a better histological quality of the repair tissue compared to tissue retrieved from microfracture patients. This study demonstrated that the first-generation cell-based repair technique (ACI) can successfully restore cartilage tissue in about 85% of cases. However, there are still many biological and technical factors that may negatively influence the clinical outcome of the ACI method. As such there remains room for improving this method by simplifying the cell implantation technique and eliminating the need for the periosteal patch.

Our research efforts have focused on improving the functional efficacy of the ACI technique and reducing the operative morbidity. In the original ACI technique, the liquid chondrocyte suspension is difficult to handle during surgery. The suspension has no structural integrity and requires a patch to hold the cells in position within the defect that is to be treated; a periosteal flap is typically used. Thus, the surgical technique is long, is technically demanding, and requires large joint exposure. These factors increase the morbidity of the ACI method and carry a high risk of joint stiffness and arthrofibrosis. Micheli et al. *(12,13)* reported a reoperation rate of up to 42% following ACI because of joint stiffness or hypertrophic changes of the implanted periosteal graft *(13)*.

When using the liquid cell suspension in ACI, another important concern is whether the chondrocytes will be homogeneously distributed in the three-dimensional space of the defect *(4)*.

In an attempt to avoid these technical problems associated with ACI, we have developed a new cell-based tissue-engineering technology that creates cartilagelike tissue using a three-dimensional culture system. We believe that this second-generation cartilage repair strategy will reduce morbidity, improve cell culture biology, and ultimately improve clinical results.

HYAFF® (FIDIA Advanced Biomaterials, Bologna, Italy) is the class of hyaluronan derivates that is obtained by esterifying the glucoronic acid group with different types of alcohols *(14)*. HYAFF-11®-based scaffolds can be used in skeletal tissue engineering both as a tissue-guiding device and as a delivery vehicle *(15)*. HYAFF-11 (nonwoven matrix) has been extensively characterized in a series of in vitro and in vivo studies, in which it has been shown to support the growth of chondrocytes effectively and to favor the expression of typical chondrocyte markers *(16)*. This three-dimensional scaffold allows the maintenance of a differentiated chondrocyte phenotype during culture and after cell-matrix implantation.

The quality of this scaffold in laboratory tests has been verified in animal studies. In a rabbit model, Grigolo et al. *(15)* demonstrated significant differences in the quality of regenerated cartilage tissue found in defects treated with grafts containing chondrocytes compared to the graft biomaterial alone (no cells). Thus, the efficacy of HYAFF-11-based scaffold for autologous chondrocyte transplantation has a strong preclinical basis in support of its use in the treatment of symptomatic articular cartilage defects.

We have started to use autologous chondrocyte implantation in association with HYAFF to treat symptomatic cartilage lesions. HYAFF possesses handling characteristics; thus, this scaffold can be implanted using a mini-open (limited arthrotomy) or arthroscopic technique *(17)*, and the use of either of these methods largely depends on the location of the defect. The HYAFF scaffold is hydrophilic, and if the HYAFF patch is correctly positioned inside a prepared defect, a tensioactive pressure facilitates a natural fixation of the patch that does not require the use of fibrin glue, sutures, or a periosteal cover. By eliminating the need for a periosteal cover, we were able to develop an arthroscopic implant procedure that simplified this two-stage procedure, reduced morbidity, and improved on the original ACI cell-based repair technique.

SURGICAL TECHNIQUE: HYAFF GRAFT IMPLANTATION

The arthroscopic surgical technique for ACI has two stages: cartilage biopsy and graft implantation. The arthroscopic biopsy of healthy cartilage for cell culture remains mandatory to evaluate the site of the lesion and cartilage quality. During the first surgery, associated problems, including meniscal injury or anterior cruciate ligament (ACL) insuffiency are addressed surgically. A small biopsy of healthy articular cartilage is obtained from the superior

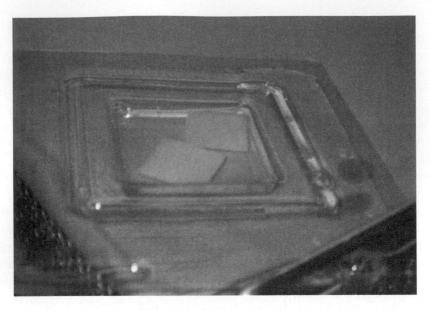

Fig. 1. Scaffold (2 × 2 cm).

femoral trochlea or femoral notch. Chondrocytes from this biopsy are expanded in culture for reimplantation on the HYAFF construct.

Harvesting Technique

A 100-mg cartilage biopsy was taken from a nonweight-bearing site of the articular surface (intercondylar notch) and sent to the processing center in a serum-free nutritional medium. The following day, the tissue was minced into smaller pieces and digested with 0.25% trypsin at 37°C for 15 min and then with 300 U/mL collagenase type II (Worthington, Lakewood, NJ) at 37°C for 4 h in Ham's F12. The digested material was centrifuged at 1000 rpm for 10 min, and the pellet was resuspended in Ham's F12 containing 10% fetal calf serum (Sigma, St. Louis, MO), 1% penicillin-streptomycin, 1% l-glutamine, 1 ng/mL transforming growth factor-α1, 1 ng/mL insulin, 1 ng/mL epidermal growth factor, and 10 ng/mL basic fibroblast growth factor (all growth factors were recombinant and of human sequence).

Typically, from 200 mg of tissue, we recovered 1–2 million cells. Cells were amplified in monolayer cultures up to three passages, then they were seeded onto HYAFF-11 scaffolds (2 × 2 cm). We suspended 8×10^6 cells in 0.4 mL medium (as above, but containing 50 mg/mL ascorbic acid); the cell suspension was pipeted onto the scaffold, and the culture was kept at 37°C, 5% $CO2$ overnight. The next day, additional medium was added to submerge the cell construct completely; medium was changed twice a week. Hyalograft C® (FIDIA Advanced Biomaterials) chondrocyte cultures are ready for shipment after 2 wk in culture. The day of shipment, the cell construct is washed exhaustively with phosphate-buffered saline, then sealed in a sterile plastic tray containing 4 mL nutritional medium (Fig. 1). The expiry time of the product is 72 h.

Open Technique

The open surgical technique includes a mini-arthrotomy, the defect preparation, the graft sizing, and successive implantation of the autologous chondrocyte culture graft. The exposure

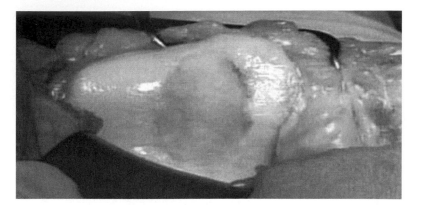

Fig. 2. Cartilage lesion of patella covered by Hyalograft C stamp.

dimension depends on the size and the location of the defect: a medial parapatellar incision for defects of the medial compartment and a lateral parapatellar exposure for lateral locations.

Complete visualization of the defect is necessary for easy preparation of the defect. The subchondral bone must be exposed, removing all damaged cartilage without damaging the subchondral layer. The subchondral bone has to be exposed, avoiding any lesion, to maintain the hemostasis in the defect area. It is fundamental to leave a sharp rim of healthy cartilage all around the defect area. The defect is then measured, and Hyalograft C graft is prepared to match the defect dimensions. The graft must be completely inside the margins of the defect to guarantee stability of the graft and avoid any possible mobilization (Fig. 2). The graft is then applied in the defect, and its stability is evaluated after cyclic bending of the knee. The wound and skin are then closed in standard manner.

ARTHROSCOPIC TECHNIQUE

The arthroscopic implant was originally developed for medial or lateral condyle lesions. With our improving expertise, we are now able to address almost every knee surface with a grade IV defect.

After the HYAFF graft construct has been seeded with chondrocytes, it is forwarded to the surgeon for implantation. A second arthroscopic procedure is then performed. At this time, the lesion is visualized and debrided to a stable rim using a motorized shaver. All unstable cartilage flaps are removed; all fibrous tissue is also removed from the base of the defect. A tourniquet may be needed at this point to prevent bleeding at the defect site as blood is toxic to articular chondrocytes. The defect is mapped and sized using a delivery device of variable diameter (6.5–8.5 mm) with a sharp edge to achieve the complete coverage of the defect (Fig. 3).

A flipped custom cannula is then inserted in the appropriate portal (anteromedial portal-medial femoral condyle; anterolateral portal-lateral femoral condyle). The cannula facilitates the removal of the fat pad from the camera's view field; this is especially helpful when the knee is positioned in a high degree of flexion. A custom cannulated low-profile drill/reamer (6.5–8.5 mm) is positioned according to the location of the defect (Fig. 4). The drill is maintained in the desired position by a Kirschner guide wire (0.9-mm diameter) that is fixed to bone. This reamer, which has a safety stop at 2 mm, has been developed specifically to avoid deep penetration of the subchondral bone, which must remain intact for successful graft implantation and function. Only the Kirschner wire passes through the subchondral plate. The

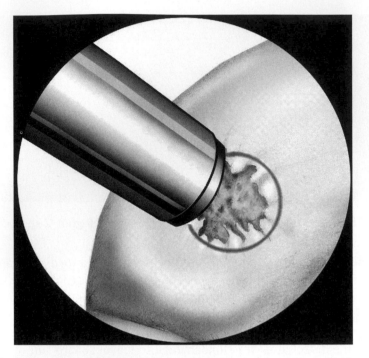

Fig. 3. With the sharp edge of delivery system, the sizing and mapping of lesion is performed.

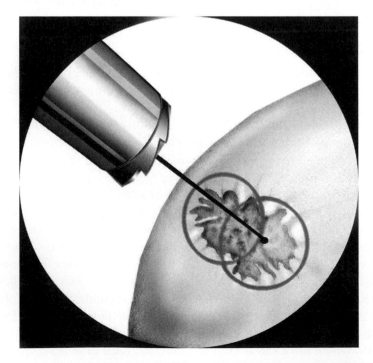

Fig. 4. With a low-profile and slow-speed drill, preparation of the area is performed, avoiding the lesion of the subchondral bone.

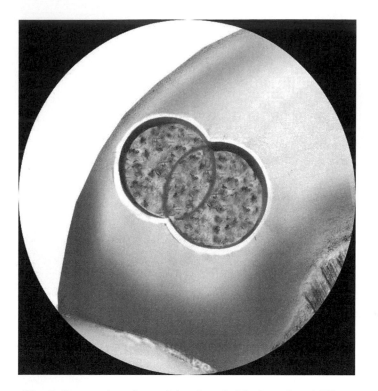

Fig. 5. Prepared surface of the chondral lesion after drilling.

low-speed reaming of the lesion surface creates a circular area with well-defined margins for graft placement (Figs. 5 and 6). This reaming step must be executed carefully to achieve stable and precise lesion contours.

Multiple HYAFF graft disks can be placed to achieve full defect coverage. As such, the reaming step is repeated to prepare the entire defect surface. It is usually possible to prepare a large defect by changing the knee flexion angle and orientation of the cannula.

After reaming, the joint is cleared of cartilage debris. The fluid inflow is then closed, and the joint is dried using suction applied through the cannula. The sharp-edge delivery system is put into contact with the hyaluronic acid (HYAFF) patch containing the autologous chondrocytes. The patch remains in the sheath of the delivery system; the patch is then transported through the cannula and positioned in the prepared defect. A delivery tamp is pushed to plug the patch precisely into the defect. The procedure is repeated until the defect is filled (Figs. 7 and 8).

It is important to cover the prepared lesion maximally without overlapping the margin of the defect with the implanted patches. When placed in such a fashion, the stamps do not move from the defect. This technique has been tested after repeated cycles of joint motion in open arthrotomy cases, with and without tourniquet, utilizing the same device.

The stability of implanted HYAFF patches is evaluated with a probe. The tourniquet is released, and the graft stability is evaluated. If swelling of the patch increases its size in such a way that the graft overlaps the defect margins, then it is possible to place a 6.5-mm patch into a prepared 8.5-mm diameter area. Although the entire area may not be covered, the graft will remain stable; again, it is important to avoid multiple overlapping of multiple grafts. Mobilization of the implanted patch has not been observed in our series.

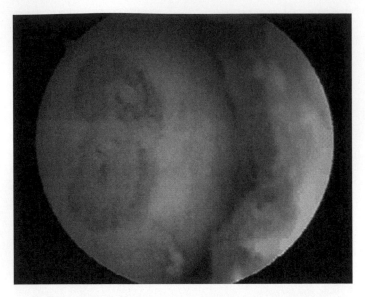

Fig. 6. Arthroscopic view of the lesion after drilling.

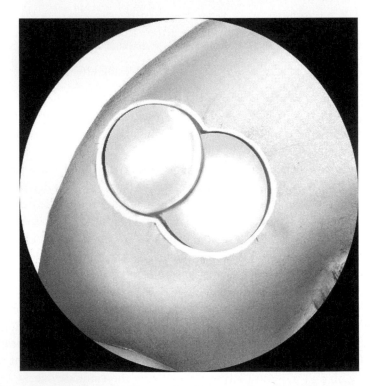

Fig. 7. Complete coverage of the defect by two implanted patches after irrigation removal from the joint.

REHABILITATION PROTOCOL

Following surgery, patients are discharged 1 d after the arthroscopic implantation procedure. In the first 2 wk after surgery, CPM is started (0–90°) on the second postoperative day to promote defect healing and joint nutrition and to prevent the development of adhesions.

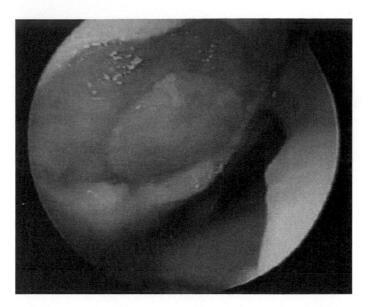

Fig. 8. Arthroscopic view of the lesion covered by tree patches of Hyalograft C.

Lower extremity stretching exercise and quadriceps contractions are allowed if tolerated. Toe-touch weight bearing is permitted during the first 4 wk following surgery. From weeks 4 to 5, weight bearing is increased gradually. Gait training in a swimming pool facilitates the recovery of normal gait phases. Muscle strengthening exercises are started at week 7. Increased strength and functional exercise are then gradually allowed. Return to sports involving contact should not be attempted before 10–12 mo.

Initial Phase (Weeks 1–3)

The initial phase starts with CPM with a range of motion of 10° and 40° to promote joint nutrition and prevent intra-articular adhesions. The range is slowly increased to 0–60° when it is accepted by the patient. Unload the operated leg with two crutches, allowing foot-touch weight bearing only. After 3 wk, the load may be increased.

Transition Phase (Weeks 4–5)

The transition phase starts with functional training with exercises, gradually increasing weight bearing in a controlled way (closed-chain exercises). Start stationary cycling with low resistance in the beginning. Start in a pool, increasing mobility and muscle strength in a controlled way. Start walking between bars and straight leg kicks when holding the pool wall. After 4 wk, low weights (1 kg maximum) may be used for straight leg raises if the knee can be fully extended.

Mid-Phase (Weeks 7–12)

Gradually increase weight bearing in walking. Start walking without crutches indoors. Increase functional daily life training. Walking, bicycling, and swimming are recommended.

Final Phase (After 12 Wk)

The same program can be continued. Emphasize those exercises that are similar to activities in daily life at home or at work. After 13 wk, start dynamic strength training and slowly increase. Patients are allowed to run after 5–6 mo; the return to competitive sport at a level that involves sudden change in direction or contact should not be attempted before 12 mo after ACI.

CLINICAL EXPERIENCE

The ACT on HYAFF scaffold has been used in Europe since 1999. At the moment, more than 3000 implants have been performed using a mini-open or arthroscopic technique. At our institution, 158 patients have been treated since 1999. Of these patients, 102 were treated arthroscopically (since November 2000). Following the approval of the Ethical Committee of the Rizzoli Orthopaedic Institute, information on clinical findings and informed consent were obtained.

All patients were clinically evaluated using the International Cartilage Repair Society score preoperatively and at 12, 24, and 36 mo following surgery. We were able to obtain computed tomography scans or magnetic resonance images for all patients at 12, 24, and 36 mo of follow-up.

Among the patients who were treated using the arthroscopic method, we reported on a group of the initial 30 patients (26 male, 4 female) who were the first to reach a minimum 2-yr follow-up interval. Twenty-nine patients presented with isolated symptomatic chondral lesions: 23 medial femoral condyle, 6 lateral femoral condyle lesions. One patient presented with multiple knee lesions (medial condyle and trochlea). All the defects were grade III–IV Outerbridge; the mean size was 2.9 cm^2 (2–4.5 cm^2). The mean age of the patients at time of surgery was 27 yr (17–46 yr). The lesion etiology was traumatic in 19 cases, osteochondritis dissecans in 2 cases, and degenerative (microtraumatic) in 9 cases. Of the 19 traumatic lesions, 9 were treated acutely (within 3 mo after traumatic event) and 10 chronically.

In 18 of the 30 patients, associated procedures were performed during the first-stage cartilage harvesting: 9 ACL reconstructions, 10 partial medial meniscectomies, 2 partial lateral meniscectomies, 2 medial meniscal and 1 lateral meniscal repairs, and 2 autologous bone grafts (patients with osteochondritis dissecans lesions).

Previous surgery in 13 of the 30 patients included 4 meniscectomies; 4 ACL reconstructions; 5 cartilage reparative operations, such as shaving and debridement of chondral lesion; and 2 mosaicplasties.

The evaluation protocol consisted of three assessments. Patients were asked for a subjective evaluation of the knee symptoms and physical function using the International Knee Documentation Committee (IKDC) Subjective Knee Evaluation Form *(18)*. According to this questionnaire, a higher score represents higher levels of function and lower levels of symptoms. Therefore, a score of 100 is interpreted to mean no limitations on daily living activities or sports and the absence of symptoms (IKDC subjective score).

A knee functional test (IKDC objective score) was performed by the surgeon according to the IKDC Knee Examination Form. The lowest ratings in effusion, passive motion deficit, and ligament examination were used to determine the final functional grade of the knee (normal, nearly normal, abnormal, or severely abnormal). Patients were also asked to evaluate their quality of life using the EuroQol EQ-5D questionnaire. This is a recognized assessment of health-related quality of life based on self-care, mobility, usual activities, pain/discomfort, and anxiety/depression dimensions. It includes a 0–100 Visual Analogue Scale (EQ-VAS) for a self-rating of the global health state, in which the 100 value represents the best imaginable health state. No complications related to the implant and no serious adverse events were observed during the treatment and follow-up period.

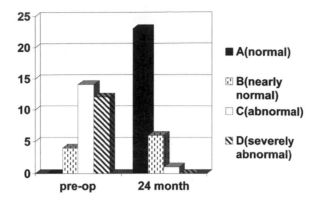

Fig. 9. IKDC scores of patients treated with ACT on the Hyaff® scaffold.

The mean preoperative IKDC subjective score obtained was 41.9 (SD = 15.6); the mean follow-up IKDC subjective scores were 75.9 (SD = 16.0) at 12 mo and 74.2 SD = 17.7) at 24 mo of follow-up. Approximately 97% of the patients experienced a subjective improvement in knee function and symptoms. Only 1 patient (3.3%) reported no improvement following surgery.

According to the IKDC objective evaluation, all the treated patients except 1 displayed knee conditions within the two best categories (normal or nearly normal) at 24-month follow-up (Fig. 9).

At 2-year follow-up, 93.4% of patients experienced an improvement in their quality of life as assessed by the EQ-VAS. Resumption of sport at the same or slightly lower level was obtained in 17 (56.7%) of 30 patients at 12-month follow-up. Eleven patients returned to the sport activity at the lower level. Only 2 patients were not able to return to sports activity by 24 months.

A second-look arthroscopy was performed in 5 patients at 12-month follow-up, and a visual check and probing for consistency of the implanted cartilage demonstrated complete healing of the defect and good quality tissue of regenerated cartilage by gross examination. The biopsy of implanted cartilage was performed in two cases, and the histological evaluation by an independent examiner showed a hyalinelike tissue with good integration within the host tissue.

CONCLUSIONS

The results of our series using Hyalograft C are comparable to the ones of the original ACI technique *(2)*. The clinical and histological results of our first patients after short- to medium-term follow-up are encouraging. Our studies demonstrate the efficiency of the HYAFF graft in improving clinical function in patients with symptomatic cartilage defects. This cell-based repair strategy appears to be free of many of the problems associated with the first-generation ACI techniques.

The arthroscopic method of graft implantation reduces the morbidity of the procedure and decreases recovery time and the length of rehabilitation. Our preliminary results suggest this method may be used for the treatment of large cartilage lesions (there is no limit in size of lesion, but it is important that the lesion is contained), including those in high-demand individuals (i.e., competitive athletes). Long-term studies are still needed to confirm the reliability of this procedure.

This cell-based cartilage repair technique represents a step forward compared to the original ACI technique. We believe that the addition of a scaffold to the ACI methodology will result in more predictable lesion fill and clinical function in treated patients.

ACKNOWLEDGMENTS

The author acknowledges the contributions of A. Montaperto, S. Bassini, A. Visani, G. Bernagozzi, M. Bonfiglioli (Biomechanics Laboratory, Rizzoli Orthopedic Institute, Bologna, Italy).

REFERENCES

1. Curl WW, Krome J, Gordon ES, Rushing J, Smith BP, Poehling GG. Cartilage injuries: a review of 31,516 knee arthroscopies. Arthroscopy 1997;13:456–460.
2. Peterson L, Minas T, Brittberg M, Nilsson A, Sjogren-Jansson E, Lindahl A. Two- to 9-year outcome after autologous chondrocyte transplantation of the knee. Clin Orthop 2000;:212–234.
3. Peterson L, Brittberg M, Kiviranta I, Akerlund EL, Lindahl A. Autologous chondrocyte transplantation. Biomechanics and long-term durability. Am J Sports Med 2002;30:2–12.
4. Ochi M, Uchio Y, Kawasaki K, Wakitani S, Iwasa J. Transplantation of cartilage-like tissue made by tissue engineering in the treatment of cartilage defects of the knee. J Bone Joint Surg Br 2002;84:571–578.
5. Steadman JR, Briggs KK, Rodrigo JJ, Kocher MS, Gill TJ, Rodkey WG. Outcomes of microfracture for traumatic chondral defects of the knee: average 11-year follow-up. Arthroscopy 2003;19:477–484.
6. Nehrer S, Spector M, Minas T. Histologic analysis of tissue after failed cartilage repair procedures. Clin Orthop August 1999;149–162.
7. Hangody L, Kish G, Karpati Z, Udvarhelyi I, Szigeti I, Bely M. Mosaicplasty for the treatment of articular cartilage defects: application in clinical practice. Orthopedics 1998;21:751–756.
8. Bentley G, Biant LC, Carrington RW, et al. A prospective, randomised comparison of autologous chondrocyte implantation vs mosaicplasty for osteochondral defects in the knee. J Bone Joint Surg Br 2003;85:223–230.
9. Brittberg M, Lindahl A, Ohlsson C, Isaksson O, Peterson L. Treatment of deep cartilage defects in the knee with autologous chondrocite transplantation. N Engl J Med 1994;331:889–895.
10. Sgaglione NA, Miniaci A, Gillogly SD, Carter TR. Update on advanced surgical techniques in the treatment of traumatic focal articular cartilage lesions in the knee. Arthroscopy 2002;18(2 suppl 1):9–32.
11. Knutsen G, Engebretsen L, Ludvigsen TC, et al. Autologous chondrocyte implantation compared with microfracture in the knee. A randomized trial. J Bone Joint Surg Am 2004;86: 455–464.
12. Micheli LJ, Browne JE, Erggelet C, et al. Autologous chondrocyte implantation of the knee: multicenter experience and minimum 3-yr follow-up. Clin J Sport Med 2001;11:223–228.
13. Anderson AF, Fu FH, Bert RM, et al. A controlled study of autologous chondrocyte implantation vs microfracture for articular cartilage lesions of the femur. Paper presented at: 70th AAOS Annual Meeting Proceedings; February 5–9, 2003; New Orleans, LA.
14. Campoccia D, Doherty P, Radice M, Brun P, Abatangelo G, Williams DF. Semisynthetic resorbable materials from hyaluronan esterification. Biomaterials 1998;19:2101–2127.
15. Grigolo B, Roseti L, Fiorini M, et al. Transplantation of chondrocytes seeded on a hyaluronan derivative (HYAFF®11) into cartilage defects in rabbits. Biomaterials 2001;22:2417–2424.
16. Brun P, Abatangelo G, Radice M, et al. Chondrocyte aggregation and reorganization into three-dimensional scaffolds. J Biomed Mater Res 1999;46:337–346.
17. Marcacci M, Zaffagnini S, Kon E, Visani A, Iacono F, Loreti I. Arthroscopic autologous chondrocyte transplantation: technical note. Knee Surg Sports Traumatol Arthrosc 2002;10:154–159.
18. ICRS Cartilage Injury Evaluation Package. 2000. Available at: http://www.cartilage.org/ Evaluation_Package/ICRS_Evaluation.pdf. (Accessed Dec., 2006)

14

Allogeneic Chondrocyte-Based Cartilage Repair Using Alginate Beads

Peter C. M. Verdonk, MD, **Karl F. Almqvist,** MD, PhD,
René Verdonk, MD, PhD, **Koenraad L. Verstraete,** MD, PhD,
and Gust Verbruggen, MD, PhD

Summary

We describe the use of enzymatically isolated human allogeneic chondrocytes embedded in an alginate matrix in combination with a periosteal flap for the treatment of chondral and osteochondral lesions. The short-term clinical results illustrate the feasibility and safety of this procedure. This concept essentially involves a one-step surgical transplantation procedure with a well-characterized cell product in a biodegradable matrix; this is hoped to result in an easier and less time-consuming surgical procedure and in a more reproducible clinical and histological outcome than first- and second-generation autologous chondrocyte transplantation.

Key Words: Alginate matrix; allogenic chondrocytes; cartilage defect; cartilage transplantation; knee.

INTRODUCTION

In 1994, the first report on autologous chondrocyte transplantation (ACT), also known as autologous chondrocyte implantation (ACI), was published by Lars Peterson and colleagues *(1)*. Since then, numerous clinical articles have documented the feasibility of this technique for the treatment of symptomatic chondral and osteochondral lesions *(1–5)*. Although only a few long-term and comparative follow-up data are available, the clinical improvement appears to persist for more than 10 yr *(6)*. For defects larger than 2 cm^2, ACT is considered by some to be superior to the microfracture technique because the initial improvement achieved with microfracture probably declines after approx 5 yr.

Several explanations have been proposed to elucidate this difference; the most important is the biochemical and biomechanical consistency and nature of the induced repair tissue. With the microfracture technique, repair tissue is induced by the creation of tiny holes in the subchondral bone plate. Bone marrow-derived mesenchymal stem cells are thus able to enter the articular cartilage defect and differentiate within this defect to fibrocartilagelike repair tissue *(4,7)*. Indeed, microfracture-induced repair tissue is thought to be unable to withstand the mechanical forces within the knee joint over time, therefore leading to degeneration. ACT, on the other hand, has been shown to result in the creation of a hyalinelike repair tissue; this fact could explain its potential to relieve symptoms and improve function for a prolonged period *(1,5,6)*.

From: *Cartilage Repair Strategies*
Edited by: Riley J. Williams © Humana Press Inc., Totowa, NJ

The first-generation ACT as described by Peterson and coworkers uses monolayer-expanded autologous chondrocytes obtained from prior biopsy specimens *(1)*. These chondrocytes are implanted as a cell suspension within the debrided defect under a periosteal flap. However, this has several possible drawbacks, resulting in variability in the presence of hyalinelike repair tissue, hypertrophy of the periosteal patch, and the need for a meticulous and time-consuming surgical procedure.

We believe that this variability is mainly induced by the application of monolayer expansion of the autologous chondrocytes to increase the cell number. Monolayer expansion of human chondrocytes has been shown to induce cell dedifferentiation, resulting in the expression of type I collagen and the progressive decline in the synthesis of type II collagen and aggrecan *(8)*. These last two extracellular molecules are indicative of the stable articular chondrocyte phenotype. It is believed that these monolayer-expanded differentiated chondrocytes regain their original phenotype once implanted into the knee joint and are exposed to the biological and biomechanical local environment. This process is called *redifferentiation* and is seldom completely observed in vitro *(8)*.

Another important variable is the quality of the patient's own cartilage biopsy. Laboratory results have shown an important interpatient variability in the quality and amount of newly synthesized matrix *(8,9)*. The use of well-characterized, quality-controlled allogeneic (allograft donor) chondrocytes might address concerns over the variability of chondrocytes obtained from individual patients.

Furthermore, the need for a biopsy itself requires the patient to undergo an additional surgical procedure to harvest articular cartilage for cellular expansion. This biopsy inflicts additional trauma to the knee articular cartilage; optimally such a procedure would be avoided.

The transplantation of the monolayer-expanded chondrocytes is performed as a cell suspension. To retain the cell suspension within the debrided defect, a periosteal or membrane patch is sutured to the defect edge in a watertight fashion to avoid leakage of cells from the defect. The first-generation ACT procedure is considered to be time consuming and tedious by most orthopedic surgeons. Thus, a technical barrier remains despite the widespread good results that have been reported with ACT. Moreover, transplanting cells as a suspension has been documented to result in variable chondrocyte distribution within the cell defect because of sedimentation of the cells according to gravity *(10)*.

To avoid these drawbacks, we have developed a modification of the ACT technique that is predicated on the use of allogeneic chondrocytes suspended in an alginate matrix (Fig. 1; *see* Color Plate 4, Following p. 206).

THE ALLOGENEIC CHONDROCYTE-ALGINATE-FIBRIN CONCEPT

Alginate Gel

The term *alginate* refers to a family of polyanionic copolymers derived from brown sea algae and comprises 1,4-linked β-D-mannuronic (M) and β-l-guluronic (G) residues in varying proportions. Sodium alginate is soluble in aqueous solutions and forms stable gels at room temperature in the presence of noncytotoxic concentrations of divalent calcium cations through the ionic interaction between the guluronic acid groups. This enables three-dimensional beads to be formed with viable chondrocytes embedded in the gel by crosslinking in noncytotoxic conditions. Furthermore, alginate can be uncrosslinked by

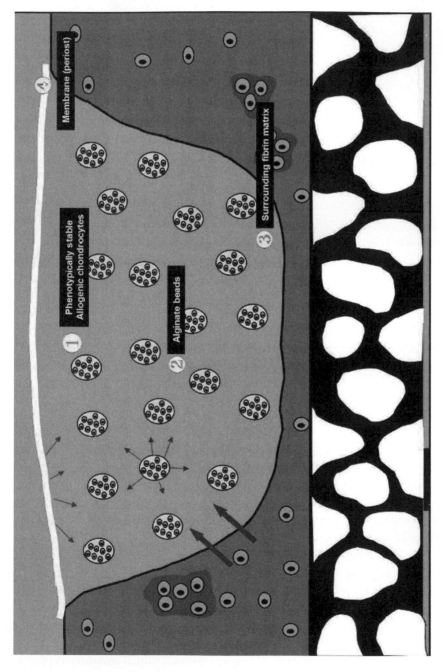

Fig. 1. (Color Plate 3, following p. 206). The allogeneic chondrocyte-alginate-fibrin concept. Allogeneic chondrocytes in alginate beads are delivered to the cartilage defect. The virtual spaces between the beads are filled by fibrin glue. The defect is covered by a periosteal patch. Allogeneic cells can grow out of the beads and colonize the fibrin glue as do periosteal-derived cells and cells derived from the defect edges. Future modifications can include the treatment of defect edges by specific biologicals, the addition of specific biologicals to the alginate matrix, and the omission of the periosteal patch.

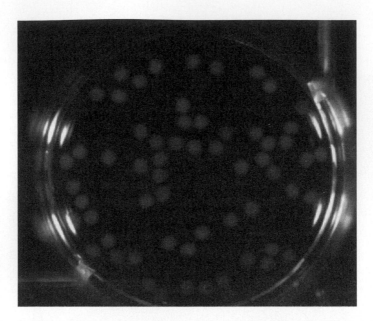

Fig. 2. Allogeneic articular chondrocytes are cultured in alginate beads.

using mild chelating agents, which can release the entrapped cells together with the cell-associated matrix. Calcium crosslinked sodium alginate has been implanted in both animals and humans. A number of animal models have demonstrated the biodegradation of calcium crosslinked alginate in vivo, although large differences in degradation times have been reported *(11)*.

The fact that articular chondrocytes do not dedifferentiate within the biodegradable alginate gels has led to the exploitation of these hydrogels for cartilage tissue engineering *(12)*.

Allogeneic Chondrocytes

Articular cartilage was harvested from the knee joint within 24 h postmortem in accordance with the currently accepted organ transplantation protocol of the hospital and with the approval of the local ethics committee. All donors had died after a short disease and were screened for transmittable diseases. None had received corticosteroids or cytostatic drugs. Human articular chondrocytes were isolated as described elsewhere *(13)* with a few modifications. The cartilage tissue was sampled from the femur condyles, diced in small fragments, and digested in a spinner bottle with a series of enzymatic solutions in Dulbecco's modified Eagle's medium (DMEM; Gibco BRL, Grand Island, NY) with 0.002 M/mL l-glutamine, antibiotics, and antimycotics (Gibco BRL). Cartilage was first treated with 0.25% (w/v) sheep testes hyaluronidase (Sigma, St. Louis, MO) for 120 min and 0.25% Pronase (*Streptomyces griseus* Pronase E; Sigma) for 90 min at 37°C. After an overnight period in DMEM supplemented with 10% autologous serum, a incubation of 3–6 h with 0.25% collagenase (*Clostridium histolyticum*; Sigma) in DMEM containing 10% autologous serum at 37°C resulted in the liberation of isolated cartilage cells. More than 95% of the cells were visible after isolation (Trypan Blue exclusion test). Depending on the condition of the tissue, $50–150 \times 10^6$ chondrocytes could be isolated from femoral condyles of one single donor.

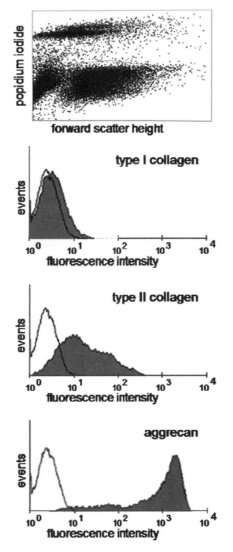

Fig. 3. Quality control by flow cytometric analysis of the extracellular matrix compounds prior to transplantation. The chondrocytes cultured in alginate gel stain positive for type II collagen and aggrecan; type I collagen is absent from the cell-associated matrix. This indicates a stabilized articular chondrocyte phenotype.

Culture of Allogeneic Chondrocytes in Alginate Gel (Fig. 2)

Chondrocyte cultures in alginate beads were prepared as described *(14)* with some modifications (Fig. 2). Chondrocytes suspended in 1 volume double-concentrated Hanks' balanced salts solution (HBSS) without calcium and magnesium (Gibco) were carefully mixed with an equal volume of 2% alginate (low-viscosity alginate from *Macrocystis pyrifera*; Sigma) in HBSS and autoclaved for 15 min. The final cell concentration was 10×10^6 chondrocytes per milliliter in 1% alginate.

The chondrocyte/alginate suspension was then slowly dripped through a 23-gage needle into a 102 mM calcium chloride solution. The beads were allowed to polymerize for 10 min at room temperature. The calcium chloride was then removed; the beads were washed three times with 0.15 M sodium chloride and finally maintained in a six-well plate in 4 mL of 6 DMEM with 10% autologous serum in an incubator at 37°C under 5% CO_2. The nutrient medium was replaced twice weekly. The chondrocytes were cultured for approx 14 d prior to transplantation. This time-period allowed us to check donor serology and to ascertain culture sterility. During this culture period, the chondrocytes assembled an extracellular matrix (ECM) rich in aggrecan and type II collagen. It is believed that this accumulated, dense mantle of ECM is able to inhibit or at least decrease the host's immunological response to these allogeneic cells.

Fibrin Gel

Fibrin gel is malleable, biodegradable, and biocompatible. When used in the implantation procedure, it would permit the temporary scaffold to adhere to the edges of the cartilage lesion, allowing transplant integration. Prior in vitro assays performed in our laboratory showed the outgrowth of articular chondrocytes from the alginate beads into the surrounding fibrin gel *(15)*. Immunohistochemistry showed a strong presence of cells staining for aggrecan and type II collagen in alginate from weeks 1 to 8 and a progressive increase of outgrowing aggrecan and type II collagen-positive cells in the surrounding fibrin gel. From these studies, it was concluded that fibrin-surrounded alginate beads could fulfill the criteria for transplantation: Phenotypically stable allogeneic chondrocytes within an alginate hydrogel can be transplanted into a cartilage defect. The alginate surrounding fibrin will serve as a temporary scaffold to allow these cells to grow out of the alginate beads. Moreover, the fibrin gel could also allow outgrowth of native articular chondrocytes from the defect edges, as well as periosteal chondroprogenitor cells from the overlying periosteal membrane.

CELL QUALITY CONTROL BY FLOW CYTOMETRY

The cell quality control procedures commonly performed by the chondrocyte expansion facilities provide the surgeon with information on proliferation potential, sterility, viability, and morphology. These parameters, however, do not give any information on the composition of the ECM produced by these cells, which is an indication of their potential to form stable hyalinelike cartilage. As mentioned, monolayer-expanded chondrocytes lose phenotypical stability; they have a more fibroblastlike morphology and an altered ECM composition (more type I collagen, decreased amounts of type II collagen and aggrecan). Alginate hydrogel culture conditions, on the other hand, preserve the native chondrocyte phenotype while still allowing proliferation, ECM production, and outgrowth into a surrounding fibrin matrix *(15)*.

Analysis of the newly synthesized ECM proteins using flow cytometry quantifies and qualifies the phenotype of the cultured chondrocytes (Fig. 3) *(8,9)*. This analysis is performed on isolated alginate-cultured articular chondrocytes prior to transplantation by dissolving the alginate with trisodium citrate dehydrate. The cell-associated matrix is subsequently stained with monoclonal antibodies (MAb) raised against type I collagen, type II collagen, and aggrecan. Fluorescence intensity is measured for each of these fluorochrome-conjugated MAb and represented by a histogram. Ideally, alginate-cultured chondrocytes produce large amounts of aggrecan and type II collagen in the cell-associated matrix, and type I collagen cannot be detected. The presence of this "mantle" of dense ECM is also considered to isolate the allogeneic cell from the immune system, thus reducing humoral and cellular immune responses.

BIOLOGICAL FREEZING

Ideally, a tissue bank containing suitable, quality-controlled allogeneic chondrocytes would allow the surgeon to perform a one-stage procedure when confronted with a cartilage lesion during arthroscopy. Therefore, we focused on the use of allogeneic chondrocytes in preliminary in vitro tests on the potential of alginate-cultured human articular chondrocytes frozen at 196°C in dimethyl sulfoxide *(16)*. Data from these studies substantiated the feasibility of this technique to store these cells for a prolonged period without significant decrease in the capacity to synthesize an appropriate ECM. Further experiments, however, are necessary to confirm these preliminary results of long-term storage of allogeneic chondrocytes.

SURGICAL TECHNIQUE

Indications and Contraindications

Comparable to the first-generation ACT, the indications for allogeneic chondrocytes in alginate are full-thickness cartilage or osteochondral lesions of the knee and talar dome; contraindications to this procedure include generalized osteoarthritis or inflammatory arthritis of any origin. The lesions should be contained, but an uncontained lesion is not considered a contraindication. So far, the treated defect area size in our series varied from 1 to 10 cm^2.

Preoperative Planning

Preoperative planning consists of a thorough clinical examination. The etiology of the cartilage lesion should be clear because this can significantly affect the treatment. Lower extremity alignment, ligament laxity, and patellar tracking should be assessed and if necessary corrected prior to or concomitant with chondrocyte transplantation. An extended magnetic resonance imaging (MRI) examination of the involved joint is routinely performed to provide the surgeon with additional information on the quality of the cartilage, menisci, subchondral bone, and ligaments.

Standing plain radiographs of the lower extremity are valuable for calculating and evaluating joint space narrowing, the subchondral bone, and axial alignment. Ultimately, it is decided during the arthroscopic examination of the involved joint whether a transplantation is indicated. The selected patient is then placed on a waiting list for an allogeneic chondrocyte transplantation. The waiting time at our institution generally varies from 1 wk to 3 mo. In the future, it will be possible to order biological frozen allogeneic chondrocytes "off the shelf," resulting in a one-stage procedure.

Donor Allogeneic Chondrocytes

As mentioned, articular cartilage chondrocytes are enzymatically isolated from intact femoral cartilage and cultured in alginate beads for a period of 10–14 d prior to transplantation. During this period, the donor is checked for transmittable diseases and sterility according to standard general organ donor procedures. In the meantime, the cultured cells accumulate a dense ECM rich in aggrecans and collagens. Prior to transplantation, a sample of the alginate-cultured chondrocytes is assayed for the ECM proteins using flow cytometry. These data are stored electronically for later analysis and correlation studies with the histological outcome.

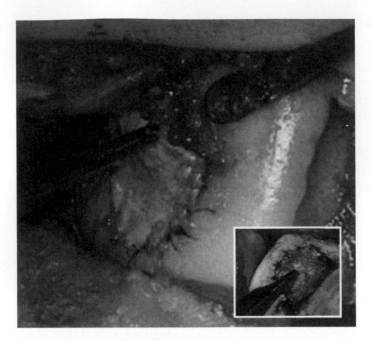

Fig. 4. (Color Plate 3, following p. 206). The cartilage defect is debrided, and a periosteal patch is sutured to the defect edges. An opening is left through which the beads are delivered to the defect by a spoon or large curette. The defect is now closed completely by suturing the periosteal patch opening circumferentially to the defect edges. One can feel the presence of the beads by palpating the overlying periosteal patch. Overfilling of the defect is generally obtained.

Surgical Procedure

A medial or lateral mini-arthrotomy is performed in a tourniquet-controlled bloodless surgical field. The cartilage lesion is identified, and all damaged, fissured, or undermined cartilage is radically excised, resulting in a cartilage defect with vertical healthy edges. Using a ring curette, the defect is carefully debrided to the subchondral bone without causing any bleeding. The size of the defect is then templated using paper or aluminum foil. Accurate sizing of the defect is essential for the harvest of the periosteal flap. This flap is generally harvested from the medial crest of the tibia, distal to the pes anserinus, through a second incision. Other harvest sites have been described. Care should be taken not to harvest too thick a flap and to remove overlying fat or fibrous tissue. The periosteal flap is elevated using a periosteal elevator. The upper side of the flap is marked using methylene blue staining because the cambium layer of the flap should face the defect.

The defect is then covered with the periosteal flap using vicryl 6-0 resorbable sutures. Classically, extreme care should be taken to obtain a watertight seal of the defect. The alginate beads approach, however, allows the surgeon to perform a quicker and less-meticulous suturing procedure because these beads prevent the leakage of cells from the defect. One side of the periosteal flap is not sutured to the edge. Using alginate hydrogel as a scaffold, the allogeneic chondrocytes are then transplanted under the periosteal flap within the defect through this opening (Fig. 4). The alginate beads are packed into the defect until filled. The opening in the periosteal flap is subsequently closed. Fibrin glue is gently injected into the defect under the periosteal flap to fill the spaces between the alginate beads.

The stability of the repair is assessed by moving the knee joint through a 0–90° motion arc prior to closure.

Concomitant Procedures

Concomitant procedures such as meniscus allograft transplantation, ACL reconstruction, varus or valgus osteotomy, and patellar realignment can be performed after debridement of the defect and harvest of the periosteal flap but prior to covering of the defect with the periosteal flap.

Postoperative Rehabilitation

Postoperative rehabilitation includes continuous passive mobilization of the joint limited to 60° of flexion and protected weight bearing during the first 3 wk, followed by partial weight bearing for another 3 wk. An unloader brace is used throughout the postoperative rehabilitation effort. The patient is allowed to walk freely at 6 wk. Full return to sports is not allowed until at least 9–12 mo.

POSTOPERATIVE MRI AND ARTHROSCOPY OF TREATED PATIENTS

The study protocol was approved by the Ethics Committee of the Ghent University Hospital, and informed consent was obtained from each patient enrolled in this study.

The patients' clinical status was evaluated at 1, 3, 6, 9, and 12 mo and yearly after using different clinical outcome as well as patient-assessed outcome scoring systems, notably the Lequesne index, the Western Ontario and McMaster University, and the Visual Analogue Scale scores.

Arthroscopic assessment of graft appearance and integrity was performed at 6 and 12 mo. An additional biopsy was taken from the center of the repair tissue at 12 mo. Histological and immunohistological assessment of the graft's cellular and biochemical composition was performed.

MRI of the operated knee joint was routinely performed in all patients at different points in time (3, 6, and 12 mo and yearly after) to evaluate the repair tissue and to describe this biological process. We obtained 3-mm sagittal proton-density and T_2-weighted images, 2-mm coronal mixed T_1-T_2-weighted DESS-3D gradient-echo images, and 1-mm sagittal fat-suppressed T_1-weighted three-dimensional spoiled gradient-echo images for optimal visualization of all portions of the menisci and for articular cartilage assessment. Early dynamic contrast-enhanced MRI after bolus injection and delayed gadolinium-enhanced MRI of the cartilage (dGEMRIC) was used to further analyze the vascularization and perfusion in different regions within the subchondral bone and cartilage and the proteoglycan content of the repair tissue and of the normal surrounding articular cartilage, respectively.

After first-generation ACT, the repair tissue heals in different stages. In the proliferative phase (0–8 wk), soft, primitive repair tissue with a signal intensity like water fills the defect. Sometimes, associated subchondral bone marrow edema and enhancement in the margin of the defect can be seen. The subchondral bone plate is usually slightly irregular, especially when small perforations have been made in the subchondral bone plate on preparation of the implantation site. The level of the defect is variable, depending on which type of defect has been filled.

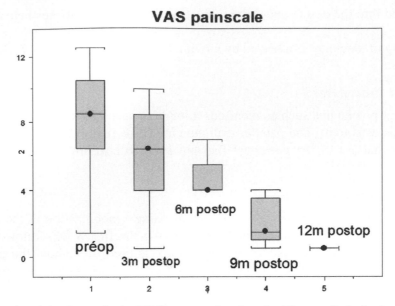

Fig. 5. Visual Analogue Scale (VAS) scores showing significant relief of pain over time.

In the transitional phase (3–6 mo), more matrix is formed, and the tissue is better defined on MRI, with a lower and sometimes inhomogeneous signal intensity. Progressive edge integration of the transplanted cartilage with the native cartilage is seen. The bone marrow edema progressively disappears. In the final, remodeling phase (6–18 mo), further matrix remodeling and maturation to repair cartilage (mixture of hyalinelike and fibrous cartilage) occur with near-normal stiffness. The signal resembles that of normal cartilage. Complete edge integration of the transplanted cartilage with the native cartilage may take as long as 2 yr *(17–19)*.

MRI can demonstrate complications such as delamination of the repair tissue, hypertrophy of the repair tissue, and rarely underfilling of the defect and formation of intra-articular adhesions attached to the ACI grafts *(18–20)*.

PRELIMINARY RESULTS OF ALLOGENEIC CHONDROCYTE-BASED CARTILAGE REPAIR USING ALGINATE BEADS

Clinical Results

Clinically, immediate or short-term major adverse reactions to the alginate/fibrin matrix seeded with the allogeneic cartilage cells were not observed. The results of the short-term clinical examination of the involved joint as well as the functional scores improved with time (Fig. 5).

Arthroscopy

Arthroscopically, good integration of the repair tissue with the defect edges was observed (Fig. 6). The consistency of the repair tissue was softer than normal articular cartilage on palpation but tended to improve with time. Frequently, overfilling of the defect was observed; the defect surface was situated higher than the surrounding native articular cartilage. The surface of the repair tissue visually appeared white but was less shiny than normal cartilage.

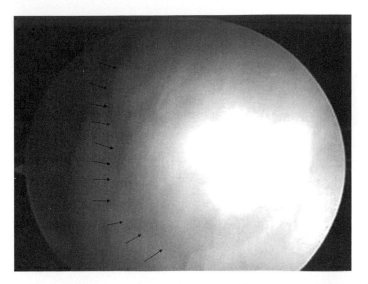

Fig. 6. Arthroscopic view of repair tissue at 12 mo. Good integration of the repair tissue with the defect edges is observed, as well as overfilling of the defect. The surface of the repair tissue appears white but less shiny than normal articular cartilage.

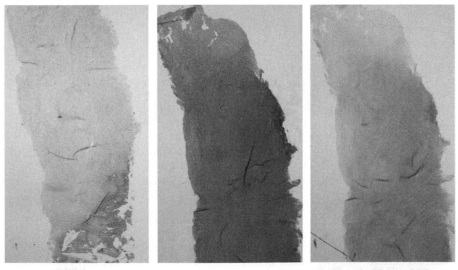

H&E   **PAS-Alcian Blue**   **Saffranin O-Fast Green**

Fig. 7. Biopsy specimen at 12 mo showing predominantly hyalinelike repair tissue. Chondrocytes are situated in lacunae surrounded by a dense extracellular matrix. Superficially, this matrix is more fibrous, reflecting the remnants of the periosteal patch. The matrix stains positive for PAS-Alcian Blue and Saffranin O, indicating the presence of proteoglycans.

Histology

The biopsies obtained at 12 mo predominantly showed hyalinelike cartilage, predominantly fibrocartilage, or a mixture of both (Fig. 7). Good vertical integration of the repair tissue with the subchondral bone was observed. Alginate particles were not found, indicating complete biodegradation of the scaffold.

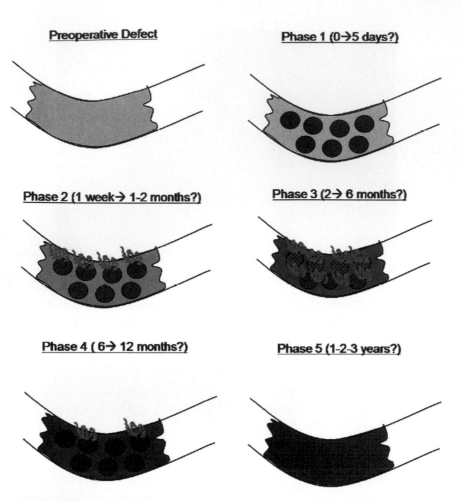

Fig. 8. Diagram showing the different stages of maturation of the repair tissue as observed with bolus dynamic contrast-enhanced MRI after bolus injection and dGEMRIC. Increased vascularity is observed early at the bottom of the reparative tissue. This vascularity progressively disappears as the regenerative tissue matures.

Magnetic Resonance Imaging

Based on dGEMRIC and the bolus study, five phases were distinguished in the evolution of the transplant area (Fig. 8) *(20)*:

Phase 1: Allograft chondrocyte implantation (0–5 days postoperatively)
Phase 2: Ingrowth of regenerative tissue and blood vessels; early matrix formation (1 wk to 1–2 mo postoperatively)
Phase 3: Maturation of regenerative tissue and increased vascularity; increased matrix formation (2–6 mo postoperatively)
Phase 4: Progressive disappearance of regenerative tissue and blood vessels; change toward fibrocartilaginous tissue (6–12 mo postoperatively)
Phase 5: Change of fibrocartilage toward hyaline(-like) cartilage (1 to 2–3 yr postoperatively)

Bone marrow edema and bone remodeling occur in the first 6 mo and then progressively disappear.

DISCUSSION

First- and second-generation ACT have become major treatment options for articular cartilage lesions. However, two major challenges remain: to improve the reproducibility of the histological results and to improve the ease of delivery of the cells to the defect. Although not always recognized as important, the major variable in the histological results is thought to be the patient; in other words, an important variability exists in the quality and repair potential of these cultured cells among patients.

To overcome this interpatient variability, we developed a surgical technique based on allogeneic articular chondrocytes. The use of allogeneic cells obviates the need for a biopsy and monolayer cell expansion. It was calculated from our donor data that approx 50 patients could in theory benefit from a single donor. A selection of appropriate donors based on the described quality control standards can thus be achieved. This approach not only could solve the reproducibility problem but also could eventually result in an off-the-shelf product and thus in a one-stage surgical procedure.

Much work is under way to improve the ease of handling and delivery of the cell product to the defect. A first- or second-generation cell suspension has the intrinsic disadvantage of leakage out of the defect and of an inhomogeneous distribution of cells within the defect *(10)*. Scaffolds or gels have been developed to overcome these drawbacks and have proven their value in animal and human models. Another possible advantage of these matrices is the possibility to enhance them by adding certain growth factors or other biologically active substances that could improve the repair potential of the treated defect.

We chose alginate as a scaffold because of its documented use in clinical practice, its ability to stabilize the chondrocytic phenotype, and its easy handling *(21)*. Reports have been published on the enhancement of alginate by adding growth factors to the matrix *(22,23)*. Alginate enables us to deliver the cells easily and homogeneously to the defect without the risk of leakage. The periosteal flap is still sutured over the defect and is considered to act as a biologically active device *(24)*. Over time, the alginate scaffold is biodegraded, as observed in the histological sections.

These short-term clinical results illustrate the feasibility and safety of the application of allogeneic chondrocytes in combination with an alginate matrix in the treatment of cartilage defects. This concept essentially involves a one-step surgical transplantation procedure with a well-characterized cell product in a biodegradable matrix and is hoped to result in an easier and less time-consuming surgical procedure and a more reproducible clinical and histological outcome. Further results and research, however, are needed to validate this type of approach in a larger setting.

REFERENCES

1. Brittberg M, Lindahl A, Nilsson A, Ohlsson C, Isaksson O, Peterson L. Treatment of deep cartilage defects in the knee with autologous chondrocyte transplantation. N Engl J Med 1994;331:889–895.
2. Richardson JB, Caterson B, Evans EH, Ashton BA, Roberts S. Repair of human articular cartilage after implantation of autologous chondrocytes. J Bone Joint Surg Br 1999;81:1064–1068.
3. Horas U, Pelinkovic D, Herr G, Aigner T, Schnettler R. Autologous chondrocyte implantation and osteochondral cylinder transplantation in cartilage repair of the knee joint. A prospective, comparative trial. J Bone Joint Surg Am 2003;85:185–192.

4. Knutsen G, Engebretsen L, Ludvigsen TC, et al. Autologous chondrocyte implantation compared with microfracture in the knee. A randomized trial. J Bone Joint Surg Am 2004;86: 455–464.
5. Peterson L, Minas T, Brittberg M, Nilsson A, Sjogren-Jansson E, Lindahl A. Two- to 9-yr outcome after autologous chondrocyte transplantation of the knee. Clin Orthop 2000; 374:212–234.
6. Peterson L, Brittberg M, Kiviranta I, Akerlund EL, Lindahl A. Autologous chondrocyte transplantation. Biomechanics and long-term durability. Am J Sports Med 2002;30:2–12.
7. Frisbie DD, Oxford JT, Southwood L, et al. Early events in cartilage repair after subchondral bone microfracture. Clin Orthop 2003;407:215–227.
8. Wang L, Verbruggen G, Almqvist KF, Elewaut D, Broddelez C, Veys EM. Flow cytometric analysis of the human articular chondrocyte phenotype in vitro. Osteoarthritis Cartilage 2001;9:73–84.
9. Wang L, Almqvist KF, Broddelez C, Veys EM, Verbruggen G. Evaluation of chondrocyte cell-associated matrix metabolism by flow cytometry. Osteoarthritis Cartilage 2001;9:454–462.
10. Sohn DH, Lottman LM, Lum LY, et al. Effect of gravity on localization of chondrocytes implanted in cartilage defects. Clin Orthop 2002;394:254–262.
11. Zimmermann U, Mimietz S, Zimmermann H, et al. Hydrogel-based non-autologous cell and tissue therapy. Biotechniques 2000;29:564–572.
12. Hauselmann HJ, Fernandes RJ, Mok SS, et al. Phenotypic stability of bovine articular chondrocytes after long-term culture in alginate beads. J Cell Sci 1994;107:17–27.
13. Kuettner KE, Pauli BU, Gall G, Memoli VA, Schenk RK. Synthesis of cartilage matrix by mammalian chondrocytes in vitro. I. Isolation, culture characteristics, and morphology. J Cell Biol 1982;93:743–750.
14. Guo JF, Jourdian GW, MacCallum DK. Culture and growth characteristics of chondrocytes encapsulated in alginate beads. Connect Tissue Res 1989;19:277–297.
15. Almqvist KF, Wang L, Wang J, et al. Culture of chondrocytes in alginate surrounded by fibrin gel: characteristics of the cells over a period of eight weeks. Ann Rheum Dis 2001;60:781–790.
16. Almqvist KF, Wang L, Broddelez C, Veys EM, Verbruggen G. Biological freezing of human articular chondrocytes. Osteoarthritis Cartilage 2001;9:341–350.
17. Recht M, White LM, Winalski CS, Miniaci A, Minas T, Parker RD. MR imaging of cartilage repair procedures. Skeletal Radiol 2003;32:185–200.
18. Alparslan L, Winalski CS, Boutin RD, Minas T. Postoperative magnetic resonance imaging of articular cartilage repair. Semin Musculoskelet Radiol 2001;5:345–363.
19. Verstraete KL, Almqvist F, Verdonk P, et al. Magnetic resonance imaging of cartilage and cartilage repair. Clin Radiol 2004;59:674–689.
20. Verstraete K, Vandenabeele V, De Cuyper C, et al. Dynamic and delayed gadolinium-enhanced MRI of cartilage and subchondral bone after alginate allograft chondrocyte implantation (ACI). Radiology Proceedings of the 90th Scientific and Annual Meeting of the Radiological Society of North America (RSNA), 2004.
21. Atala A, Kim W, Paige KT, Vacanti CA, Retik AB. Endoscopic treatment of vesicoureteral reflux with a chondrocyte-alginate suspension. J Urol 1994;152:641–643.
22. Genes NG, Rowley JA, Mooney DJ, Bonassar LJ. Effect of substrate mechanics on chondrocyte adhesion to modified alginate surfaces. Arch Biochem Biophys 2004;422:161–167.
23. Rowley JA, Madlambayan G, Mooney DJ. Alginate hydrogels as synthetic extracellular matrix materials. Biomaterials 1999;20:45–53.
24. Brittberg M, Sjogren-Jansson E, Thornemo M, et al. Clonal growth of human articular cartilage and the functional role of the periosteum in chondrogenesis. Osteoarthritis Cartilage 2005;13:146–153.

15

The Role of Knee Osteotomy in the Setting of Articular Cartilage Repair

Keith M. Baumgarten, MD and Thomas L. Wickiewicz, MD

Summary

Knee osteotomies were initially used to treat degenerative arthritis of the knee. Over time, indications have become stricter, and now knee osteotomies are primarily used to correct varus or valgus malalignment associated with unicompartmental osteoarthritis. Knee osteotomies redistribute the load from the diseased compartment to the more normal compartment. Knee osteotomies can be used for primary treatment of knee pain and tibiofemoral malalignment, or they can be combined with cartilage repair procedures to provide a chondroprotective effect. By correcting the tibiofemoral malalignment, joint reactive forces are decreased in the diseased compartment, allowing for improved survival of meniscal transplants and cartilage resurfacing procedures.

Key Words: Cartilage; knee; osteoarthritis; osteotomy; tibia.

HISTORY

Osteotomy for treatment of osteoarthritis of the knee was first reported by J. P. Jackson in 1958 at the Joint Meeting of the Orthopaedic Associations *(1)*. Jackson presented 14 patients, 6 with tibial osteotomies and 8 with femoral osteotomies, for lateral deformity of the knee associated with osteoarthritis. Jackson stated that, "There was a reasonable chance of relieving pain and retaining a useful range of motion" in the knees with osteoarthritis of the lateral compartment treated with a corrective osteotomy *(1)*.

Jackson and Waugh were the first to publish their results on the treatment of osteoarthritis of the knee with a tibial osteotomy *(2)*. They reported that they were inspired by the success of an intertrochanteric osteotomy for relieving pain in the osteoarthritic hip. Fourteen patients underwent a ball-and-socket tibial osteotomy at the level of the tibial tubercle with a concurrent midfibula osteotomy for either valgus or varus deformity of the knee secondary to osteoarthritis. After a mean follow-up of approx 3 yr, they reported that all patients had either complete or considerable pain relief and "recovery of movement after the operation has been easy."

In 1962, Wardle described a transverse osteotomy performed distal to the tibial tubercle for treatment of degenerative arthritis of the knee *(3)*. In 1964, Gariepy *(4)* described a closing wedge technique that was further modified and popularized by Coventry in his classic paper published in 1965 *(5)*.

Coventry described a closing wedge lateral-based tibial osteotomy performed proximal to the tibial tubercle *(5)*. This was advantageous because it was near the site of deformity and

From: *Cartilage Repair Strategies*
Edited by: Riley J. Williams © Humana Press Inc., Totowa, NJ

involved rapidly healing cancellous bone. Performing the osteotomy proximal to the tibial tubercle also allowed compression across the osteotomy site by the action of the extensor mechanism. In addition, its proximity to the joint line allowed the surgeon to perform an arthrotomy through the same incision to allow for intra-articular exploration. Coventry suggested that the surgeon should fully correct and even overcorrect the varus or valgus deformity. Most of the patients in this series were treated with a valgus osteotomy for a varus deformity. After a minimum of 1 yr, 18 knees had a satisfactory result, defined as at least 90°s of flexion, full extension, only intermittent swelling, and no catching sensations. The remaining 4 knees had unsatisfactory results. Coventry noted on radiographs that the degenerated joint space usually widened after osteotomy.

Originally, knee osteotomies were used to treat tricompartmental osteoarthritis. Several studies showed that knee osteotomies had poor outcomes when used as such a treatment (6–8). With the development of total knee arthroplasty, knee osteotomies fell out of favor as a treatment for tricompartmental osteoarthritis. However, knee osteotomies continue to be an efficacious treatment for unicompartmental arthritis and tibiofemoral malalignment.

THEORY

In the typical human knee, 60% of weight-bearing forces are transmitted through the medial compartment and 40% through the lateral compartment (9). In a knee with unicompartmental arthritis, limb alignment is altered, and subsequently more load is distributed to the affected compartment, causing further degenerative changes and angular deformity. The rationale for high tibial osteotomy or distal femoral osteotomy is to correct the abnormal loads on the articular surface of the knee that are caused by the deformity in the tibiofemoral axis (10,11). In essence, these osteotomies transfer the weight-bearing loads from the diseased compartment to the unaffected compartment.

Historically, knee osteotomies have been performed to postpone the need for total knee arthroplasty and prolong the lifespan of the native knee. This procedure is especially important in younger patients with unicompartmental osteoarthritis because there is a high probability of failure of total knee arthroplasty in younger, high-demand patients. Young patients who require total knee arthroplasty are likely to need multiple revision arthroplasties within their lifetime. In contrast, knee osteotomies allow patients to pursue higher demand activities that are often contraindicated after total joint arthroplasty because of the increased risk for arthroplasty failure.

KNEE OSTEOTOMIES AND CARTILAGE REGENERATION

Progressive joint space widening and bone remodeling has been observed after high tibial osteotomies (12–17). This finding led to the belief that high tibial osteotomy created a mechanical environment in the knee that allowed for articular cartilage regeneration. An animal study showed that the decreased load on the medial condyle after osteotomy led to increased proteoglycan and collagen concentrations and reduced the amount of cartilage fibrillation (18).

Several clinical studies have shown that a layer of fibrocartilage regenerates over areas of prior cartilage injury after high tibial osteotomy (19,20). Koshino et al. showed that 2 yr after high tibial osteotomy for varus gonarthrosis, most knees regenerated a mixture of fibrocartilage and hyaline cartilage over areas of prior articular cartilage loss (16). Mature cartilage regeneration was seen more often in knees that had greater than 5° of anatomic valgus after osteotomy compared to those that were undercorrected. In addition, there was a correlation with improved knee scores in knees with cartilage regeneration compared to knees without cartilage regeneration. Other studies have shown that cartilage regeneration was thicker and more complete when osteotomy was combined with additional abrasio-arthroplasty *(15,21)*.

Wakabayashi et al. demonstrated that knees with full-thickness cartilage defects had more complete cartilage regeneration compared to knees with partial-thickness defects or fibrillation after high tibial osteotomy *(22)*. Although the arthroscopic findings showed that the healing potential of fibrillated cartilage was inferior to that of eburnated bone, histological findings showed that most of the fibrillated cartilage appeared to be hyaline cartilage; in contrast, eburnated bone was repaired with fibrocartilage. The authors hypothesized that eburnated bone underwent fibrocartilage repair via mesenchymal cell transformation from the subchondral bone. In contrast, fibrocartilage repair was not promoted in fibrillated cartilage. Instead, further degeneration of the fibrillated cartilage was prevented by the correction of the mechanical axis.

One second-look arthroscopy study noted improvements in medial meniscal morphology in tears identified at the index arthroscopy *(23)*. The authors stated that the "ruptured meniscus regained a smooth inner margin or a desirable continuity as a result of a decrease in articular compressive stress" and suggested that high tibial osteotomy may improve meniscal repair. They also noted that the time course for ulcerated articular lesions to be thoroughly covered with fibrous tissue was approx 18 mo.

THE ROLE OF KNEE OSTEOTOMIES IN CARTILAGE REPAIR

Knee osteotomies have been combined with cartilage-resurfacing procedures such as mosaicplasty, autologous chondrocyte implantation (ACI), and osteochondral allografts *(24–30)*. Cartilage repair is at risk for failure if the tibiofemoral or patellofemoral axis remains malaligned after the repair procedure. Osteochondral allografts have been shown to have poor results when placed into a malaligned knee *(24)*.

Oakeshott et al. examined 18 knees that failed cartilage resurfacing with an osteochondral allograft *(30)*. Of these knees, 15 had tibiofemoral malalignment at the time of allograft implantation. Ghazavi et al. demonstrated that there was a correlation between appropriate alignment and successful clinical and radiographic results. In this study, 43% of malaligned knees failed osteochondral allograft resurfacing compared to 9% of well-aligned knees *(26)*. Shasha et al. showed that osteochondral allograft surgery was successful when realignment osteotomies preceded or were coincident with the allograft surgery *(28)*. Patients who had realignment osteotomies had equally successful outcomes up to 10 yr following allograft surgery compared to patients with normal alignment *(29)*. Although no studies have evaluated ACI or mosaicplasty regarding successful results in the presence of tibiofemoral malalignment, it is intuitive from these studies that ACI or mosaicplasty in the malaligned knee is predisposed to early failure, and strong consideration should be given to performing a concurrent realignment osteotomy.

Knee osteotomies have also been performed concurrently with meniscal allograft transplantation *(31–33)* (Fig. 1). Studies have shown that the results of meniscal transplantation are clinically more successful in patients with normal alignment compared to patients with a malaligned knee *(34,35)*. Thus, malalignment should be corrected with an osteotomy before or at the time of meniscal transplantation.

Cameron and Saha reported an 86.6% success rate in 36 patients treated with a meniscal allograft and a concurrent knee osteotomy *(31)*. They hypothesized that the higher contact

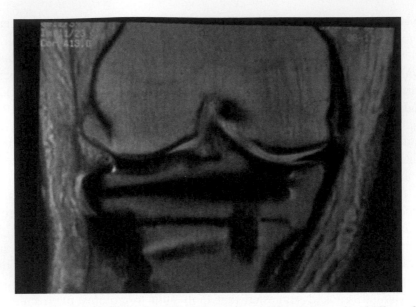

Fig. 1. MRI of combined high tibial osteotomy and medial meniscal allograft.

stresses in the diseased compartment caused by the tibiofemoral malalignment leads to vascular damage and allograft degeneration and loosening. After combined osteotomy and a cartilage-resurfacing procedure or meniscal transplantation, it is difficult to determine if the success is because of the osteotomy or the synergistic effect of the combined procedures.

TYPES OF KNEE OSTEOTOMIES

Knee osteotomies are described regarding the location of the osteotomy and site of the correction. Most knee osteotomies are performed in the proximal tibia and are termed *high tibial osteotomies*. Knee osteotomies are also performed in the distal femur. These are indicated mainly to correct valgus deformities.

High Tibial Osteotomies

Closing Wedge Osteotomies

Coventry popularized the closing wedge high tibial osteotomy (Fig. 2) as a treatment for both varus and valgus deformity. The closing wedge is based laterally to treat varus deformity. Coventry described using either a transverse or longitudinal incision based over the fibular head and lateral knee joint line to expose the osteotomy site *(5)*. He then dissected out the fibular head subperiosteally while protecting the peroneal nerve. The fibular collateral ligament and biceps femoris tendon were dissected off the fibular head, and the proximal fibula was removed to expose the lateral aspect of the tibia. Next, the proximal end of the tibia was exposed subperiosteally. A Kirschner wire was inserted at the epiphyseal scar proximal to the tibial tubercle, and roentgenograms were obtained to confirm the location and depth of the osteotomy.

Coventry embraced the technique of Bauer et al. *(36)* in determining the size of the bone wedge to achieve proper correction *(7)*. For each degree of angular correction needed, 1 mm of lateral cortex was removed. The osteotomy was made 2 cm distal and parallel to the articular surface. The osteotomy was not completed through the far cortex to leave an intact hinge

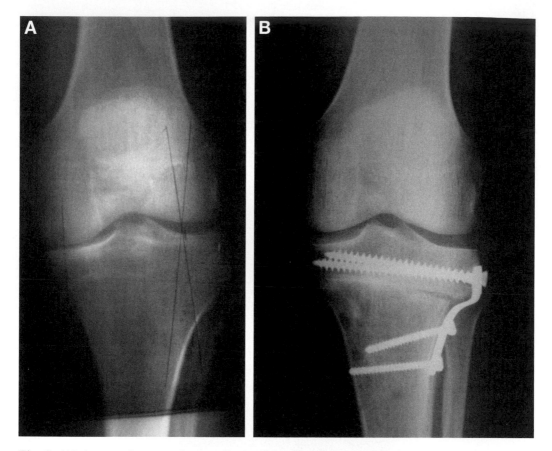

Fig. 2. (A) An anterior-posterior standing radiograph of a varus malaligned knee. The mechanical axis has been drawn over the medial compartment. The anticipated, corrected mechanical axis (62% coordinate) is drawn over the lateral compartment. **(B)** The same knee after a valgus-producing closing wedge high tibial osteotomy.

to maintain rotational stability. Instead, Coventry used a 6.4-mm osteotome to perforate the opposite cortex in several places *(7)*. Next, a valgus force was placed on the tibia, breaking the medial cortex in a greenstick manner to bring the osteotomized edges together. The osteotomy was held together with one or two staples in the lateral cortex. The common insertion of the biceps femoris tendon and the fibular collateral ligament was sutured to the remaining portion of the fibular head or to the iliotibial band near its insertion. The patient was placed into a cylinder cast with the knee in extension once the wound was healed. The patient remained in the cast, partially weight bearing, for 4–6 wk until there was evidence of radiographic union.

To treat valgus deformity, Coventry used a medial approach and closing wedge osteotomy to apply a varus correction *(7)*. The knee was flexed to 90°, and the medial collateral ligament and the pes anserinus were retracted medially. Similar to the lateral closing wedge technique, a wedge of bone was removed from the tibia, and the osteotomy site was closed down, in this situation with a varus force, and held with staples and cast immobilization. Unlike the lateral closing wedge technique, the fibula was not osteotomized. The medial collateral ligament was imbricated if it became lax after the medial closing wedge osteotomy.

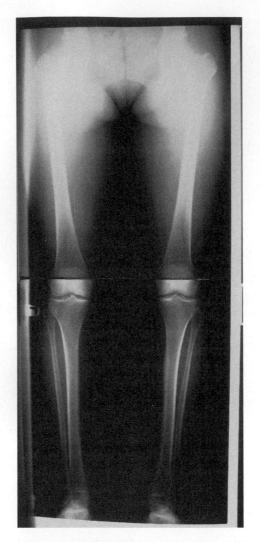

Fig. 3. Standing long-cassette radiographs of the bilateral lower extremities.

The closing wedge high tibial osteotomy has evolved since Coventry's description in 1965. Several studies have shown that Bauer et al.'s technique of determining the angular correction was imprecise, and this method has been largely abandoned *(6,37–39)*. Prefabricated calibrated jigs are now used to provide more accurate correction *(40,41)*. Fibular head resection has been replaced by tibiofibular capsule division or fibular shaft osteotomy to decrease the risk of postoperative lateral instability or peroneal nerve injury *(40–42)*. Rigid internal fixation and early motion have replaced staple and cast fixation *(40,41,43)*. The availability of intraoperative fluoroscopy has increased the accuracy of correction and improved efficiency and speed of surgery *(44)*. Standing, long-cassette radiographic films are used to determine preoperative correction *(12)* (Fig. 3).

Opening Wedge Osteotomies

Opening wedge osteotomies are performed on the medial aspect of the proximal tibia to correct varus deformities and lateral aspect of the proximal tibia to correct valgus deformities *(9)*.

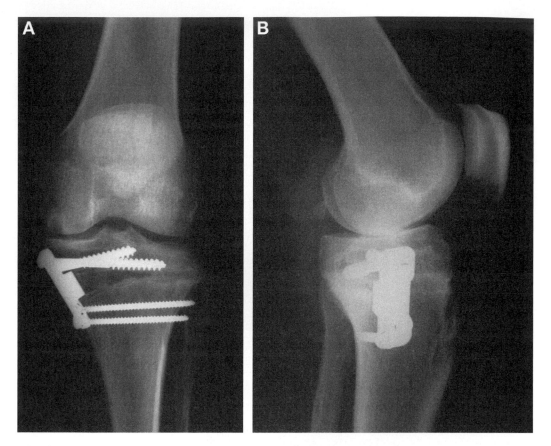

Fig. 4. (A) Anterior-posterior standing radiograph of a valgus-producing opening wedge high tibial osteotomy. **(B)** Lateral radiograph of a valgus-producing opening wedge high tibial osteotomy.

Opening wedge osteotomies are appealing because multiplanar correction can be readily obtained. In addition, opening wedge osteotomies may be technically easier to perform than closing wedge osteotomies because they require only one bone cut. Unlike closing wedge osteotomies, opening wedge osteotomies add bone to the diseased, collapsed side instead of removing bone from the more normal side *(45)*. In addition, it is not necessary to disrupt the proximal tibiofibular joint or osteotomize the fibula *(46,47)*.

Opening wedge osteotomies are performed by adding autologous bone graft, allogenic bone graft, or bone graft substitutes in combination with rigid internal fixation to correct the varus deformity *(45)* (Fig. 4). Distraction lengthening with external fixation is another technique used to perform an opening wedge osteotomy *(47,48)*.

The disadvantages of opening wedge osteotomies include the potential need for either autogenous bone graft with harvest site morbidity or allogenic bone with the potential for disease transmission, the potential increased risk for delayed or nonunion, an increased length of restricted weight bearing, and pin site infections when external fixation is used. In one study, approx 40% of patients had pin site infections requiring antibiotic treatment.

A randomized, prospective study compared closing wedge high tibial osteotomy to opening wedge osteotomy by hemicallotasis. Although there were no clinically significant differences in pain or function between the two groups, patients treated with the opening wedge

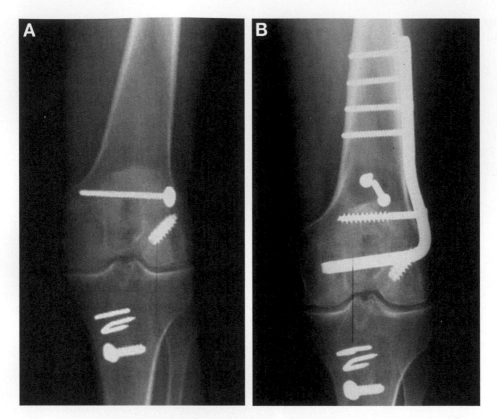

Fig. 5. (A) Preoperative standing radiograph showing valgus malalignment of the left knee. The pencil mark represents the weight bearing line or mechanical axis. **(B)** Postoperative anterior-posterior radiograph of distal femoral osteotomy with the corrected mechanical axis depicted over the medial tibial spine.

technique had a decreased length of convalescence and hospital stay and a more precise and predictable angular correction. However, the authors did acknowledge that the pin tract infections associated with the opening wedge technique could be detrimental if a total knee arthroplasty was indicated in future treatment *(49)*.

Distal Femoral Osteotomy

Coventry believed that the ability to transfer load medially using a tibial closing wedge osteotomy to treat valgus deformity was limited by the anatomical valgus alignment of the femur. Coventry suggested that patients with greater than 12° of preoperative varus angulation or patients with a calculated, postoperative joint line obliquity of greater than 10° should be treated with a distal femoral osteotomy instead of a medial-based tibial closing wedge osteotomy *(50)* (Fig. 5).

Coventry described a medial-based closing wedge distal femoral osteotomy *(7)*. A medial incision was made over the distal femur, and the rectus femoris and the vastus medialis were separated exposing the medial femoral condyles. Kirshner wires and roentgenograms were used to localize the appropriate placement for the osteotomy at the junction of the femoral shaft and the medial femoral condyle. A reciprocating saw was used to perform the osteotomy, and fixation was obtained using a blade plate. Once the incision healed, patients were placed in a cylinder cast and were allowed to bear weight with crutches for 5 wk.

OUTCOMES

The Varus Knee

In Coventry's initial study of predominantly valgus osteotomies, he showed 75% satisfactory results. Since that landmark paper, there have been many studies that have evaluated the long-term outcomes of closing wedge osteotomies for treatment of the varus knee. Nearly all of these studies demonstrated that the clinical success of the osteotomy deteriorates with time.

Insall et al. reported that the passage of time was the most important single determinant of the result *(42)*. Keene and Dyreby showed 79% excellent and good results after 32 mo *(51)*. Miniaci et al. found 83% excellent and good results at 35 mo *(52)*. Aglietti et al. demonstrated a 68% excellent and good results at 6.5-yr follow up *(53)*. Berman et al. found 57% excellent and good results at 8.5 yr *(6)*. Yasuda et al. showed 63% satisfactory results at 11-yr follow-up *(54)*. Rinonapoli et al. demonstrated 55% good and excellent results at a mean 15-yr follow-up *(8)*. Survivorship of closing wedge high tibial osteotomy has ranged from 50 to 87% at 5 yr, 28 to 74% at 10 yr, 15 to 39% at 15 yr and was 30% at 20 yr *(41,43,44,55,56)*. In one study, 38% of the patients required conversion to a total knee arthroplasty at a mean of 5 yr after the initial osteotomy *(41)*.

The long-term follow-up studies include many first-generation osteotomies (no or minimal internal fixation, cast immobilization, excision of fibular head, correction of deformity determined using Bauer et al.'s technique). It is reasonable to anticipate that long-term follow-up of second-generation osteotomies (stricter indications, rigid internal fixation, initiation of early postoperative range of motion, osteotomies by calibrated jigs) will show improved and more durable outcomes. One such study showed that osteotomies performed with tibial cutting jigs, rigid internal fixation, and postoperative continuous passive range of motion had fewer complications compared to osteotomies performed using Bauer's technique of angular correction, staple fixation, and casting for 6 wk *(40)*.

There have been fewer studies evaluating opening wedge high tibial osteotomies for treatment of the varus knee than those for closing wedge osteotomies. Sterett and Steadman demonstrated a 96% survivorship at 3 yr and 84% survivorship at 5 yr *(47)*, whereas Amendola showed that more than 90% of patients were subjectively improved and satisfied *(45)*.

The Valgus Knee

The first description of knee osteotomies for treatment of the degenerative knee addressed valgus deformity *(1)*. Coventry examined 31 knees that underwent varus closing wedge tibial osteotomy for valgus deformity of the knee at a follow-up of 9 yr *(50)*. Of these patients, 77% had major pain relief, and there was no significant loss in preoperative range of motion. The chief complication of valgus osteotomy was recurrence of valgus deformity. Recurrence of valgus deformity was not noticed in knees that were overcorrected to 0° of anatomical tibiofemoral alignment. Patients with a postoperative joint line obliquity of greater than 10° were found to have poor results. Coventry hypothesized that correcting too large a preoperative valgus deformity with a tibial osteotomy results in excessive tibial obliquity, leading to instability and a poor result. As a result, he suggested that valgus deformities greater than 12° should be corrected with a distal femoral osteotomy.

Marti et al. reported on a laterally based opening wedge varus-producing osteotomy of the proximal tibia for valgus deformities in 36 knees *(9)*. After 11 yr, 88% of knees had excellent and good results; 9% had an apraxia of the peroneal nerve that resolved spontaneously.

FACTORS AFFECTING OUTCOME

Amount of Initial Correction

The recommended amount of intraoperative correction varies. For varus knees, Coventry suggested a femoral-tibial angle (FTA) of 167–170° (10–13° of valgus) *(5,7)*. Others have recommended correction ranging from 164 to 177°s *(11,36,53,54,57)*. The mechanical axis passes through the center of the knee when the FTA is 171.7° (8.3° anatomic valgus) *(58)*.

The amount of initial correction is an important predictor of outcome after osteotomy. Multivariate Cox regression modeling showed that 1-yr postoperative alignment was the most significant factor influencing survival for valgus-producing osteotomies *(43)*. Failure to correct or maintain a valgus alignment at 1 yr after osteotomy was correlated with an increased risk of early failure *(56)*. The FTA at 10-yr follow-up was significantly correlated with the FTA at 1-yr follow-up and clinical outcome *(54)*.

Studies have shown that the degree of valgus correction correlates with the amount of cartilage regeneration found at second-look arthroscopy *(23,59)*. Knees that were overcorrected into valgus alignment had the best clinical and radiographic results *(8,11,14,42,44,51,60,61)*.

Improvements in knee function score decreased when the FTA increased. Aglietti et al. showed that an alignment of 6–15° of valgus achieved the best clinical results, and both undercorrected and overcorrected knees had less-satisfactory results *(53)*. Undercorrected knees tended to progress further into varus and had more progression of medial compartment narrowing when compared to knees corrected into 6–15° of valgus.

Coventry showed that survivorship was dependent on the amount of correction. Knees with less than 5° of valgus angulation had a 63% survival at 10 yr; knees with 6–7° of valgus angulation had an 87% survival rate, and knees with 8° or more of valgus angulation had a 94% survival at 10 yr *(55)*.

Sprenger and Doerzbacher showed that a valgus alignment of 8–16° at 1 yr postoperatively significantly improved knee scores, patient subjective satisfaction, and increased survivorship at 5 yr (95 vs 80%), 10 yr (90 vs 55%), and 15 yr (72 vs 34%) compared to corrections of less than 8° or greater than 17° of valgus *(43)*.

Several studies have suggested that good pain relief and functional results occurred from extreme valgus alignment (10–16° valgus), but some patients have not been satisfied with the appearance of the leg *(42,43,54,61,62)*.

For varus-producing osteotomies for valgus deformity, Coventry reported that a final alignment between 5° of valgus and 4° of varus was reasonable, but the optimal alignment was 0° of varus/valgus *(50)*. He noted that the most common complication of valgus osteotomy was recurrent valgus deformity, which did not occur in his series of patients who were overcorrected to 0° of varus/valgus alignment.

Loss of Initial Correction

A common complication of closing wedge osteotomies was the loss of the initial correction, which ranged from 1.5 to 3.3° *(8,41,54,55,63,64)*. Progression of osteoarthritis and the return of pain was more prevalent in knees that had a loss of initial correction compared to knees that maintained the correction *(8,42,64)*. Rinonapoli et al. showed that the number of knees with loss of correction increased with length of follow-up *(8)*. Shaw et al. hypothesized that loss of correction was caused by the adduction moment on the knee during gait, which resulted in residual medial compartment loading, causing further bone collapse *(65)*. Future studies evaluating the results of osteotomies stabilized with rigid internal fixation may show a decreased incidence of loss of correction and more durable clinical results.

Degree of Preoperative Deformity and Osteoarthritis

The outcome of closing wedge high tibial osteotomies is dependent on preoperative deformity. Rinonapoli et al. demonstrated that knees with less than 10° of varus preoperatively were 88% successful compared to a 66% success rate in knees with 10–15° preoperative varus and an 11% success rate in knees with greater than 15° of varus preoperatively *(8)*. When a lateral closing wedge tibial osteotomy is performed to correct angular deformities greater than 15°, the lateral collateral ligament may become lax and nonfunctional *(65)*. Thus, under varus loads such as those experienced during gait, the knee may fall back in varus and negate the correction afforded by the osteotomy. Several studies suggested that a preoperative valgus deformity of greater than 10° is an indication for a total knee arthroplasty *(8,42)*.

Multiple investigators have demonstrated that the clinical outcomes deteriorated as the preoperative grade of arthrosis became more severe *(7,14,53,57,61)*. Berman et al. demonstrated that knees with preoperative bicompartmental disease had only fair or poor results and concluded that high tibial osteotomy was not indicated to treat generalized osteoarthritis of the knee and should be reserved for unicompartmental osteoarthritis *(6)*. Rinonapoli et al. also listed concomitant lateral compartment osteoarthritis as a contraindication to high tibial valgus osteotomy *(8)*. Patients with prior lateral meniscectomy did poorly after valgus-producing high tibial osteotomies *(66)*. However, Keene and Dyreby showed that subradiographic evidence of lateral compartment articular degeneration diagnosed by arthroscopy did not affect clinical outcomes at a mean follow-up of 32 mo *(51)*.

The presence of patellofemoral arthritis as a contraindication for high tibial osteotomy has been debated. Several studies suggested that moderate-to-severe patellofemoral arthritis was not a contraindication to high tibial valgus osteotomy *(14,51)*. In contrast, Rudan and Simurda showed that high tibial osteotomy produced the best results when there was minimal evidence of patellofemoral arthritis *(61)*. Knees with no or mild patellofemoral arthrosis had statistically higher postoperative scores and good-to-excellent results when compared with knees with moderate or severe patellofemoral arthrosis diagnosed by radiographs.

Preoperative Instability

Many studies list preoperative collateral ligament instability as a contraindication to knee osteotomies *(7,8,56,63)*. Insall et al. demonstrated that 13 of 51 knees had a persistent thrust after high tibial osteotomy *(63)*. Shoji and Insall showed that 30 of 49 knees had a persistent medial thrust after a high tibial osteotomy performed for valgus deformity, and 21 of these knees had persistent pain *(67)*. It is important to note that patients with preoperative instability tend to have higher degrees of angular deformity, which also puts them at an increased risk for failure when treated with an osteotomy.

Anterior cruciate ligament (ACL) insufficiency in the setting of medial compartment arthritis and varus deformity is not a contraindication to surgery. The ACL can be reconstructed at the same time as the osteotomy procedure or can be done in a staged fashion. Based on the Hospital for Special Surgery (HSS) knee score, Williams et al. demonstrated

100% excellent results in patients treated with combined high tibial osteotomy and concurrent ACL reconstruction *(68)*. In addition, 68% of ACL-deficient patients treated with high tibial osteotomy alone for varus malalignment with medial arthritis had improvement of their instability symptoms.

Age

There is some debate regarding the effect of age on the outcome of high tibial osteotomy for the treatment of varus gonarthrosis. Insall et al. showed that patients older than 60 yr had 52% good and excellent results compared to 74% good and excellent results in patients younger than 60 yr *(42)*. Naudie et al. showed that patients older than 50 yr were at increased risk for early failure of high tibial osteotomy *(56)*. In the study by Berman et al., patients with good results averaged 52 yr of age, patients with fair results averaged 58 yr of age, and those with poor results averaged 62 yr of age *(6)*. The 30- and 40-yr-old patients had approx 70% satisfactory results up to 10 yr after high tibial osteotomy *(66,69)*.

In contrast, several studies did not demonstrate a correlation with increased age and worse outcome after high tibial osteotomy *(8,14,43,54)*. Nevertheless, with the good long-term outcomes of total knee arthroplasty and the improving outcomes of unicompartmental arthroplasty, there are few indications for knee osteotomies in patients over 60 yr of age with degenerative arthritis. The exception to this would be a very high-demand sexagenarian who wished to keep participating in high-impact activities, such as jogging, which might lead to early arthroplasty failure.

Weight

Several studies have correlated increased weight and obesity with a higher probability of failure *(44,55)*. However, one study revealed that there was a significant association between a low body mass index (<25 kg/m^2) and the probability of early failure of a high tibial osteotomy *(56)*. This may be related to the higher demand placed on the osteotomies performed in lighter, more active patients.

Preoperative Range of Motion

Coventry stated that flexion less than 90° was a contraindication to an osteotomy *(5)*. Naudie et al. found that preoperative flexion less than 120°s was a risk factor for early failure *(56)*. Kettelkamp et al. were unable to determine a correlation between preoperative range of motion and postoperative outcome *(11)*. Several studies have shown that patients lose range of motion after a high tibial osteotomy *(6,44)*. This may be because of the creation of a patella baja that has been shown to occur in some patients after high tibial osteotomy *(8,70,71)*.

Rheumatoid Arthritis

Coventry's initial study included four patients with rheumatoid arthritis who had satisfactory results at short-term follow-up after knee osteotomy *(5)*. However, his follow-up study revealed that 45% of patients with quiescent rheumatoid arthritis had fair or poor results *(7)*. A more recent study by Coventry revealed that all eight patients who underwent varus osteotomy for lateral deformity had persistent pain and instability even though the angular deformity was corrected *(50)*. Poor results were found in other studies evaluating the use of knee osteotomy in patients with rheumatoid arthritis *(6,12,44)*. In general, rheumatoid arthritis is not an indication for knee osteotomies.

Gait

Gait studies have shown that high tibial osteotomies reduced the peak adduction moment that occurred with walking. Patients with a low preoperative adduction moment at the knee during walking had a better result after the osteotomy and maintained the postoperative alignment better than did patients with a high adduction moment *(72,73)*. Wang et al. demonstrated an association between the adduction moment at the knee and the inversion moment at the ankle and hypothesized that patients can reduce the adduction moment at the knee through changes in placement of the foot during gait *(73)*. This adaptation may be an important mechanism for reducing the load at the knee and improving the survivorship of high tibial osteotomy.

DEVELOPMENT OF LATERAL COMPARTMENT OSTEOARTHRITIS AFTER VALGUS-PRODUCING OSTEOTOMIES

Several studies have noted the development of osteoarthritis in the lateral compartment after overcorrected valgus-producing high tibial osteotomies *(8,62,63)*. However, these studies did not show a correlation with development of lateral osteoarthritis and deterioration of clinical results.

ACTIVITY AFTER KNEE OSTEOTOMIES

Knee osteotomies are often done in young, high-demand patients who are not suitable candidates for knee arthroplasty. Thus, improved postoperative function and the ability to return to premorbid activities are important for these patients. Holden et al. reported that many patients with good and excellent results returned to some type of sporting activities, but they were unable to return to cutting or jumping sports *(69)*. The patients who resumed running were only able to return on a limited basis.

Nagel et al. polled osteotomy patients to determine their postoperative levels of function *(74)*. The best predictor of postoperative activity was the preoperative level of activity. In general, postoperative activity level plateaued at a level lower than the preoperative level and then gradually decreased with time. Of the patients, 79% were able to stand for longer than 4 h, 91% of patients could walk over a mile, 76% were able to perform manual labor, 87% were able to ride a bicycle, and 50% of patients were able to kneel.

Williams et al. showed a mean 1.1 increase in Tegner Activity Scores after high tibial osteotomy *(68)*. Preoperatively, 56% of the patients were able to participate in competitive or recreational sports. After high tibial osteotomy, 92% of patients were able to participate in competitive or recreational sports.

PREFERRED APPROACH

Our preferred approach to treating the varus malaligned knee is to perform a high tibial osteotomy in the coronal plane (Fig. 6). Unlike other osteotomies, the coronal plane osteotomy does not distort the architecture of the proximal tibia and does not cause a change in limb length. The coronal plane osteotomy is indicated in the treatment of the painful knee with either varus or valgus femoral-tibial alignment. We also use this procedure as an adjunct procedure to ligament reconstruction in the leg with malaligned knee (Fig. 7). Uncorrected malalignment after ACL or posterolateral corner reconstruction can predispose the knee to early failure. The coronal plane osteotomy is also used in combination with meniscal allografts, mosaicplasty,

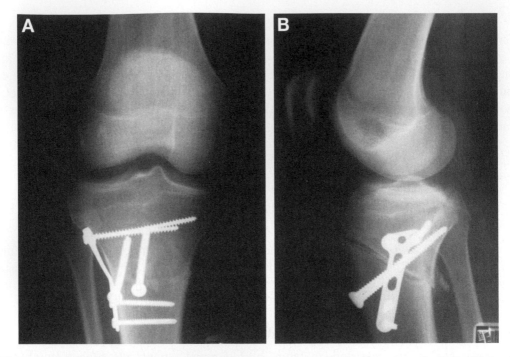

Fig. 6. (**A**) Anterior-posterior radiograph of a valgus-producing coronal plane high tibial osteotomy. (**B**) Lateral radiograph of a valgus-producing coronal plane high tibial osteotomy.

osteochondral allografts, and ACI to correct malalignment that may lead to failure of the index procedure (Fig. 8).

A history and physical examination is performed on all potential candidates for coronal plane osteotomy. Functional age rather than chronological age is used to determine the suitability of an osteotomy. Decisions to proceed with osteotomy over unicompartmental or total knee arthroplasty are determined on a case-by-case basis, taking into consideration the patient's lifestyle demands and desires. Patients with inflammatory knee arthritis are excluded from consideration. Obesity is not a contraindication to osteotomy. Patients with less than 90° of flexion or a significant flexion contracture are not considered for coronal plane osteotomy because the procedure will not correct the loss of motion. The patient's gait is assessed because tibiofemoral malalignment in the presence of a thrust is a significant indication for coronal plane osteotomy. Knees are assessed for ligamentous instability that might require concomitant reconstruction during the osteotomy.

The preoperative radiographic workup includes anterior-posterior, lateral, Merchant, and Rosenberg radiographic projections. The radiographic presence of bicompartmental osteoarthritis is a contraindication to coronal plane osteotomy. Significant, symptomatic, radiographic patellofemoral arthritis is a contraindication to the coronal plane osteotomy.

A full-length, bilateral lower extremity standing radiograph is obtained to evaluate the mechanical and anatomic axes. Patients with a mechanical axis passing through the medial compartment or a TFA of greater than 180° are candidates for coronal plane osteotomy. Preoperative planning for angular correction is determined by the method of Dugdale et al. (*75*).

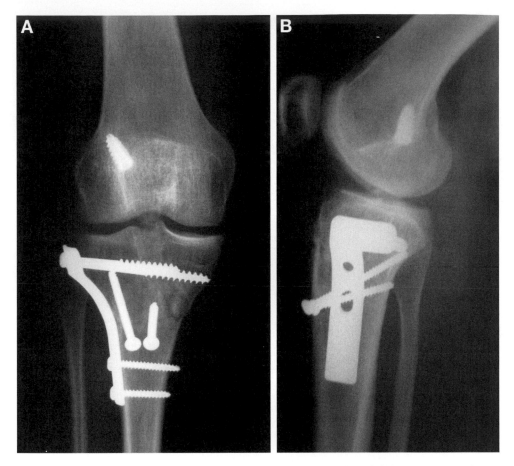

Fig. 7. (A) Anterior-posterior radiograph of a coronal plane high tibial osteotomy with anterior cruciate ligament reconstruction. **(B)** Lateral radiograph of a coronal plane high tibial osteotomy with anterior cruciate ligament reconstruction.

Intraoperative Procedure

Preoperative antibiotics are administered to the patient. Regional anesthesia is induced by the anesthesiologists. The patient is placed supine on a radiolucent operating table. A non-sterile tourniquet is placed over the proximal thigh. An electrocardiograph lead is placed over the center of the femoral head with the use of fluoroscopic guidance. The patient's affected lower extremity is prepped in draped sterile fashion. The lower extremity is exsanguinated by gravity. The tourniquet is raised to 300 mmHg. Arthroscopy is indicated if there are loose bodies present or the patient is having locking sensations.

A 2-cm incision is made over the proximal, midshaft fibula. Dissection is performed down to the fibula, and the periosteum is split. Two retractors are placed subperiosteally around the fibula. A fibular osteotomy is made with a sagittal saw in a superolateral-to-inferomedial direction to allow for a valgus angulation to occur after tibial osteotomy.

Next, a 6- to 8-cm incision is made from the inferior pole of the patella to just distal to the tibial tubercle. Electrocautery is used to incise the fascia over the tibia. An elevator is used to dissect subperiosteally. A deep retractor is placed lateral and posterior to the tibia, retracting

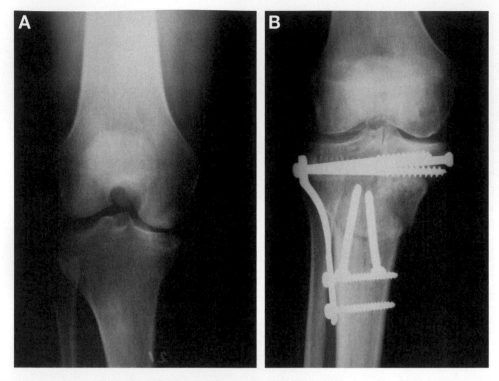

Fig. 8. (A) Flexion posterior-anterior radiograph of a varus malaligned knee with a medial tibial plateau osteochondral defect. **(B)** Anterior-posterior radiograph of a coronal plane high tibial osteotomy with a medial tibial plateau osteochondral allograft.

the anterior compartment. The oblique coronal plane osteotomy is started anteriorly, proximal to the tibial tubercle, and is extended distal and posterior. Two preliminary drill holes are drilled in the distal aspect of the osteotomy with the 4.5-mm drill bit prior to creation of the osteotomy. A sagittal saw is used to start the osteotomy, and osteotomes are used to complete it. Just prior to completion of the osteotomy, a smooth Steinman pin is temporarily placed across the osteotomy site to act as a pivot and provide rotational control.

After completion of the osteotomy, a varus or valgus force is placed on the distal piece, and the angular correction is performed. A bone-holding forceps is used to hold the proximal and distal fragments stable once the appropriate correction is made. The electrocautery cord is placed over the electrocardiograph lead, across the tibiofemoral joint, down to the center of the tibiotalar joint to recreate the mechanical axis. Fluoroscopy is used to confirm appropriate correction of the mechanical axis. For a valgus-producing osteotomy, the goal is to have the mechanical axis pass through the 62nd percentile of the joint line *(75)*. For a varus-producing osteotomy, the goal is to have the mechanical axis pass through the medial tibial spine.

Two 4.5-mm cortical screws are used to compress and stabilize the osteotomy site in an anterior-to-posterior direction. An L-plate is used as a neutralization plate and is placed laterally on the tibia. Initially, we used a small fragment plate, but we have now modified the technique to a large fragment plate for increased rigidity at the osteotomy site. The wounds are irrigated vigorously. The fascia and skin are closed in standard fashion, and a soft, sterile dressing is applied. Patients are placed in a hinged knee brace, which is initially locked in extension.

Postoperatively, all patients remain non-weight bearing until there is both clinical and radiographic evidence of healing, ranging from 6 to 8 wk. Range of motion is started on the operative day using a continuous passive motion machine. Continuous passive motion is used for the first 2 wk and is combined with a physical therapy regimen to focus on regaining range of motion. Patients are gradually progressed to closed-chain strengthening exercises. More strenuous exercise is allowed after 5 mo.

Outcomes

A short-term follow-up study revealed that the coronal plane high tibial osteotomy provided both good clinical and good radiographic results (S. Fealy and T. L. Wickiewicz, unpublished data, 2004). Patients were corrected from a mean preoperative 4.6° of varus to 6.3° of valgus. The mean range of motion at final follow-up was 1.6° of extension to 123° of flexion. Visual analog pain scores decreased from 7.8 to 2.6 at a minimum 2-year follow-up. The mean Lysholm score was 84.3 (good). There were no failures that required a revision procedure.

SUMMARY

The high tibial osteotomy and the distal femoral osteotomy are effective methods for correcting tibiofemoral malalignment. Isolated knee osteotomies have been shown to stimulate cartilage repair. Knee osteotomies can be used for primary treatment of knee pain and tibiofemoral malalignment, or they can be combined with cartilage repair procedures to improve long-term results. Length of follow-up and the amount of tibiofemoral correction are important predictors for outcome. We have found the coronal plane high tibial osteotomy to be a straightforward procedure with good short-term results.

REFERENCES

1. Jackson JP. Osteotomy for osteoarthritis of the knee. J Bone Joint Surg Br 1958;40B:826.
2. Jackson JP, Waugh W. Tibial osteotomy for osteoarthritis of the knee. J Bone Joint Surg Br 1961;43-B:746–751.
3. Wardle EN. Osteotomy of the tibia and fibula. Surg Gynecol Obstet 1962;115:61–64.
4. Gariepy G. Genu varum treated by high tibial osteotomy. In Proceedings of the Joint Meeting of the Orthopaedic Associations. JBJS 1964;46-B:783–784.
5. Coventry MB. Osteotomy of the upper portion of the tibia for degenerative arthritis of the knee. A preliminary report. J Bone Joint Surg Am 1965;47:984–990.
6. Berman AT, Bosacco SJ, Kirshner S, Avolio A Jr. Factors influencing long-term results in high tibial osteotomy. Clin Orthop Relat Res 1991;272:192–198.
7. Coventry MB. Osteotomy about the knee for degenerative and rheumatoid arthritis. J Bone Joint Surg Am 1973;55:23–48.
8. Rinonapoli E, Mancini GB, Corvaglia A, Musiello S. Tibial osteotomy for varus gonarthrosis. A 10- to 21-year followup study. Clin Orthop Relat Res 1998;353:185–193.
9. Marti RK, Verhagen RA, Kerkhoffs GM, Moojen TM. Proximal tibial varus osteotomy. Indications, technique, and 5- to 21-yr results. J Bone Joint Surg Am 2001;83-A:164–170.
10. Papachristou G. Photoelastic study of the internal and contact stresses on the knee joint before and after osteotomy. Arch Orthop Trauma Surg 2004;124:288–297.
11. Kettelkamp DB, Wenger DR, Chao EY, Thompson C. Results of proximal tibial osteotomy. The effects of tibiofemoral angle, stance-phase flexion-extension, and medial-plateau force. J Bone Joint Surg Am 1976;58:952–960.

12. Harris WR, Kostuik JP. High tibial osteotomy for osteo-arthritis of the knee. J Bone Joint Surg Am 1970;52:330–336.
13. Maquet P. The treatment of choice in osteoarthritis of the knee. Clin Orthop Relat Res 1985;192:108–112.
14. Tjornstrand BA, Egund N, Hagstedt BV. High tibial osteotomy: a 7-yr clinical and radiographic follow-up. Clin Orthop Relat Res 1981;160:124–136.
15. Schultz W, Gobel D. Articular cartilage regeneration of the knee joint after proximal tibial valgus osteotomy: a prospective study of different intra- and extra-articular operative techniques. Knee Surg Sports Traumatol Arthrosc 1999;7:29–36.
16. Koshino T, Wada S, Ara Y, Saito T. Regeneration of degenerated articular cartilage after high tibial valgus osteotomy for medial compartmental osteoarthritis of the knee. Knee 2003;10: 229–236.
17. Akamatsu Y, Koshino T, Saito T, Wada J. Changes in osteosclerosis of the osteoarthritic knee after high tibial osteotomy. Clin Orthop Relat Res 1997;334:207–214.
18. Wei L, Hjerpe A, Brismar BH, Svensson O. Effect of load on articular cartilage matrix and the development of guinea-pig osteoarthritis. Osteoarthritis Cartilage 2001;9:447–453.
19. Matsui N, Moriya H, Kitahara H. The use of arthroscopy for follow-up in knee joint surgery. Orthop Clin North Am 1979;10:697–708.
20. Odenbring S, Egund N, Lindstrand A, Lohmander LS, Willen H. Cartilage regeneration after proximal tibial osteotomy for medial gonarthrosis. An arthroscopic, roentgenographic, and histologic study. Clin Orthop Relat Res 1992;277:210–216.
21. Akizuki S, Yasukawa Y, Takizawa T. Does arthroscopic abrasion arthroplasty promote cartilage regeneration in osteoarthritic knees with eburnation? A prospective study of high tibial osteotomy with abrasion arthroplasty vs high tibial osteotomy alone. Arthroscopy 1997;13:9–17.
22. Wakabayashi S, Akizuki S, Takizawa T, Yasukawa Y. A comparison of the healing potential of fibrillated cartilage vs eburnated bone in osteoarthritic knees after high tibial osteotomy: an arthroscopic study with 1-yr follow-up. Arthroscopy 2002;18:272–278.
23. Fujisawa Y, Masuhara K, Shiomi S. The effect of high tibial osteotomy on osteoarthritis of the knee. An arthroscopic study of 54 knee joints. Orthop Clin North Am 1979;10:585–608.
24. McDermott AG, Langer F, Pritzker KP, Gross AE. Fresh small-fragment osteochondral allografts. Long-term follow-up study on first 100 cases. Clin Orthop Relat Res 1985;197:96–102.
25. Hangody L, Fules P. Autologous osteochondral mosaicplasty for the treatment of full-thickness defects of weight-bearing joints: 10 yr of experimental and clinical experience. J Bone Joint Surg Am 2003;85-A(suppl 2):25–32.
26. Ghazavi MT, Pritzker KP, Davis AM, Gross AE. Fresh osteochondral allografts for post-traumatic osteochondral defects of the knee. J Bone Joint Surg Br 1997;79:1008–1013.
27. Beaver RJ, Mahomed M, Backstein D, et al. Fresh osteochondral allografts for post-traumatic defects in the knee. A survivorship analysis. J Bone Joint Surg Br 1992;74:105–110.
28. Shasha N, Krywulak S, Backstein D, Pressman A, Gross AE. Long-term follow-up of fresh tibial osteochondral allografts for failed tibial plateau fractures. J Bone Joint Surg Am 2003; 85-A(suppl 2):33–39.
29. Aubin PP, Cheah HK, Davis AM, Gross AE. Long-term followup of fresh femoral osteochondral allografts for posttraumatic knee defects. Clin Orthop Relat Res 2001;391(suppl):S318–S327.
30. Oakeshott RD, Farine I, Pritzker KPH, Langer F, Gross AE. A clinical and histologic analysis of failed fresh osteochondral allografts. Clin Orthop 1988;233:283–294.
31. Cameron JC, Saha S. Meniscal allograft transplantation for unicompartmental arthritis of the knee. Clin Orthop Relat Res 1997;337:164–171.
32. Verdonk R. Alternative treatments for meniscal injuries. J Bone Joint Surg Br 1997;79:866–873.
33. Graf KW Jr, Sekiya JK, Wojtys EM. Long-term results after combined medial meniscal allograft transplantation and anterior cruciate ligament reconstruction: minimum 8.5-yr follow-up study. Arthroscopy 2004;20:129–140.
34. van Arkel ERA, de Boer HH. Human meniscal transplantation. Preliminary results at 2- to 5-yr follow-up. J Bone Joint Surg Br 1995;77-B:589–595.

35. de Boer HH, Koudstaal J. Failed meniscus transplantation. A report of three cases. Clin Orthop Relat Res 1994;306:155–162.
36. Bauer GC, Insall J, Koshino T. Tibial osteotomy in gonarthrosis (osteo-arthritis of the knee). J Bone Joint Surg Am 1969;51:1545–1563.
37. Kettelkamp DB, Leach RE, Nasca R. Pitfalls of proximal tibial osteotomy. Clin Orthop Relat Res 1975;106:232–241.
38. Waugh W. Tibial osteotomy in the management of osteoarthritis of the knee. Clin Orthop Relat Res 1986;210:55–61.
39. Paley D, Maar DC, Herzenberg JE. New concepts in high tibial osteotomy for medial compartment osteoarthritis. Orthop Clin North Am 1994;25:483–498.
40. Hofmann AA, Wyatt RW, Beck SW. High tibial osteotomy. Use of an osteotomy jig, rigid fixation, and early motion vs conventional surgical technique and cast immobilization. Clin Orthop Relat Res 1991;271:212–217.
41. Billings A, Scott DF, Camargo MP, Hofmann AA. High tibial osteotomy with a calibrated osteotomy guide, rigid internal fixation, and early motion. Long-term follow-up. J Bone Joint Surg Am 2000;82:70–79.
42. Insall JN, Joseph DM, Msika C. High tibial osteotomy for varus gonarthrosis. A long-term follow-up study. J Bone Joint Surg Am 1984;66:1040–1048.
43. Sprenger TR, Doerzbacher JF. Tibial osteotomy for the treatment of varus gonarthrosis. Survival and failure analysis to 22 yr. J Bone Joint Surg Am 2003;85-A:469–474.
44. Matthews LS, Goldstein SA, Malvitz TA, Katz BP, Kaufer H. Proximal tibial osteotomy. Factors that influence the duration of satisfactory function. Clin Orthop 1988:193–200.
45. Amendola A. Unicompartmental osteoarthritis in the active patient: the role of high tibial osteotomy. Arthroscopy 2003;19(suppl 1):109–116.
46. Amendola A, Fowler PJ, Litchfield R, Kirkley S, Clatworthy M. Opening wedge high tibial osteotomy using a novel technique: early results and complications. J Knee Surg 2004;17:164–169.
47. Sterett WI, Steadman JR. Chondral resurfacing and high tibial osteotomy in the varus knee. Am J Sports Med 2004;32:1243–1249.
48. Catagni MA, Guerreschi F, Ahmad TS, Cattaneo R. Treatment of genu varum in medial compartment osteoarthritis of the knee using the Ilizarov method. Orthop Clin North Am 1994;25:509–514.
49. Magyar G, Ahl TL, Vibe P, Toksvig-Larsen S, Lindstrand A. Open-wedge osteotomy by hemicallotasis or the closed-wedge technique for osteoarthritis of the knee. A randomised study of 50 operations. J Bone Joint Surg Br 1999;81:444–448.
50. Coventry MB. Proximal tibial varus osteotomy for osteoarthritis of the lateral compartment of the knee. J Bone Joint Surg Am 1987;69:32–38.
51. Keene JS, Dyreby JR, Jr. High tibial osteotomy in the treatment of osteoarthritis of the knee. The role of preoperative arthroscopy. J Bone Joint Surg Am 1983;65:36–42.
52. Miniaci A, Ballmer FT, Ballmer PM, Jakob RP. Proximal tibial osteotomy. A new fixation device. Clin Orthop Relat Res 1989;246:250–259.
53. Aglietti P, Rinonapoli E, Stringa G, Taviani A. Tibial osteotomy for the varus osteoarthritic knee. Clin Orthop Relat Res 1983;176:239–251.
54. Yasuda K, Majima T, Tsuchida T, Kaneda K. A 10- to 15-year follow-up observation of high tibial osteotomy in medial compartment osteoarthrosis. Clin Orthop Relat Res 1992;282:186–195.
55. Coventry MB, Ilstrup DM, Wallrichs SL. Proximal tibial osteotomy. A critical long-term study of 87 cases. J Bone Joint Surg Am 1993;75:196–201.
56. Naudie D, Bourne RB, Rorabeck CH, Bourne TJ. Survivorship of the high tibial osteotomy: A 10- to 22-yr followup study. Clin Orthop 1999;367:18–27.
57. Vainionpaa S, Laike E, Kirves P, Tiusanen P. Tibial osteotomy for osteoarthritis of the knee. A 5- to 10-yr follow-up study. J Bone Joint Surg Am 1981;63:938–946.
58. Koshino T, Morii T, Wada J, et al. High tibial osteotomy with fixation by a blade plate for medial compartment osteoarthritis of the knee. Orthop Clin North Am 1989;20:227–243.

59. Kanamiya T, Naito M, Hara M, Yoshimura I. The influences of biomechanical factors on cartilage regeneration after high tibial osteotomy for knees with medial compartment osteoarthritis: clinical and arthroscopic observations. Arthroscopy 2002;18:725–729.
60. Ivarsson I, Myrnerts R, Gillquist J. High tibial osteotomy for medial osteoarthritis of the knee. A 5- to 7- and 11-yr follow-up. J Bone Joint Surg Br 1990;72:238–244.
61. Rudan JF, Simurda MA. High tibial osteotomy. A prospective clinical and roentgenographic review. Clin Orthop Relat Res 1990;255:251–256.
62. Hernigou P, Medevielle D, Debeyre J, Goutallier D. Proximal tibial osteotomy for osteoarthritis with varus deformity. A 10- to 13-yr follow-up study. J Bone Joint Surg Am 1987;69:332–354.
63. Insall J, Shoji H, Mayer V. High tibial osteotomy. A 5-yr evaluation. J Bone Joint Surg Am 1974;56:1397–1405.
64. Stuart MJ, Grace JN, Ilstrup DM, et al. Late recurrence of varus deformity after proximal tibial osteotomy. Clin Orthop Relat Res 1990;260:61–65.
65. Shaw JA, Dungy DS, Arsht SS. Recurrent varus angulation after high tibial osteotomy: an anatomic analysis. Clin Orthop Relat Res 2004;420:205–212.
66. Morrey BF. Upper tibial osteotomy for secondary osteoarthritis of the knee. J Bone Joint Surg Br 1989;71:554–559.
67. Shoji H, Insall J. High tibial osteotomy for osteoarthritis of the knee with valgus deformity. J Bone Joint Surg Am 1973;55:963–973.
68. Williams R Jr, Kelly BT, Wickiewicz TL, Altchek DW, Warren RW. The short-term outcome of surgical treatment for painful varus arthritis in association with chronic ACL deficiency. J Knee Surg 2003;16:9–16.
69. Holden DL, James SL, Larson RL, Slocum DB. Proximal tibial osteotomy in patients who are 50 yr old or less. A long-term follow-up study. J Bone Joint Surg Am 1988;70:977–982.
70. Kaper BP, Bourne RB, Rorabeck CH, Macdonald SJ. Patellar infera after high tibial osteotomy. J Arthroplasty 2001;16:168–173.
71. Scuderi GR, Windsor RE, Insall JN. Observations on patellar height after proximal tibial osteotomy. J Bone Joint Surg Am 1989;71:245–248.
72. Prodromos CC, Andriacchi TP, Galante JO. A relationship between gait and clinical changes following high tibial osteotomy. J Bone Joint Surg Am 1985;67:1188–1194.
73. Wang JW, Kuo KN, Andriacchi TP, Galante JO. The influence of walking mechanics and time on the results of proximal tibial osteotomy. J Bone Joint Surg Am 1990;72:905–909.
74. Nagel A, Insall JN, Scuderi GR. Proximal tibial osteotomy. A subjective outcome study. J Bone Joint Surg Am 1996;78:1353–1358.
75. Dugdale TW, Noyes FR, Styer D. Preoperative planning for high tibial osteotomy. The effect of lateral tibiofemoral separation and tibiofemoral length. Clin Orthop Relat Res 1992;274:248–264.

16

Management of Osteochondritis Dissecans

Mininder S. Kocher, MD, MPH and Joseph J. Czarnecki, MD

Summary

Osteochondritis dissecans (OCD) is an acquired condition affecting subchondral bone that manifests as a pathologic spectrum including softening of the overlying articular cartilage with an intact articular surface, early articular cartilage separation, partial detachment of an articular lesion, and osteochondral separation with loose bodies. The etiology of OCD remains speculative; however. repetitive microtrauma is a common association. Nonoperative initial management is indicated for stable lesions in skeletally immature patients given the potential for healing with normal subsequent function and radiographs. Nonoperative treatment options range from "watchful waiting" and activity modification to nonweightbearing and immobilization with trials lasting from 6 to 18 months. Operative treatment is indicated for detached or unstable lesions, adult OCD lesions or juvenile patients approaching epiphyseal closure, and failure of nonoperative management. Surgical options depend on the involved pathology and include drilling, curettage, bone grafting, internal fixation, open or arthroscopic reduction of a loose fragment with internal fixation, fragment removal, autologous or allogeneic osteochondral grafting, and autologous chondrocyte implantation. This chapter is an overview of the etiology, clinical presentation, diagnostic studies, nonoperative treatment, and operative treatment of OCD of the knee.

Key Words: Adolescents; articular cartilage; children; osteochondral fracture; osteochondritis dissecans.

INTRODUCTION

Osteochondritis dissecans (OCD) is relatively common cause of knee pain and dysfunction in the child, adolescent, and young adult. OCD is an acquired condition affecting subchondral bone that manifests as a pathological spectrum, including softening of the overlying articular cartilage with an intact articular surface, early articular cartilage separation, partial detachment of an articular lesion, and osteochondral separation with loose bodies (1–7).

The etiology of OCD remains speculative; however, repetitive microtrauma is commonly described as a potential mechanism (1–3,6). OCD of the knee has been classified based on anatomic location, surgical appearance, scintigraphic findings, and age (1–3,6,8,9). OCD of the knee is often subcategorized into a juvenile form and an adult form depending on the status of the distal femoral physis. The majority of adult OCD cases are thought to be persistence of a juvenile OCD lesion that did not heal, although *de novo* adult OCD lesions have been described (1). Juvenile OCD has a much better prognosis than adult OCD, with over 50% of juvenile cases demonstrating healing within 6–18 mo from detection (9–13). Adult OCD, on the other hand, infrequently heals without operative intervention (10). Adult OCD lesions and juvenile OCD lesions that do not heal have potential for developing osteoarthritis (14,15).

From: *Cartilage Repair Strategies*
Edited by: Riley J. Williams © Humana Press Inc., Totowa, NJ

The management of juvenile OCD is controversial. Nonoperative initial management is indicated for stable lesions in skeletally immature patients *(1,3,10,16)*. Nonoperative treatment options range from observation and activity modification to limiting weight bearing and joint immobilization. Such joint protection trials can last from 6 to 18 mo. Operative treatment is indicated for unstable lesions, symptomatic OCD lesions in juvenile patients who are near skeletal maturity, symptomatic adult OCD lesions, and those patients who fail nonoperative management *(1)*. Surgical options include drilling, curettage, bone grafting, lesion fixation, reduction of the OCD fragment with internal fixation, fragment removal, autologous or allograft osteochondral transplantation, and autologous chondrocyte implantation.

This chapter reviews the etiology, clinical presentation, diagnostic studies, nonoperative treatment, and operative treatment of OCD of the knee.

ETIOLOGY

The etiology of OCD remains unclear. Chronic inflammation, genetic predisposition, bone ischemia, ossification, and repetitive trauma have been implicated. The terminology regarding osteochondral lesions of the knee overlaps and may contribute to inconsistency regarding the diagnosis, management, and prognosis of OCD. OCD lesions may present and appear like other cartilage lesions (acute chondral fracture, osteonecrosis). OCD is thought to be an acquired condition that affects subchondral bone. This loss of underlying support results in myriad clinical findings that include softening of the overlying articular cartilage with an intact articular surface, early articular cartilage separation, partial detachment of an articular lesion, and osteochondral separation with loose bodies *(1–3,6)*.

An inflammatory etiology was suggested by König in 1887, by his coining of the condition "osteochondritis dissecans" *(17)*. However, further studies into the etiology of OCD lesions did not support inflammation as a primary cause of OCD. OCD was attributed to an ossification abnormality of the distal femoral epiphysis by Ribbing in 1955 *(18)*. Although abnormalities in ossification are not thought to be the etiology for the majority of cases of OCD, some lateral femoral condyle lesions in younger children that resolve spontaneously may represent an ossification variant.

Ischemia was proposed as an etiology of OCD by Green and Banks based on anatomic and histological findings *(11)*. However, pathologic analysis of OCD lesions has failed to demonstrate avascular necrosis of the OCD fragment or a relative ischemic watershed of the lateral aspect of the medial femoral condyle *(16,19–21)*.

There may also be a genetic predisposition for the development of OCD as families with numerous cases of OCD have been described. Mubarak and Carroll reported on 12 members of a family over four generations who had OCD *(22)*. Petrie, however, found OCD in only 1 of 86 first-degree relatives, and current thought holds that the common form of OCD is not predictably familial *(23)*.

OCD has also been described in association with endocrinopathy, ligamentous laxity, lower limb malalignment, apophysitis, epiphyseal dysplasia, and other osteochondropathies.

The etiology of OCD in most cases includes repetitive trauma. In 1933, Fairbanks proposed that "violent rotation inwards of the tibia, driving the tibial spine against the inner condyle" caused OCD *(24)*. Although anterior tibial spine impingement on the distal femur may not be the cause of OCD lesions of the posterior medial femoral condyle, the frequent occurrence of OCD lesions in patients who are involved in sports with repetitive impact supports the notion of a repetitive trauma etiology. Repetitive trauma is thought to cause a stress reaction of bone, which may then further progress to a stress fracture of the subchondral bone. If such repetitive loading persists and impairs the ability of the subchondral bone to heal following the described insult, then bone necrosis could occur and eventually lead to articular cartilage fragmentation, dissection, and separation.

EPIDEMIOLOGY

The incidence of OCD is unknown. Hughston et al. reported an incidence of 15–21 cases per 100,000 (25). Linden reported an incidence of 18 per 100,000 in females and 29 per 100,000 in males (26). The incidence of OCD appears to be increasing with increased participation in more competitive levels of sports by children at younger ages (1). In addition, the mean age of OCD appears to be decreasing, and more females seem to affected according to some authors (1). Increasing suspicion of serious knee problems in the pediatric population, the availability of magnetic resonance imaging (MRI), and the frequent use of arthroscopy in treating knee problems has resulted in greater recognition of OCD lesions. Current trends in youth sports, including the loss of free play, early sport specialization, multiple leagues in a single sport, and intensive training may also be contributing factors.

CLINICAL PRESENTATION

Because most children and adolescents with OCD have a stable lesion, the presenting complaints are generally vague. The most common complaints are joint ache and activity-related knee pain localized to the anterior aspect of the knee. The symptom complex often overlaps with the complaints heard for other causes of anterior knee pain, such as chondromalacia patella and patellofemoral malalignment. In both cases, there may be pain when climbing hills or stairs. There is usually not a sense of knee instability.

On physical examination, children and adolescents with stable OCD lesions may walk with a subtle antalgic gait. With careful palpation, a point of maximum tenderness can often be located over the anterior medial aspect of the knee through varying amounts of knee flexion. This tender area will correspond to the lesion, which is most commonly on the lateral aspect of the distal medial femoral condyle. In stable lesions, there is usually not a knee effusion, crepitus, or much pain through a range of normal motion. Wilson's sign may be helpful but is often not present (27,28). This test is performed by starting with the knee flexed to 90°. The tibia is then internally rotated as the knee is extended from 90° toward full extension. A positive Wilson's test will elicit pain at about 30° of knee flexion. This pain is thought to result from contact of the medial tibial eminence with the OCD lesion. Pain is located over the anterior aspect of the medial femoral condyle. Ipsilateral quadriceps atrophy may be noted if the patient has been having pain for more than a few weeks.

In the unusual circumstance in which the child or adolescent presents with an unstable lesion, mechanical symptoms may be more pronounced. An antalgic gait is common. There is usually a knee effusion, possibly associated with crepitus as the knee is taken through a range of motion. In both stable and unstable presentations, both knees should be examined as the condition may be bilateral.

DIAGNOSTIC STUDIES

Several goals must be considered when imaging a child or adolescent presenting with signs and symptoms suggestive for OCD. Successful imaging will characterize the lesion,

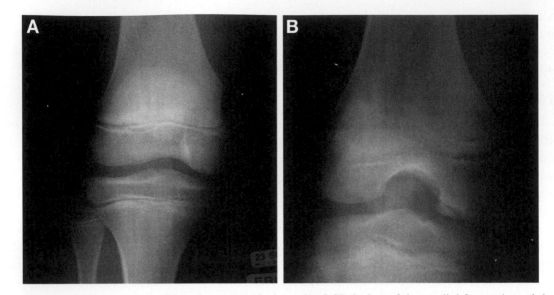

Fig. 1. AP (**A**) and notch (**B**) radiographs of a juvenile OCD lesion of the medial femoral condyle. The lesion can be difficult to see on the AP radiograph but is often more apparent on the notch radiograph, which images the more posterior aspect of the femoral condyle with the knee in flexion.

determine the prognosis of nonoperative management, and possibly determine the ultimate healing of the lesion. Because the success of nonoperative management is somewhat unpredictable in juvenile OCD, many studies have investigated various OCD imaging protocols. An ideal imaging strategy should guide the surgeon in determining which cases should be treated immediately with surgical management and which cases will heal with nonoperative means. Technetium bone scanning, MRI, and MR arthrography have been studied, but to date there is no single imaging protocol that reliably predicts the success of nonoperative management.

Radiographs should always be obtained; anteroposterior (AP) and lateral views of the knee are taken. Tunnel views are also valuable as OCD in the typical location (the posterior lateral portion of the medial femoral condyle) may be difficult to see on a typical AP view (Fig. 1). Merchant or skyline view should be added when patellar OCD is a possibility. These radiographs should facilitate characterization and localization of the lesion. In children younger than 7 yr, irregularities of the distal femoral epiphyseal ossification center may simulate the appearance of OCD. In older children, the status of the physis (open, closing, or closed) should be assessed as this has major implications in the prognosis for healing. The location of the lesion can be described as per Cahill and Berg (8), and a general estimate of size can also be obtained from the plain films.

MRI has become a routine part of the diagnostic evaluation of OCD (29). The initial MRI can give an accurate estimation of the size of the lesion and the status of the cartilage in the subchondral bone (Figs. 2 and 3). The extent of bony edema, the presence of a high signal zone beneath the fragment, and the presence of other loose bodies are also important findings on the initial MRI (Table 1).

For more than a decade, MRI has been studied extensively with the hope that certain MR findings would have definitive prognostic value in determining if an OCD lesion in the skeletally

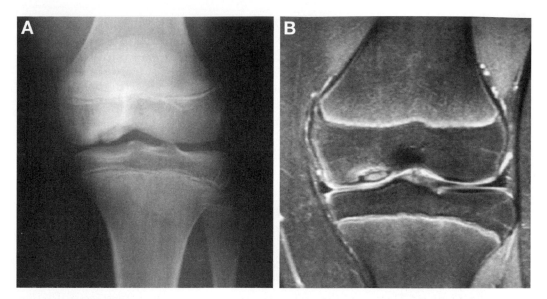

Fig. 2. AP radiograph (**A**) and coronal (**B**) MRI of a stage 2 juvenile OCD lesion of the medial femoral condyle. The lesion is clearly demarcated from the underlying subchondral bone without evidence of healing; however, the articular surface appears intact.

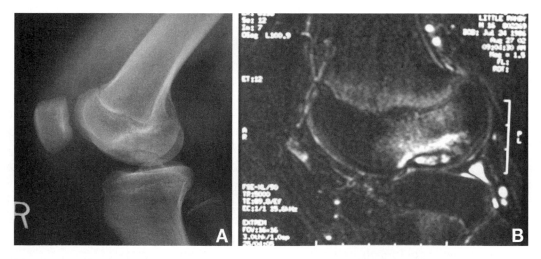

Fig. 3. Lateral radiograph (**A**) and sagittal (**B**) MRI of a stage 3 juvenile OCD lesion of the medial femoral condyle. The lesion is clearly demarcated from the underlying subchondral bone, with apparent separation of the articular surface anteriorly.

immature patient will heal with nonoperative treatment *(30)*. De Smet et al. *(31)* described four MRI criteria on T_2 weighted images:

1. A line of high signal intensity at least 5 mm long between the OCD lesion and the underlying bone.
2. An area of increased homogeneous signal at least 5 mm in diameter beneath the lesion.
3. A focal defect of 5 mm or more in the articular surface.
4. A high signal line traversing the subchondral plate into the lesion.

Table 1
MRI Classification of Juvenile OCD Lesions (29)

Stage 1	Small change of signal without clear margins of fragment.
Stage 2	Osteochondral fragment with clear margins but without fluid between fragment and underlying bone.
Stage 3	Fluid is visible partially between fragment and underlying bone.
Stage 4	Fluid is completely surrounding the fragment, but the fragment is still *in situ*.
Stage 5	Fragment is completely detached and displaced (loose body).

Of these signs, De Smet et al. *(31)* found that the high signal line behind the fragment was most predictive as it was found in 72% of all unstable lesions.

Pill et al. *(32)* attempted to predict the success of nonoperative treatment using both MRI and clinical criteria. These investigators applied De Smet et al.'s four signs and found that the high signal line was the most common of the signs to be present in the patients who failed nonoperative treatment. The size of the lesion and the maturity of the patient were also important predictors of the failure of nonoperative treatment in this study.

O'Connor et al. *(33)* compared MRI and arthroscopic findings, focusing specifically on the prognostic value of De Smet et al.'s high signal line behind the fragment. These authors and others believe that this high signal line can represent either healing vascular granulation tissue or articular fluid that has collected beneath the subchondral bone (implying a break in the articular surface). In this study, the investigators could improve the staging accuracy from 45 to 85% when they interpreted the high signal line on T_2 as a predictor of instability only when it was accompanied by a breach in the cartilage as seen on MRI T_1 imaging.

With several studies suggesting that unenhanced MRI does not have definitive prognostic value in juvenile OCD, some investigators have explored the value of gadolinium. Bohndorf *(30)* found intravenous gadolinium helpful. After intravenous gadolinium, enhancement of the high signal line behind the fragment indicated healing granulation tissue and not fluid from the joint. However, Vonstein et al. showed no correlation between gadolinium enhancement and healing in juvenile OCD *(34)*. These investigators found that the lesion size was still the main determinant of healing. Kramer et al. studied MR arthrography with gadolinium. Although they did not look at the prognostic value in terms of healing, they did determine that this technique could reliably show a breach in the articular cartilage *(35)*.

Technetium bone scans have also been evaluated in hopes that they would provide information about the biological capacity of an OCD lesion to heal. Cahill and Berg *(8)* proposed a protocol of static serial technician bone scans every 6 wk until evidence of healing (Table 2). Litchman et al. *(36)* found that patients with more than 2 mo of symptoms from an OCD who had increased blood flow quantified on technician scans healed their lesions spontaneously. Paletta et al. *(37)* looked at quantitative bone scans in a small series (12 patients) and found that increased activity predicted healing in those patients with open physis but not in adolescents with closing physis. This is unfortunate because it is this latter group in whom healing is most difficult to predict. Despite this information, serial bone scanning has not been widely adopted in the management of OCD lesions, perhaps because of the length of the test, the need for intravenous access, and the perceived risk of the radiotracer injection.

Table 2
Bone Scan Classification of Juvenile OCD Lesions (11)

Stage 0	Normal radiographic and scintigraphic appearance.
Stage 1	The lesion is visible on plain radiographs, but bone scans reveal normal findings.
Stage 2	The scan reveals increased uptake in the area of the lesion.
Stage 3	In addition, there is increased isotopic uptake in the entire femoral condyle.
Stage 4	In addition, there is uptake in the tibial plateau opposite the lesion.

Considering the results of work published to date, current diagnostic imaging recommendations for OCD begin with AP, lateral, and tunnel and Merchant views of the involved knee at presentation. An initial MRI is usually obtained to study the lesion for its size, the status of the cartilage and the subchondral bone, the presence of a high signal zone beneath the lesion, the extent of surrounding bony edema, as well as the possible presence of loose bodies or any other pathology within the knee. Smaller lesions with intact cartilage are much more likely to respond to nonoperative treatment, especially in skeletally immature patients. Unstable lesions, or knees with loose bodies, torn menisci, or any other operative intra-articular pathology, warrant initial arthroscopic evaluation and treatment.

NONOPERATIVE MANAGEMENT

Because the natural history of stable OCD lesions is generally favorable in a child with open physes, there is widespread agreement that initial nonoperative management is indicated *(13)*. However, there has been a debate about whether immobilization is therapeutic or detrimental. This controversy centers on which tissue is considered most important in the healing process. Those who focus on the injured subchondral bone argue that initially the knee should be protected in a cast or knee immobilizer, just as a fracture would be. Conversely, those focused on the cartilage cite the literature on the value of continuous passive motion for cartilage health. Because the failure of the cartilage surface probably follows the failure of the underlying bone, most have embraced some sort of rest or immobilization protocol.

Immobilization can be successfully achieved in a cast or brace. Some authors prefer the protocol of partial weight bearing in a cylinder cast in slight flexion. This allows some compressive forces across the lesion while minimizing shear. This same protocol can usually be accomplished with a standard knee immobilizer. However, although bathing and other activities are easier, compliance with full-time immobilizer use in a young athlete can be a problem. Some have used a hinged, unloader-type brace that allows motion. This treatment has not yet been proven efficacious and has problems with compliance and expense. Further studies are needed to determine the optimal immobilization protocol.

The nonoperative management protocol should consist of three phases. The first phase involves immobilization of the knee for 6 wk with partial weight bearing. At the end of this period, the child should be pain free. Radiographs are repeated. In phase 2 (weeks 6–12), weight bearing as tolerated is permitted without immobilization. A physical therapy protocol is initiated, emphasizing knee range of motion and low-impact quadriceps and hamstring strengthening. If the patient remains pain free, phase 3 begins at 3 mo after diagnosis. This

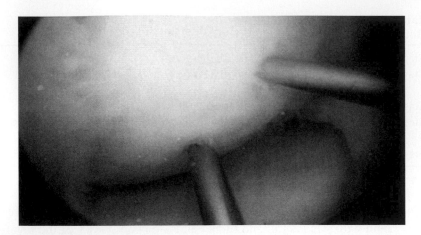

Fig. 4. Arthroscopic image of retrograde transarticular drilling of a stable OCD lesion of the medial femoral condyle with an intact articular surface.

final phase includes close observation of the pediatric athlete at the beginning of running, jumping, and cutting sports. Such high-impact and -shear activities should be restricted until the child has several months of pain-free, low-impact conditioning, and the radiographs show healing. An MRI may be repeated in phase 3 to assess healing.

If the symptoms return or if radiographs show any progression, then a repeat of immobilization can be considered. However, although immobilization alone is often successful in juvenile OCD, it may be completely intolerable to a young athlete and the athlete's parents. The art of dealing with these impatient and frustrated young athletes includes counseling on the risks and benefits of continued nonoperative treatment vs moving on to drilling or other surgical management.

OPERATIVE MANAGEMENT

Although patients with juvenile OCD have a better prognosis for healing than those with adult OCD, not all lesions in skeletally immature knees heal. Operative treatment should be considered in those patients with detached or unstable lesions and in those patients approaching epiphyseal closure whose lesions have been unresponsive to nonoperative management *(1,4,38,39)*.

Because OCD affects the subchondral bone and can secondarily compromise the overlying articular cartilage, the goal of treatment is to encourage healing of the subchondral bone. Additional goals of operative treatment are to restore joint congruity, to rigidly fix unstable fragments, and to replace osteochondral defects with cells that can replace and grow cartilage *(12)*. It is important both to have an ample supply of cartilage and to restore a stable construct of subchondral bone.

For patients with a symptomatic but stable OCD lesion with an intact articular surface, bony drilling offers the potential to create channels for revascularization and healing (Fig. 4). Options include retrograde drilling or antegrade (transarticular) drilling. Retrograde drilling avoids damaging the articular surface; however, this method is associated with the technical challenges of maintaining accuracy in localizing the lesion, verifying adequate depth of penetration, and physeal violation. Antegrade drilling is accurate and technically straightforward, although this method creates articular cartilage channels, which may heal with fibrocartilage *(40)*.

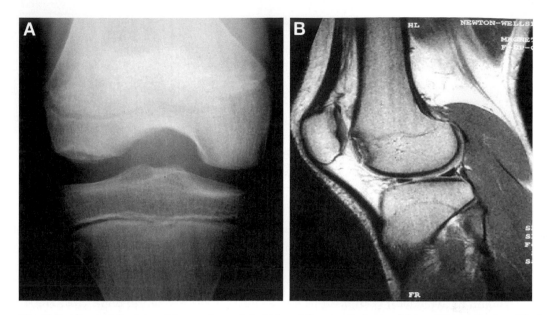

Fig. 5. Lesions of the lateral femoral condyle **(A)** and the patellofemoral joint **(B)** may be less likely to heal with nonoperative treatment or arthroscopic drilling than medial femoral condyle lesions.

A number of authors have found arthroscopic antegrade drilling to be effective in the treatment of OCD lesions in skeletally immature patients. Aglietti et al. noted healing on the AP as well as lateral radiographs in 16 knees in 14 patients studied after drilling, and all patients were asymptomatic at an average follow-up of 4 yr *(41)*. Bradley and Dandy performed this technique and noted radiographic healing and pain relief in 9 of 11 knees within 1 yr *(42)*. All lesions were located at the lateral aspect of the medial femoral condyle. One knee was healed within 2 yr, and a nonunion developed with loose body formation in another knee *(42)*.

Anderson and colleagues performed transarticular drilling in 17 patients with open physes and in 4 patients with closed physes. In the skeletally immature group, 18 of 20 lesions healed; in the skeletally mature group, only 2 of 4 healed at an average follow up of 5 yr *(40)*. Transarticular drilling was performed on 51 knees in 49 patients up to 18 yr of age by Ganley et al. *(43)*. Drilling was effective in skeletally immature patients and was curative in 83% of adolescents with open physes, in contrast to 75% of adolescents with closed physes. Factors associated with inadequate healing despite drilling included lesions in atypical locations (Fig. 5), multiple lesions, and patients with underlying medical conditions *(43)*.

Kocher et al. reviewed functional and radiographic outcomes using this technique *(44)*. They studied 23 skeletally immature patients and 30 affected knees with lesions at the classic lateral aspect of the medial femoral condyle location for an average follow-up of 3.9 yr. There was significant improvement in the mean Lysholm score, and radiographic healing was achieved in all patients at an average of 4.4 mo after drilling. Younger age was also noted to be an independent multivariate predictor of Lysholm score using linear regression analysis.

In patients with unstable flap lesions, fibrous tissue can be found between the fragments and underlying bone. The fibrous tissue should be removed; removal of significant portions of underlying bone from the fragment and from the subchondral bone at the base of the

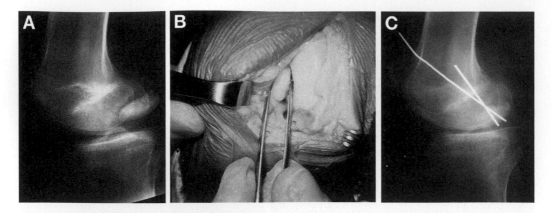

Fig. 6. Unstable OCD lesion in a patient approaching skeletal maturity (**A**) treated with arthrotomy (**B**), bone grafting, and K wire fixation (**C**, 3 months postoperative).

lesion should be avoided. If partially unstable lesions with subchondral bone loss exist, then autogenous bone graft can be packed into the craters prior to reduction and fixation (Fig. 6). In patients with unstable lesions that have subchondral bone attached and that have an appropriate match of the size of the defect and the fragment, fixation can be performed by a variety of methods arthroscopically or via open incisions.

Rapid relief of pain has led some authors to theorize that increased pressure at the line of separation between the fragment and the epiphysis may be a source of pain *(42,45,46)*. Navarro et al. recently used cortical strips of bone from the metaphysis of the tibia to treat OCD lesions most of which were partially dislocated *(47)*. All 11 patients returned to strenuous, activities although 1 patient required an arthroscopy for synovitis 4 mo postoperatively before returning to sports. Although Herbert screws and cannulated screws have been used successfully (Figs. 7 and 8), second surgeries may be required for removal *(48,49)*. Kivisto et al. used a metal staple that was placed arthroscopically and did not require removal; however, broken staples were observed in 9 of 25 knees treated *(50)*.

Despite the emergence and use of a variety of bioabsorbable screws and pins (Fig. 9) as well as bone and osteochondral plugs, a number of authors have described complications associated with these treatments *(51–54)*. Scioscia et al. and Friederichs et al., in separate reports, noted loosening and failure of bioabsorbable screws, which had backed out, causing damage to adjacent articular surfaces, and unabsorbed screw heads found as intra-articular loose bodies *(52,54)*. Kim and Shin described loose bodies as a complication of osteochondral allograft treatment for OCD *(53)*. The donor site was seen as the origin of the loose body formation.

For large, unsalvageable fragments (Fig. 10), a variety of techniques have been developed to attempt to closely replace the defect with subchondral bone calcified tidemark and overlying cartilage. Drilling and abrasion arthroplasty as well as microfracturing using picks serve to recruit pluripotential cells from marrow elements *(32,55)*. The recruited cells differentiate primarily into fibrocartilage, which typically does not respond to shearing forces as effectively as native hyaline cartilage. Smaller lesions can be effectively resurfaced using these techniques; however, the results for large lesions have been shown to deteriorate with time because of decreased resilience and stiffness of the fibrocartilage *(56)*. Agletti et al. reported that removal of the fragment and debridement of the crater alone were viable options; however, one-grade worsening of Fairbanks changes was found in 45% of weight-bearing AP

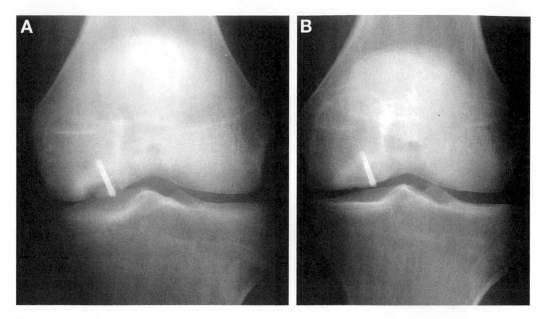

Fig. 7. Unstable OCD lesion in a patient approaching skeletal maturity treated with arthroscopic fixation using a variable-pitch screw: **(A)** 3 wk postoperative; **(B)** 3 mo postoperative.

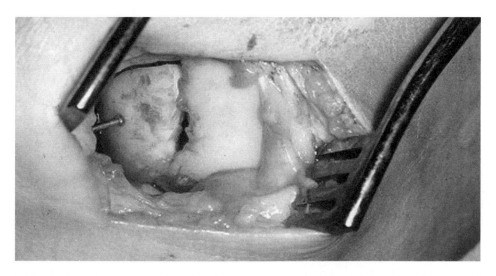

Fig. 8. Loose body lesion treated with arthrotomy, fragment reshaping, bone grafting, and fixation.

radiographs at an average follow-up of 9 yr *(57,58)*. Results of this technique were better in lesions less than 2 cm.

Periosteum can be used with transplantation of the cambium layer down into the defect to produce a cartilaginous extracellular matrix. Although Neidermann reported successful results after periosteal transplantation for knee OCD at 1 yr, Angermann et al. reported disappointing results in 14 patients with adult OCD of the femoral condyle at 6- to 9-yr follow-up *(32)*. Madsen et al. studied the long-term results of periosteal transplantation without chondrocyte grafting in OCD of the knee *(59)*. The median age was 19 yr among the 18

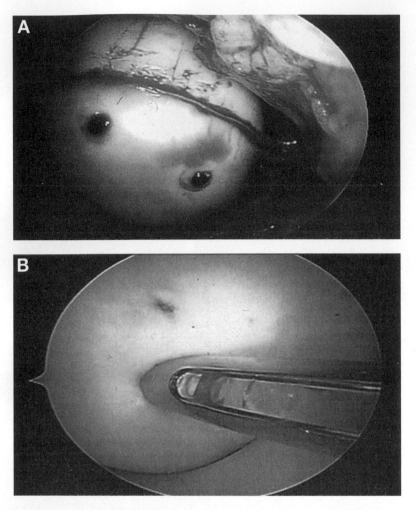

Fig. 9. Bioabsorbable fixation for OCD lesions: (**A**) bioabsorbable pins; (**B**) bioabsorbable tack.

patients studied, and 8 patients required reoperations up to 8 yr postoperatively. Periosteum alone was found to be unsatisfactory because of the number of reoperations and continued knee pain in most patients.

Other techniques have been developed to address the weaker structural properties of reparative fibrocartilage. Transplantation of autologous osteochondral plugs has also been used for defect replacement (60,61). These plugs are obtained from non-weight-bearing regions of the knee, such as the edge of the intercondylar notch or the upper outer trochlea, and are inserted into the defect. Outerbridge reported good results using osteochondral grafts harvested from the lateral facet of the patella to treat 10 patients with large femoral OCD lesions (62). Yoshizumi et al. reported on a successful osteochondral graft treatment for OCD lesions in 3 patients 18 yr of age and younger with closed growth plates (63). The authors noted the potential disadvantages of donor site morbidity and congruent articular fit and the advantages of biological internal fixation.

Autologous chondrocyte implantation has been used for isolated large femoral defects in younger patients with no lower extremity malalignment. The chondrocytes are generally

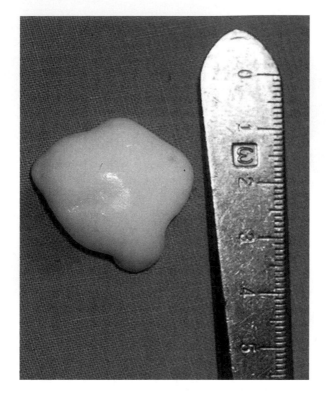

Fig. 10. Excision of chronic loose body.

harvested arthroscopically from a healthy articular cartilage surface and grown in vitro. These grown chondrocytes are injected into the defect and beneath a periosteal patch, which is usually harvested from the ipsilateral tibial metaphysis.

Peterson et al. reported on the treatment of OCD at 2–10 yr using autologous chondrocyte transplantation *(64)*. Although the mean age was 26.4 yr in the 48 patients treated, 7 patients received surgery at less than 18 yr of age, and 35 patients had the onset of OCD as juveniles. These authors found that the procedure produced an integrated repair tissue and noted successful clinical results in over 90% of patients.

King et al. evaluated autologous chondrocyte transplantation for the treatment of large defects in articular cartilage of the distal femur in adolescent patients and noted outcomes slightly better than previous reported results for adult patients *(65)*. It was theorized that this was because of presumed superior articular substance in the adjacent regions of the knee in those without malalignment.

Secondary reconstruction with bone-articular surface allografts has been described, with success in patients with significant surface defects in OCD, although no long-term results in skeletally immature patients are yet available *(66)*.

PREFERRED APPROACH

Our algorithm for management is shown in Fig. 11.

In the initial evaluation of a patient with OCD, attention is paid to the duration of symptoms, the amount and types of activities, and the presence of swelling and mechanical symptoms. Radiographs (AP, lateral, skyline, notch) are taken to document the lesion and to

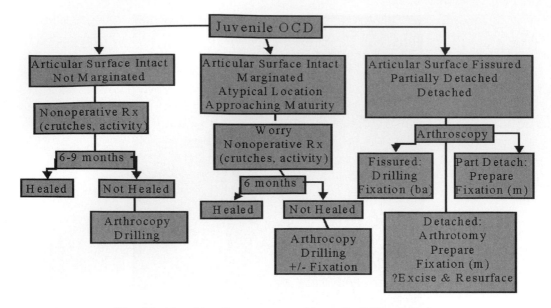

Fig. 11. Algorithm for treatment of juvenile OCD of the knee.

classify the patient as adult OCD vs juvenile OCD. A radiograph of the left hand and wrist can be useful to determine skeletal age, and full-length lower extremity radiographs can be useful to determine mechanical axis deviations. An MRI scan is routinely obtained to stage the OCD lesion (Table 1).

For adult OCD lesions, surgical management is recommended as healing potential with nonoperative management is minimal. For juvenile OCD lesions that are stable with an intact articular surface, nonoperative treatment is recommended for 6–9 mo. The emphasis of non-operative treatment is the cessation of impact activities. Protected weight bearing and bracing are used intermittently for patients with limping or pain with walking. Care is taken to watch for signs of depression or adjustment disorder in these very active adolescent athletes treated with activity restriction. Repeat MRI is performed at 6 mo if the lesion has not healed. For stable juvenile OCD lesions (stages 1 and 2) that have not healed with 6 mo of nonoperative management or for juvenile OCD lesions that are unstable (stages 3–5), surgical management is recommended.

For stable lesions with an intact articular surface, arthroscopic retrograde transarticular drilling is performed. Postoperatively, patients are maintained with touch-down weight bearing with a postoperative brace limiting motion from 0 to 90° for 6 wk. Healing typically occurs by 4 mo postoperatively per radiographs and clinical examination. For stable lesions with a fissured articular surface, bioabsorbable fixation tacks are added to transarticular drilling.

Unstable hinged lesions that are not chronic are treated with arthroscopic fixation using a variable-pitch screw or a cannulated screw. Postoperatively, patients are maintained with touch-down weight bearing with a postoperative brace limiting motion from 0 to 90° for 6 wk. Healing typically occurs by 6 mo postoperatively per radiographs and clinical examination. The hardware is routinely removed after healing.

Unstable chronic hinged lesions and acute loose bodies are treated with arthrotomy, bone grafting of the lesion base from bone graft obtained from the proximal tibia, and fixation with variable-pitch or cannulated screws. Postoperatively, patients are maintained with touch-down weight bearing for 3 mo postoperatively. Healing typically occurs by 6 mo postoperatively per radiographs and clinical examination. The hardware is routinely removed after healing.

Chronic loose bodies are treated with arthrotomy and fixation of the fragment if technically possible as mentioned. For chronic loose bodies with minimal or avascular bone, mismatch in size and shape between lesion and base, or maceration of the loose body, fixation may not be possible. In these cases, chondral resurfacing is performed. Microfracture is performed initially; however, it may be technically suboptimal as the subchondral bone plate is absent. Patients with persistent symptoms and full-thickness chondral defect after microfracture are treated with autologous chondrocyte implantation.

SUMMARY

OCD of the knee is seen with increasing frequency in the pediatric patient. Early recognition is essential because early stable juvenile OCD lesions with an intact articular surface have the potential to heal with nonoperative treatment. The mainstay of nonoperative treatment is the cessation of repetitive impact loading. The value of adjunctive immobilization, protected weight bearing, and unloader bracing has not been established. For stable lesions that have not healed with 6–9 mo of nonoperative treatment, consideration should be given to arthroscopic drilling to affect healing before the lesion progresses to an unstable lesion, which requires more involved treatment and has a less-sanguine prognosis. MRI may allow earlier prediction of lesion healing potential. Unstable lesions and acute loose bodies require fixation and possible bone grafting. The majority of these lesions will heal; however, the long-term prognosis is not clear. Chronic loose bodies can be difficult to fix and may have poor healing potential. The results of excision of large lesions alone is poor; the addition of chondral resurfacing techniques may decrease the risk of subsequent arthrosis.

REFERENCES

1. Cahill BR. Osteochondritis dissecans of the knee: treatment of juvenile and adult forms. J Am Acad Orthop Surg 1995;3:237–247.
2. Clanton TO, DeLee JC. Osteochondritis dissecans. History, pathophysiology and current treatment concepts. Clin Orthop Relat Res 1982;167:50–64.
3. Glancy GL. Juvenile osteochondritis dissecans. Am J Knee Surg 1999;12:120–124.
4. Iobst C, Kocher MS. Cartilage injury in the skeletally immature athlete. In Mirzayan R, ed., Cartilage Injury in Athlete. New York, Thieme; 2006:134–145.
5. Kocher MS, Micheli L. The pediatric knee: evaluation and treatment. In Insall JN, Scott WN, eds., Surgery of the Knee. New York: Churchill-Livingstone; 2001:1356–1397.
6. Pappas AM. Osteochondrosis dissecans. Clin Orthop Relat Res 1981;158:59–69.
7. Wall E, Von Stein D. Juvenile osteochondritis dissecans. Orthop Clin North Am 2003; 34:341–353.
8. Cahill BR, Berg BC. 99m-Technetium phosphate compound joint scintigraphy in the management of juvenile osteochondritis dissecans of the femoral condyles. Am J Sports Med 1983; 11:329–335.
9. Hefti F, Beguiristain J, Krauspe R, et al. Osteochondritis dissecans: a multicenter study of the European Pediatric Orthopedic Society. J Pediatr Orthop B 1999;8:231–245.
10. Cahill BR, Phillips MR, Navarro R. The results of conservative management of juvenile osteochondritis dissecans using joint scintigraphy. A prospective study. Am J Sports Med 1989;17: 601–605; discussion 605–606.

11. Green WT, Banks HH. Osteochondritis dissecans in children. J Bone Joint Surg Am 1953;35-A: 26–47; passim.
12. Smillie IS. Treatment of osteochondritis dissecans. J Bone Joint Surg Br 1957;39-B:248–260.
13. Van Demark RE. Osteochondritis dissecans with spontaneous healing. J Bone Joint Surg Am 1952;35A:143–148.
14. Linden B. Osteochondritis dissecans of the femoral condyles: a long-term follow-up study. J Bone Joint Surg Am 1977;59:769–776.
15. Twyman RS, Desai K, Aichroth PM. Osteochondritis dissecans of the knee. A long-term study. J Bone Joint Surg Br 1991;73:461–464.
16. Chiroff RT, Cooke CP 3rd. Osteochondritis dissecans: a histologic and microradiographic analysis of surgically excised lesions. J Trauma 1975;15:689–696.
17. Konig F. Ueber freie Korper in den Gelenken. Dtsch Z Chir 1887;27:90–109.
18. Milgram JW. Radiological and pathological manifestations of osteochondritis dissecans of the distal femur. A study of 50 cases. Radiology 1978;126:305–311.
19. Koch S, Kampen WU, Laprell H. Cartilage and bone morphology in osteochondritis dissecans. Knee Surg Sports Traumatol Arthrosc 1997;5:42–45.
20. Reddy AS, Frederick RW. Evaluation of the intraosseous and extraosseous blood supply to the distal femoral condyles. Am J Sports Med 1998;26:415–419.
21. Rogers WM, Gladstone H. Vascular foramina and arterial supply of the distal end of the femur. J Bone Joint Surg Am 1950;32(A:4):867–874.
22. Mubarak SJ, Carroll NC. Familial osteochondritis dissecans of the knee. Clin Orthop Relat Res 1979;140:131–136.
23. Petrie PW. Aetiology of osteochondritis dissecans. Failure to establish a familial background. J Bone Joint Surg Br 1977;59:366–367.
24. Fairbanks HAT. Osteochondritis dissecans. Br J Surg 1933;21:67–82.
25. Hughston JC, Hergenroeder PT, Courtenay BG. Osteochondritis dissecans of the femoral condyles. J Bone Joint Surg Am 1984;66:1340–1348.
26. Linden B. The incidence of osteochondritis dissecans in the condyles of the femur. Acta Orthop Scand 1976;47:664–667.
27. Conrad JM, Stanitski CL. Osteochondritis dissecans: Wilson's sign revisited. Am J Sports Med 2003;31:777–778.
28. Wilson JN. A diagnostic sign in osteochondritis dissecans of the knee. J Bone Joint Surg Am 1967;49:477–480.
29. Kocher MS, DiCanzio J, Zurakowski D, Micheli LJ Diagnostic performance of clinical examination and selective magnetic resonance imaging in the evaluation of intraarticular knee disorders in children and adolescents. Am J Sports Med 2001;29:292–296.
30. Bohndorf K. Osteochondritis (osteochondrosis) dissecans: a review and new MRI classification. Eur Radiol 1998;8:103–112.
31. De Smet AA, Ilahi OA, Graf BK. Untreated osteochondritis dissecans of the femoral condyles: prediction of patient outcome using radiographic and MR findings. Skeletal Radiol 1997; 26:463–467.
32. Pill SG, Ganley TJ, Milam RA, Lou JE, Meyer JS, Flynn JM. Role of magnetic resonance imaging and clinical criteria in predicting successful nonoperative treatment of osteochondritis dissecans in children. J Pediatr Orthop 2003;23:102–108.
33. O'Connor MA, Palaniappan M, Khan N, Bruce CE. Osteochondritis dissecans of the knee in children. A comparison of MRI and arthroscopic findings. J Bone Joint Surg Br 2002;84: 258–262.
34. Vonstein DW, Nosir H, Laor T, Emery K. Juvenile osteochondritis dissecans of the knee: healing prognosis based on x-ray and gadolinium enhanced MRI. Pediatric Orthopaedic Society of North America. Amelia Island, FL; 2003.
35. Kramer J, Stiglbauer R, Engel A, Prayer L, Imhof H. MR contrast arthrography (MRA) in osteochondrosis dissecans. J Comput Assist Tomogr 1992;16:254–260.

36. Litchman HM, McCullough RW, Gandsman EJ, Schatz SL. Computerized blood flow analysis for decision making in the treatment of osteochondritis dissecans. J Pediatr Orthop 1988;8:208–212.

37. Paletta GA Jr, Bednarz PA, Stanitski CL, Sandman GA, Stanitski DF, Kottamasu S. The prognostic value of quantitative bone scan in knee osteochondritis dissecans. A preliminary experience. Am J Sports Med 1998;26:7–14.

38. Ewing JW, Voto SJ. Arthroscopic surgical management of osteochondritis dissecans of the knee. Arthroscopy 1988;4:37–40.

39. Guhl JF. Arthroscopic treatment of osteochondritis dissecans. Clin Orthop Relat Res 1982;167:65–74.

40. Anderson AF, Richards DB, Pagnani MJ, Hovis WD. Antegrade drilling for osteochondritis dissecans of the knee. Arthroscopy 1997;13:319–324.

41. Aglietti P, Buzzi R, Bassi PB, Fioriti M. Arthroscopic drilling in juvenile osteochondritis dissecans of the medial femoral condyle. Arthroscopy 1994;10:286–291.

42. Bradley J, Dandy DJ. Results of drilling osteochondritis dissecans before skeletal maturity. J Bone Joint Surg Br 1989;71:642–644.

43. Ganley TJ, Amro RR, Gregg JR, Halpern KV. Antegrade drilling for osteochondritis dissecans of the knee. Pediatric Orthopaedic Society of North America. 2002.

44. Kocher MS, Micheli LJ, Yaniv M, Zurakowski D, Ames A, Adrignolo AA. Functional and radiographic outcome of juvenile osteochondritis dissecans of the knee treated with transarticular arthroscopic drilling. Am J Sports Med 2001;29:562–566.

45. Johnson LL, Uitvlugt G, Austin MD, Detrisac DA, Johnson C. Osteochondritis dissecans of the knee: arthroscopic compression screw fixation. Arthroscopy 1990;6:179–189.

46. Thomson NL. Osteochondritis dissecans and osteochondral fragments managed by Herbert compression screw fixation. Clin Orthop Relat Res 1987;224:71–78.

47. Navarro R, Cohen M, Filho MC, da Silva RT. The arthroscopic treatment of osteochondritis dissecans of the knee with autologous bone sticks. Arthroscopy 2002;18:840–844.

48. Cugat R, Garcia M, Cusco X, et al. Osteochondritis dissecans: a historical review and its treatment with cannulated screws. Arthroscopy 1993;9:675–684.

49. Zuniga RS, Blasco L, Grande M. Arthroscopic use of Herbert screws in osteochondritis dissecans of the knee. Arthroscopy 1993;9:668–670.

50. Kivisto R, Pasanen L, Leppilahti J, Jalovaara P. Arthroscopic repair of osteochondritis dissecans of the femoral condyles with metal staple fixation: a report of 28 cases. Knee Surg Sports Traumatol Arthrosc 2002;10:305–309.

51. Dervin GF, Keene GC, Chissell HR. Biodegradable rods in adult osteochondritis dissecans of the knee. Clin Orthop Relat Res 1998;356:213–221.

52. Friederichs MG, Greis PE, Burks RT. Pitfalls associated with fixation of osteochondritis dissecans fragments using bioabsorbable screws. Arthroscopy 2001;17:542–545.

53. Kim SJ, Shin SJ. Loose bodies after arthroscopic osteochondral autograft in osteochondritis dissecans of the knee. Arthroscopy 2000;16:E16.

54. Scioscia TN, Giffin JR, Allen CR, Harner CD. Potential complication of bioabsorbable screw fixation for osteochondritis dissecans of the knee. Arthroscopy 2001;17:E7.

55. Steadman JR, Briggs KK, Rodrigo JJ, Kocher MS, Gill TJ, Rodkey WG. Outcomes of microfracture for traumatic chondral defects of the knee: average 11-yr follow-up. Arthroscopy 2003;19:477–484.

56. Mandelbaum BR, Browne JE, Fu F, et al. Articular cartilage lesions of the knee. Am J Sports Med 1998;26:853–861.

57. Aglietti P, Ciardullo A, Giron F, Ponteggia F. Results of arthroscopic excision of the fragment in the treatment of osteochondritis dissecans of the knee. Arthroscopy 2001;17:741–746.

58. Anderson AF, Pagnani MJ. Osteochondritis dissecans of the femoral condyles. Long-term results of excision of the fragment. Am J Sports Med 1997;25:830–834.

59. Madsen BL, Noer HH, Carstensen JP, Normark F. Long-term results of periosteal transplantation in osteochondritis dissecans of the knee. Orthopedics 2000;23:223–226.

60. Bentley G, Biant LC, Carrington RW, et al. A prospective, randomised comparison of autologous chondrocyte implantation vs mosaicplasty for osteochondral defects in the knee. J Bone Joint Surg Br 2003;85:223–230.
61. Berlet GC, Mascia A, Miniaci A. Treatment of unstable osteochondritis dissecans lesions of the knee using autogenous osteochondral grafts (mosaicplasty). Arthroscopy 1999;15:312–316.
62. Outerbridge RE. Osteochondritis dissecans of the posterior femoral condyle. Clin Orthop Relat Res 1983;175:121–129.
63. Yoshizumi Y, Sugita T, Kawamata T, Ohnuma M, Maeda S. Cylindrical osteochondral graft for osteochondritis dissecans of the knee: a report of three cases. Am J Sports Med 2002;30: 441–445.
64. Peterson L, Minas T, Brittberg M, Lindahl A. Treatment of osteochondritis dissecans of the knee with autologous chondrocyte transplantation: results at 2 to 10 yr. J Bone Joint Surg Am 2003;85-A(suppl 2):17–24.
65. King PJ, Lou JE, Gregg JR. Autologous chondrocyte transplantation for the treatment of large defects in the articular cartilage of the distal femur in adolescent patients. American Academy of Orthopaedic Surgeons. New Orleans, LA; 2003.
66. Garrett JC. Osteochondritis dissecans. Clin Sports Med 1991;10:569–593.

17

Meniscus Transplantation and Cartilage Resurfacing
Considerations, Indications, and Approach

Scott A. Rodeo, MD

Summary

Many knees with articular cartilage pathology have concomitant meniscus loss. I consider four structural factors when evaluating knees with meniscus and cartilage injury: (1) hyaline cartilage condition, (2) ligament stability, (3) lower extremity alignment, and (4) meniscus status. All of these factors need to be considered when evaluating a patient for cartilage repair. Surgical intervention for articular cartilage problems often involves addressing meniscus deficiency and malalignment. In this chapter, I discuss my rationale and approach to meniscus transplantation with concomitant osteotomy and cartilage resurfacing.

Key Words: Meniscus; allograft; osteotomy; chondral injury.

INTRODUCTION

Basic Indications for Meniscus Transplantation

Meniscus replacement is indicated for the treatment of symptoms (typically pain and swelling) of early arthrosis in the meniscus-deficient compartment. An important goal of meniscus transplantation is to forestall further degenerative changes that are known to occur following meniscectomy. Most authors currently recommend limiting transplantation to those patients with no more than partial-thickness cartilage loss as the results of meniscus transplantation are much less predictable in knees with advanced degenerative changes *(1,2)*. Alignment must be normal or corrected by osteotomy (discussed in a separate section).

Meniscus transplantation may also be considered for knee stability. The medial meniscus is a secondary restraint to anterior tibial translation in the anterior cruciate ligament (ACL)-deficient knee *(3,4)*. A cadaveric study found significant increases in the *in situ* forces in an ACL graft in medial meniscus-deficient knees compared to meniscus-intact knees *(5)*. These studies suggest that medial meniscus transplantation at the time of ACL reconstruction may help to protect the ACL graft.

Clinical evidence for the role of the medial meniscus in knee stability was provided by Shelbourne and Gray, who demonstrated greater knee laxity, as measured with KT-1000 arthrometry following ACL reconstruction, in patients that had undergone previous medial meniscectomy compared to knees with intact menisci *(6)*. Also, Garrett reported significantly improved KT-1000 arthrometer results for ACL reconstructions performed with concomitant medial meniscus transplantation compared to a group of patients who underwent isolated ACL reconstruction with persistent medial meniscus deficiency *(7)*.

From: *Cartilage Repair Strategies*
Edited by: Riley J. Williams © Humana Press Inc., Totowa, NJ

A less-common consideration regarding knee stability is the contribution of the menisci to varus-valgus stability. The absence of both the medial and lateral menisci may result in slightly increased varus-valgus rotation, and meniscus transplantation may be considered in this setting if collateral ligament repair or reconstruction is performed. It has been noted in such patients that replacing both the medial and lateral meniscus may help improve varus and valgus laxity. Support for this strategy comes from Markolf et al., who demonstrated greater varus-valgus laxity in the ACL-deficient and medial meniscus-deficient knee compared to the ACL-deficient knee with an intact medial meniscus *(8)*.

Another important indication for meniscus transplantation is "prophylactic" transplantation in the asymptomatic patient following meniscectomy to prevent the known sequelae of meniscectomy. This is not currently recommended for the asymptomatic patient with normal articular surfaces. However, I consider meniscus transplantation in the asymptomatic patient once early articular cartilage degeneration is present. Articular cartilage degeneration is associated with the elevated articular contact stress known to occur following even partial meniscus resection. The rationale is to detect early cartilage degeneration before advanced structural changes occur and attempt to prevent these changes by restoring functional meniscus tissue to the affected compartment. The development of an effusion is an early sign of cartilage degeneration. I currently use cartilage-sensitive magnetic resonance imaging to detect early cartilage degeneration in patients following meniscectomy. Advanced imaging techniques, such as measurement of T_2 relaxation times, will improve the ability to detect the early onset of cartilage breakdown.

CONTRAINDICATIONS TO MENISCUS TRANSPLANTATION

Absolute contraindications to meniscus transplantation include the presence of diffuse subchondral bone exposure, remodeling of the femoral condyle that has resulted in flattening, and uncorrected malalignment (Fig. 1) *(1)*. An important purpose of this chapter is to consider how correction of malalignment (with osteotomy) or chondral degeneration (with a resurfacing procedure) may render the knee suitable for meniscus transplantation. There is currently very little information available about the efficacy of combined meniscus transplantation and cartilage resurfacing. For example, although it is known that extensive chondral degeneration is a contraindication to meniscus transplantation, the location of chondral lesions is probably as important as size and depth.

Because most failures of meniscus transplantation occur because of progressive degeneration of the posterior part of the transplanted meniscus, the presence of full-thickness articular cartilage lesions on the flexion weight-bearing zone of the femoral condyle or tibia that are greater than 10–15 mm in width or length is currently considered a contraindication to meniscus transplantation *(9)*. In addition to articular cartilage degeneration, the clinician should consider changes in subchondral bone morphology. Uncorrected knee instability is also a contraindication to meniscus transplantation.

WHEN SHOULD MENISCUS TRANSPLANTATION BE CONSIDERED?

The contact stresses on articular cartilage increase proportionately with meniscus loss *(10,11)*. Although it is well established that elevated contact stresses adversely affect hyaline cartilage, the threshold level of contact stress that initiates progressive cartilage degeneration is unknown. It is felt that absence of the posterior horn of the meniscus will lead to more rapid arthritis progression because the posterior horn bears a greater load in knee flexion *(12)*. In

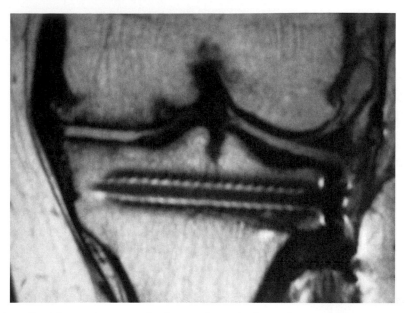

Fig. 1. This patient has undergone closing wedge osteotomy for medical compartment arthosis. The flattening of the femoral condyle and associated full-thickness loss of hyaline cartilage contraindicate meniscus transplantation.

support of this, a study found that the point of greatest articular contact stress moved posteriorly with progressive knee flexion in the lateral compartment (because of internal tibial rotation with flexion) *(13)*. It is also well established that the lateral meniscus transmits a greater proportion of the load in the lateral compartment during weight bearing than does the medial meniscus in the medial compartment. These experimental findings are supported by clinical studies that have found more rapid onset of degenerative changes following lateral meniscectomy compared to medial meniscectomy *(14,15)*.

For these reasons, more aggressive replacement of the lateral meniscus should be considered, and I recommend lateral meniscus transplantation once more than 50% of the posterior horn of the meniscus has been removed. On the medial side, meniscus replacement should be considered once more than 60–70% of the posterior horn of the meniscus has been removed (Fig. 1).

Another consideration is the pattern of meniscus loss: An irreparable radial tear that extends from the inner rim to the capsule is functionally tantamount to total meniscectomy. The disruption of the circumferential collagen fibers that is observed in full-thickness radial tears of the meniscus eliminates the ability of the meniscus to develop hoop stresses and transmit load. Meniscus transplantation should be considered in this setting.

No studies have examined how elevated contact stresses in the meniscectomized knee affect healing of a resurfacing procedure. It is reasonable that elevated contact stresses could adversely affect healing and remodeling of an articular surface implant. Articular contact stress would not be expected to affect the initial healing of a resurfacing procedure in the early postoperative period because the patient is typically nonweight bearing during that time. However, patients will advance to full weight bearing prior to complete healing, incorporation, and remodeling of the articular surface implant; thus, abnormal articular contact stresses in the meniscectomized knee may adversely affect healing of a resurfacing procedure. These considerations support meniscus transplantation in this setting if the meniscus is absent.

OSTEOTOMY AND MENISCUS TRANSPLANTATION

Axial alignment needs to be considered in the evaluation of any knee with articular cartilage pathology. Significant malalignment should be corrected prior to or in conjunction with meniscus transplantation or cartilage resurfacing. Failure rates are higher when these procedures are performed in the setting of axial malalignment. Weight-bearing hip-to-ankle radiographs on a long cassette are required for accurate determination of the mechanical axis of the limb.

In a normal knee, the mechanical axis generally passes through or just medial to the center of the knee (between the tibial spines). I measure the width of the tibial plateau and determine the 50% point (middle of the tibial width). I will accept no more than 10% deviation into the involved compartment (i.e., the mechanical axis should pass between 40 and 60% of the tibial width). This generally corresponds to the area between the tibial spines. The mechanical axis of the uninvolved knee should also be measured and taken into account. In treatment of an acute cartilage injury, I will accept greater deviation of the mechanical axis if it is symmetric with the contralateral, uninvolved knee.

Combination of Meniscus Transplantation With Osteotomy Guidelines

It is established that symptomatic arthritis can recur after 5–10 yr following realignment osteotomy *(16)*. These findings are based on reports in the literature on long-term follow-up studies of osteotomy in patients who underwent osteotomy following prior meniscectomy. It is not known if concomitant meniscus transplantation will delay the recurrence of symptoms following osteotomy. It makes theoretical sense that restoration of the meniscus would be beneficial. However, there is little evidence in the literature to support combined meniscus transplantation and osteotomy.

Cameron and Saha reported on 34 knees that received a meniscal allograft in combination with a valgus high tibial osteotomy, varus high tibial osteotomy, or varus distal femoral osteotomy to correct for preoperative varus or valgus deformities, with 29 (85%) attaining good-to-excellent results *(17)*. There is no way to determine how much of the clinical improvement can be attributed to the meniscus transplant and how much to the osteotomy. Long-term studies will be required to determine if osteotomy combined with meniscus transplantation results in improved survivorship compared to osteotomy alone.

I consider meniscus transplantation with concomitant osteotomy if two conditions are satisfied: (1) There are no architectural changes on the femoral condyle (flattening); and (2) there are no areas of full-thickness cartilage loss greater than 10 mm on the meniscus weight-bearing zone of the femoral or tibial condyles.

As osteotomy techniques improve, I believe that osteotomy can be used earlier in the course of degenerative joint disease and can be combined with meniscus transplantation or cartilage resurfacing. In this setting, often only a small correction in alignment may be required to optimize the mechanical axis for meniscus transplantation or cartilage resurfacing. Correction of the mechanical axis with osteotomy is not likely to make the compartment suitable for meniscus transplantation if there is condylar flattening.

Knee osteotomy should be performed prior to, or in conjunction with, meniscus transplantation or cartilage resurfacing. Osteotomy and meniscus transplantation can be performed as a single-stage procedure. If a cartilage resurfacing procedure is also planned with meniscus transplantation and osteotomy, consideration may be made for staging the procedures by doing the osteotomy first followed by combined meniscus transplantation and cartilage resurfacing.

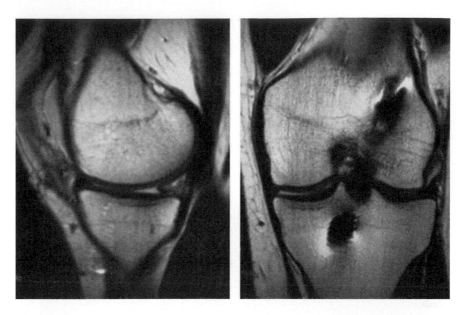

Fig. 2. Sagittal and coronal MR images of 23-yr-old patient who has undergone prior ACL reconstruction and subtotal medial meniscectomy.

Various types of osteotomy (opening wedge, closing wedge, dome, or coronal plane) may be used to correct the mechanical axis. The technique with which the surgeon has the greatest familiarity should generally be used, taking into consideration the location of bone tunnels or troughs for the meniscus transplant and their relationship to internal fixation devices used for the osteotomy. A valgus-producing osteotomy will be combined with medial meniscus replacement; a varus-producing osteotomy will be combined with lateral meniscus replacement.

Medial Meniscus Transplantation and Valgus-Producing Osteotomy

When combining medial meniscus transplantation with osteotomy, I recommend use of a lateral closing wedge or a tibial coronal plane osteotomy as described by Wickiewicz *(18)* (Fig. 3). Surgical planning requires consideration of the technique to be used for meniscus transplantation. The recommendation is to transplant the meniscus with bone plugs attached to the anterior and posterior horns. Biomechanical studies demonstrate better restoration of contact mechanics following medial meniscus transplantation using bone plugs compared to suture fixation in drill holes *(19)*. The location of bone tunnels for the bone plugs and any internal fixation devices for the osteotomy needs to be carefully planned. The coronal plane osteotomy technique retains adequate bone stock for placement of drill tunnels for the bone plugs (Fig. 4). A disadvantage of the lateral closing wedge technique is loss of proximal tibial bone stock, which may compromise future conversion to total knee arthroplasty. For this reason, the closing wedge technique should not be used for corrections greater than 10–15°.

I do not recommend the use of the opening wedge osteotomy method in combination with meniscal allograft transplantation for several reasons. Opening wedge techniques have been shown to increase the sagittal slope of the tibia, which may also increase the contact stresses on the articular cartilage. The opening wedge needs to be protected from weight bearing for a longer period of time to allow healing compared to a closing wedge technique. Prolonged avoidance of weight bearing is undesirable because it is usually easier to establish full range

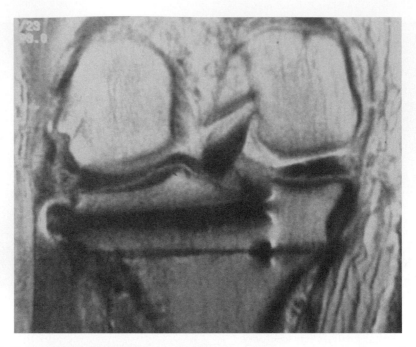

Fig. 3. Medial meniscus transplantation combined with lateral closing wedge, valgus-producing osteotomy.

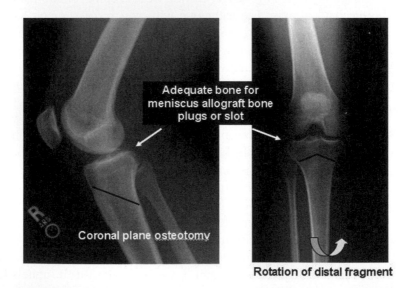

Fig. 4. An obliquely oriented osteotomy is made in the coronal plane of the tibia. There is adequate bone above the osteotomy site to allow for bone attached to a meniscus allograft.

of motion once full weight bearing is allowed; this is usually possible earlier following a closing wedge osteotomy compared to an opening wedge technique. Also, use of an opening wedge technique requires that the bone plug tunnels be proximal to the osteotomy (between the joint surface and the osteotomy). This may be difficult to do as the tunnel for the posterior horn bone plug is usually made more distally. If the opening wedge osteotomy is done proximal to the tibial tuberosity, then the patella will be translated distally, resulting in increased patellofemoral contact pressures. Last, a study from my institution found that the opening wedge technique results in obligatory external rotation of the distal tibial fragment as the osteotomy is opened because of tethering by the intact fibula *(20)*. This rotation may alter tibiofemoral contact mechanics. Such external rotation would be especially undesirable in the setting of concomitant posterolateral ligament laxity.

LATERAL MENISCUS TRANSPLANTATION AND VARUS-PRODUCING OSTEOTOMY

When combining lateral meniscus transplantation with osteotomy, I recommend use of a tibial coronal plane osteotomy (as discussed above) a lateral femoral opening wedge. Alternative approaches include a lateral tibial opening wedge or a medial femoral closing wedge. If the degenerative changes in the knee have developed secondary to lateral menis-cectomy and the planned correction is less than 12°, the osteotomy may be done on the tibial side. Primary lateral compartment osteoarthritis typically results in deformity on the lateral femoral condyle, so varus-producing osteotomy has traditionally been done on the femur. The advantage of the coronal plane tibial technique is that the healing process is more predictable because of the presence of large, opposing cancellous surfaces that are fixed in compression. However, a potential disadvantage of the coronal plane varus-producing tibial technique is the risk of delayed union of the fibular osteotomy that is performed as part of this osteotomy. The varus moment leads to distraction at the fibular osteotomy and may result in delayed healing. The opening wedge techniques have the disadvantage of potentially slower healing of the opened wedge and the requirement for bone graft.

Lateral meniscus transplantation is performed using a bone slot technique that connects the anterior and posterior horns of the meniscus (Fig. 5). The recipient slot is cut in the proximal tibia using commercially available instruments (Arthrex Dovetail or Keyhole, Naples, FL) or freehand using a burr. This technique requires that the placement of internal fixation devices for concomitant tibial osteotomy be planned appropriately to accommodate the bone slot for meniscus transplantation.

COMBINED MENISCUS TRANSPLANTATION AND CARTILAGE RESURFACING

The majority of knees in which meniscus transplantation is considered will have articular cartilage injury of varying degrees. It is likely that the size and location of a hyaline cartilage lesion plays an important role in the fate of a meniscus transplant. There is little information available about the effect of the size, location, and depth of articular cartilage lesions on the biologic incorporation and mechanical function of a meniscus transplant. For example, a small, focal lesion may permit load bearing around its periphery and thus not present a dele-terious mechanical environment. There are usually varying degrees of cartilage damage on different parts of the articular surfaces, making it difficult to grade such surfaces accurately and difficult to interpret published reports.

Many patients with meniscus deficiency demonstrate focal erosive lesions on the flexion weight-bearing (posterior) zone of the femur and tibia *(21)*. Such lesions may result in early joint space narrowing on flexion weight-bearing radiographs. Because the posterior aspect of the meniscus is loaded in flexion *(12)*, the presence of focal erosive lesions on the flexion weight-bearing zone of the femur and the posterior tibia should be carefully evaluated.

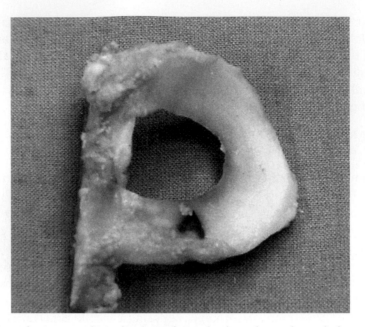

Fig. 5. Lateral meniscus transplantation is performed using a bone slot technique that connects the anterior and posterior horns of the meniscus.

Although meniscus transplantation may be particularly advantageous in an individual with articular cartilage degeneration in the meniscal weight-bearing zone of the femoral condyle or tibial plateau, loss of cartilage in these areas predisposes the meniscus transplant to failure. This is the setting in which concomitant cartilage resurfacing may be considered.

Cartilage resurfacing in conjunction with meniscus transplantation is indicated for treatment of a focal chondral defect. I use the microfracture technique for a chondral defect up to 8–10-mm diameter that is surrounded by essentially normal cartilage. Microfracture can only be used if the chondral defect is well contained. I prefer use of osteochondral tissue for lesions greater than 10 mm in diameter. Autograft tissue is used for lesions up to 25 mm in diameter. Osteochondral allograft tissue is recommended for lesions greater than 25 mm in diameter. The advantage of transferring osteochondral tissue is that the lesion is immediately covered with hyaline cartilage, compared to lesion repair using the microfracture or autologous chondrocyte implantation techniques, which requires time and maturation of the repaired cartilage surface. If microfracture or autologous chondrocyte implantation is performed with meniscus transplantation, then I recommend a conservative postoperative regimen with a longer period of protected weight bearing (8–12 wk) to protect the healing articular surface. Alternatively, the meniscus transplantation may be done as a staged procedure following the cartilage resurfacing (typically 6 mo).

There is little information in the literature on the outcome of combined meniscus transplantation and osteochondral resurfacing procedures. Noyes et al. reported on 40 cryopreserved meniscal transplants in 38 patients. Sixteen patients also received a concomitant osteochondral autograft. A comparison of patients who had a concomitant osteochondral autograft transfer procedure with those who underwent only meniscus transplantation did not reveal any difference regarding clinical pain symptoms, daily and sports activities, complications, the rate of reoperations, or the patient's perception of the knee condition *(1)*.

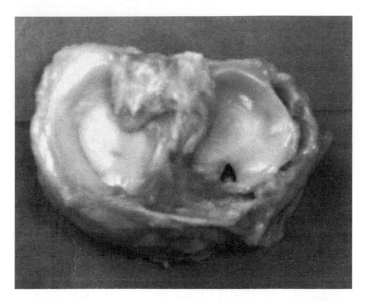

Fig. 6. An osteochondral allograft with attached meniscus can be used to replace an extensively damaged tibial plateau completely.

MANAGEMENT OF TIBIAL PLATEAU OSTEOCHONDRAL DEFORMITY FOLLOWING FRACTURE

Severe damage to the lateral tibial plateau can occur following fracture, especially in patients with excessive preexisting valgus alignment. If there is extensive damage to the tibial plateau and lateral meniscus, then an osteochondral allograft with an attached lateral meniscus is used to replace the damaged segment completely (Fig. 6). Fresh-frozen and cold-stored fresh (viable) osteochondral tissue is available for use in the United States. The height of the graft is approx 15–20 mm, with the resection made just above Gerdy's tubercle (maintaining the native attachment of the iliotibial band to Gerdy's tubercle). The lateral capsule is reattached to the allograft bone. The graft can be secured with a lateral tibial plateau buttress plate. Valgus alignment of the limb must be corrected prior to or in conjunction with the osteochondral tibial plateau reconstruction. The meniscus is attached to the native lateral capsule using standard meniscus repair suture techniques.

REHABILITATION CONSIDERATIONS

A conservative postoperative regimen is typically prescribed following chondral resurfacing procedures. A minimum of 6 wk of nonweight bearing is prescribed following microfracture and osteochondral autograft transfer, with progression to full weight bearing by approx 8 wk. Up to 12 wk of protected weight bearing may be considered for a large osteochondral allograft. Healing of a concomitant osteotomy (by radiographic criteria) must be established before progressing to full weight bearing. The addition of a meniscus transplant does not change these recommendations. Early active-assisted and passive motion is prescribed following both meniscus transplantation and chondral resurfacing. Flexion is limited to 90° for the first 4 wk following meniscus transplantation because flexion places a load on the posterior horn of the meniscus *(22)*. No significant limitations in eventual flexion achieved have resulted from this regimen.

SUMMARY

The knee surgeon must consider many issues, including meniscal volume, articular cartilage condition, and knee alignment when developing a treatment plan for the symptomatic patient with chondral injury. The menisci are important in distributing the normal contact forces associated with joint function. Meniscal deficiency increases these contact forces and ultimately results in articular cartilage degeneration over time. As such, the restoration of functional meniscal tissue and the correction of knee malalignment may be necessary when a cartilage repair procedure is planned. Ultimately, meniscal transplantation (with or without the use of knee osteotomy) may increase the likelihood of clinical success in patients who present with symptomatic articular cartilage lesions and a meniscal injury.

REFERENCES

1. Noyes FR, Barber-Westin SD, Rankin M. Meniscal transplantation in symptomatic patients less than 50 yr old. J Bone Joint Surg 2004;86A:1392–1404.
2. Van Arkel ERA, de Boer HH. Human meniscal transplantation. Preliminary results at 2- to 5-yr follow-up. J Bone and Joint Surg 1995;77B:589–595.
3. Allen CR, Wong EK, Livesay GA, Sakane M, Fu FH, Woo SL. Importance of the medial meniscus in the anterior cruciate ligament-deficient knee. J Orthop Res 2000;18:109–115.
4. Levy IM, Torzilli PA, Warren RF. The effect of medial meniscectomy on anterior-posterior motion of the knee. J Bone Joint Surg 1982;64A:883–888.
5. Papageorgiou CD, Gil JE, Kanamori A, Fenwick JA, Woo SL, Fu FH. The biomechanical interdependence between the anterior cruciate ligament replacement graft and the medial meniscus. Am J Sports Med 2001;29:226–231.
6. Shelbourne KD, Gray T. Results of anterior cruciate ligament reconstruction based on meniscus and articular cartilage status at the time of surgery. Five- to 15-yr evaluations. Am J Sports Med 2000;28:446–452.
7. Garrett JC. Meniscal transplantation: a review of 43 cases with 2- to 7-yr follow-up. Sports Med Arthrosc Rev 1993;1:164–167.
8. Markolf KL, Kochan A, Amstutz HC. Measurement of knee stiffness and laxity in patients with documented absence of the anterior cruciate ligament. J Bone Joint Surg 1984;66A:242–253.
9. Rodeo SA Meniscal allografts—where do we stand? Am J Sports Med 2001;29:246–261.
10. Cox JS, Nye CE, Schaefer WW, Woodstein IJ. The degenerative effects of partial and total resection of the medial meniscus in dogs' knees. Clin Orthop Relat Res 1975;109:178–183.
11. Kurosawa H, Fukubayashi T, Nakajima H. Load-bearing mode of the knee joint: physical behavior of the knee joint with or without menisci. Clin Orthop Relat Res 1980;149:283–290.
12. Walker PS, Erkman MJ. The role of the menisci in force transmission across the knee. Clin Orthop Relat Res 1975;109:184.
13. Li G, DeFrate LE, Park SE, Gill TJ, Rubash HE. In vivo articular cartilage contact kinematics of the knee: an investigation using dual-orthogonal fluoroscopy and magnetic resonance image-based computer models. Am J Sports Med 2005;33:102–107.
14. Johnson RJ, Kettelkamp DB, Clark W, Leaverton P. Factors effecting late results after meniscectomy. J Bone Joint Surg 1974;56A:719–729.
15. Yocum LA, Kerlan RK, Jobe FW, et al. Isolated lateral meniscectomy. A study of 26 patients with isolated tears. J Bone Joint Surg 1979;61A:338–342.
16. Holden DL, James SL, Larson RL, Slocum DB. Proximal tibial osteotomy in patients who are 50 yr old or less. A long-term follow-up study. J Bone Joint Surg 1988;70:977–982.
17. Cameron JC, Saha S. Meniscal allograft transplantation for unicompartmental arthritis of the knee. Clin Orthop Relat Res 1997;337:164–171.
18. Wickiewicz TL. Advantages of coronal plane osteotomy. Paper presented at: Interim Meeting of the American Orthopaedic Society for Sports Medicine; February 2005; Washington, DC.

19. Alhalki MM, Howell SM, Hull ML. How three methods for fixing a medial meniscal autograft affect tibial contact mechanics. Am J Sports Med 1999;27:320–328.
20. Baumgarten KM, Fealy S, Wickiewicz TL. The coronal plane high tibial osteotomy. Unpublished manuscript.
21. Fairbank TJ. Knee joint changes after meniscectomy. J Bone Joint Surg 1948;3OB:664–670.
22. Thompson WO, Thaete FL, Fu FH, Dye SF. Tibial meniscal dynamics using three-dimensional reconstruction of magnetic resonance images. Am J Sports Med 1991;19:210–215.

18

Articular Cartilage Repair Strategies in the Ankle Joint

Monika Volesky, MD, Timothy Charlton, MD, and Jonathan T. Deland, MD

Summary

Osteochondral lesions of the talus represent a significant source of disability to those affected. An understanding of the common mechanisms of injury and a high index of suspicion leads to early diagnosis and treatment. Most osteochondral lesions are a sequel of trauma; the exact etiology of others is unclear and may be multifactorial and related to microtrauma, genetic predisposition, or metabolic factors. Definitive imaging of osteochondral lesions consists of imaging with magnetic resonance, which is useful for qualitative analysis of the bony changes and the condition of the overlying cartilage. Just over half of patients with symptomatic osteochondral lesions of the talus will improve with nonoperative treatment. Failure of conservative therapy mandates operative treatment; surgical options include arthroscopy with debridement, drilling or microfracture of the lesion, mosaicplasty or osteochondral autografting, or autologous chondrocyte transplantation. The future for treating cartilage defects in the ankle is likely to involve implants that allow cartilage regrowth and are positioned by minimally invasive surgical techniques.

Key Words: Ankle; cartilage repair; microfracture; mosaicplasty; osteochondral grafting; osteochondral lesion; talus.

BACKGROUND

In the literature, the terms osteochondritis dissecans (OCD), transchondral fracture, osteochondral fracture, osteochondral lesion of the talus (OLT) have been used interchangeably to refer to separation of a fragment of articular cartilage from its talar bed along with some subchondral bone *(1)*. OCD was first described by Pare in 1840 *(2)*, and the name was coined by Konig in 1888 *(3)*. The presence of this pathology in the ankle was first published by Kappis in 1922 *(4)*. The true prevalence in the ankle is unknown as many are thought to be asymptomatic *(5)*.

Cartilage has limited ability for repair or regeneration as it is hypocellular and avascular. Acute osteochondral fragments, when diagnosed in a timely fashion, can be replaced and internally fixed. The strategies for treating chronic osteochondral defects are designed to stimulate healing either by induction of fibrocartilage or by transplantation of bone and cartilage or cartilage alone. The goals of all treatment methods are to provide a stable, congruent joint surface, restore function, and prevent the evolution of osteoarthritis in the injured joint. Long-term results have indicated that few lesions unite when treated nonoperatively *(6)*.

From: *Cartilage Repair Strategies*
Edited by: Riley J. Williams © Humana Press Inc., Totowa, NJ

PRESENTATION

Osteochondral lesions of the talus should be suspected following ankle sprains that have continued symptoms and pain following standard treatment *(7)*. Loomer et al.'s report on 92 patients with symptomatic osteochondral lesions of the talus revealed that all patients reported pain as their primary symptom, and that over 94% had pain with activity *(8)*. Failure to recognize these injuries can lead to long-term disability, with pain from recurrent synovitis, loose bodies, or altered joint mechanics. An understanding of the common mechanisms of injury and a high index of suspicion leads to early diagnosis and treatment. Details that should raise one's index of suspicion include a history of a flexion-inversion injury, exercise-related ankle pain, persistent swelling, as well as mechanical symptoms such as clicking and catching *(9)*.

Although it is thought that most osteochondral lesions are a sequel of trauma *(10–12)*, the exact etiology of others is unclear and may be multifactorial and related to microtrauma, genetic predisposition, or metabolic factors *(13)*. Many patients cannot relate their symptoms specifically to a trauma. Most studies agree that lateral side lesions are almost exclusively posttraumatic *(6,14)*; medial side lesions are related to trauma only 64–80% of the time. The postulated mechanisms of injury according to Berndt and Harty are the combination of plantar flexion, inversion, and external tibial torsion for medial lesions; a combination of inversion, dorsiflexion, and internal tibial rotation is thought to cause lateral lesions *(15,16)*.

Although there are partial- and full-thickness chondral lesions without bone involvement that occur in the ankle, these do not comprise the majority of symptomatic lesions *(7,17)*. Ankle fractures have been associated with cartilage lesions. Loren and Ferkel identified that fractures with syndesmotic disruption have a particularly high incidence of talar cartilage injury *(18)*. As well, in their arthroscopic evaluation of 288 patients with ankle fractures, Hintermann and coworkers found that 79% had cartilage lesions, most commonly on the talus (69%), but also on the distal tibia (69%), fibula (45%), and medial malleolus (41%) *(19)*.

The association of cartilage injuries with chronic ankle instability has also been investigated in detail. In their arthroscopic evaluation of 54 patients undergoing lateral ligament reconstruction for chronic instability, Komenda and Ferkel determined that 93% had intra-articular abnormalities, including a 25% incidence of chondral injuries such as talar osteochondral lesions and chondromalacia *(20)*. This is contrasted to the study by Taga and colleagues, who arthroscopically examined 31 ankles with lateral ligament injury and found chondral lesions in 89% of freshly injured ankles and 95% of ankles with chronic instability, mostly on the anteromedial edge of the tibial plafond *(7)*.

The appearance of the osteochondral lesion during arthroscopy depends on the stage and the size of the lesion. The lesion may appear as a softening or fissuring of the cartilage, a cartilaginous flap, or a defect devoid of cartilage. Osteochondral lesions are most often found posteromedially and less commonly in the anterolateral zones of the talar dome (Fig. 1). Although medial osteochondral lesions are usually deep, cup-shaped, and symmetric, the lateral lesions tend to be shallower in nature. In a retrospective look at 31 ankles, Canale and Belding noted that lateral lesions were associated with inversion or inversion-dorsiflexion trauma, were morphologically shallow, and were more likely to become displaced in the joint and to have persistent symptoms. Medial lesions were both traumatic and atraumatic in origin, morphologically deep, and less symptomatic. Cases of mirror image defects on the tibia and talus have also been described *(21)*.

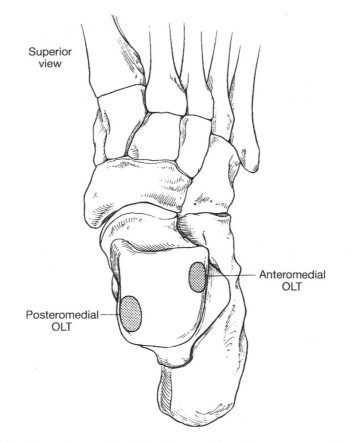

Fig. 1. Typical locations of osteochondral lesions of the talus: posteromedial and anterolateral. (Reprinted from ref. *59* with permission from Elsevier.)

WORKUP

On physical examination, tenderness is most often located along the anterior joint line medially or laterally, depending on the location of the lesion. Interestingly, symptoms and findings can actually be on the side opposite the lesion because of altered weight-bearing patterns.

If an osteochondral lesion is suspected based on clinical examination, investigations begin with plain radiographs of the ankle, including anteroposterior, mortise, and lateral views (Fig. 2A,B). The lesion may not be visualized on these films, but additional antero-posterior films in dorsiflexion may aid in demonstrating lateral lesions; ankle plantar flexion views may demonstrate medial lesions *(22)*. When plain radiographs of the ankle are relied on for the diagnosis of an osteochondral fracture of the talus, many lesions remain undiagnosed. In a study by Loomer et al., fewer than 50% of lesions were seen prospectively on radiographs, and still only 66% were identified retrospectively *(8)*. In addition, if ankle instability is suspected clinically, then stress radiographs can be undertaken to confirm or refute this diagnosis.

If a lesion is suspected but not seen on the plain radiographs, then more sensitive imaging modalities include bone scan and magnetic resonance imaging (MRI). Bone scan is an excellent

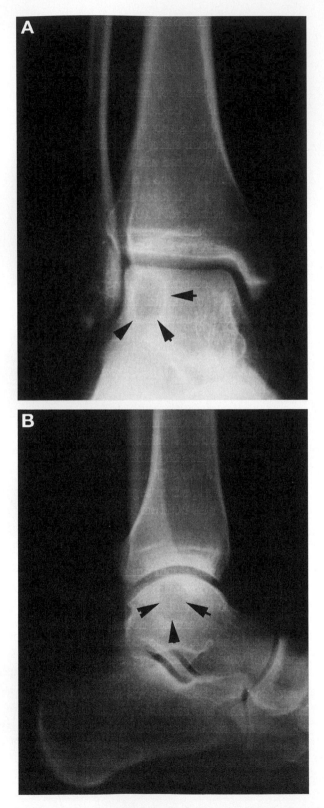

Fig. 2. Large lateral cystic osteochondral talar lesion on **(A)** mortise radiograph and **(B)** lateral radiograph.

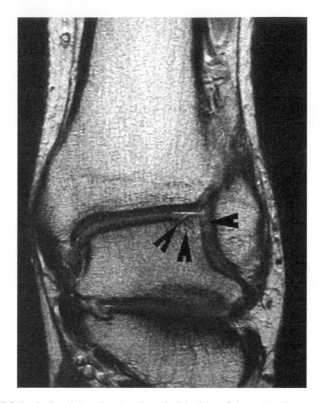

Fig. 3. Coronal MRI depicting lateral osteochondral lesion of the talus (large arrows) with overlying cartilage damage.

screening tool for patients with chronic ankle pain and has 94–99% sensitivity in depicting osteochondral lesions, with a specificity of approx 76% *(8,23)*. Although the bone scan is sensitive in detecting these lesions, unlike the MRI, it cannot be used to stage the lesions and is therefore used less and less frequently.

Definitive imaging of osteochondral lesions consists of imaging with magnetic resonance, which is useful for qualitative analysis of the bony changes and the condition of the overlying cartilage. Computed tomography will show the borders of the bony defect, but MRI is preferred because it can add details about the soft tissues as well as outline areas of bony edema. Studies with arthroscopic correlation have shown that MRI can be used to evaluate the articular cartilage covering osteochondral lesions of the talus with a high degree of accuracy *(24)*. Studies have also shown that magnetic resonance of the ankle can be used to assess talar osteochondral lesion stability accurately *(25–27)*. Current protocols consist of cartilage imaging in three planes, including a fat-suppression sequence to characterize bony edema and a moderate TE fast spin-echo pulse sequence to best delineate the cartilage damage *(24,28,29)* (Fig. 3).

The value of MRI in postoperative follow-up has garnered some attention. To evaluate the appearance and outcome of cartilage repair procedures noninvasively, the MRI with cartilage-specific sequences has become the modality of choice *(30)*. As well, after the drilling or fixation of lesions, Higashiyama et al. have postulated that the disappearance of signal rims in postoperative T_2-weighted images indicates bone union and healing with an obliteration of the interface between the osteochondral fragment and the talar bed *(31)*.

Table 1
Berndt and Harty *(15)*: Radiographic Classification of Osteochondritis Dissecans

Stage 1	Local and circumstricted compression of subchondral bone
Stage 2	Delimitation and partial detachment of a fragment from the chondral surface
Stage 3	Total detachment of the fragment, which remains in site of injury
Stage 4	Fragment is totally detached with loose body in joint

STAGING

A classification for staging OCD of the ankle, based on plain radiographs, was first proposed by Berndt and Hardy *(15)*. Their experiments on cadaveric specimens and their comprehensive review of literature greatly advanced knowledge about the topic (Table 1).

Although staging by computed tomography and MRI is comparable, some studies have found that MRI is most useful, especially when radiographs and clinical findings are not diagnostic *(32)*. Several studies have ascertained that MRI can accurately predict the grade of the lesion, as verified by arthroscopy *(24–26,33)*. With the popularity of MRI, multiple staging systems have been developed that make use of the information gained by this imaging modality. In 1989, Anderson and colleagues proposed a classification for grading osteochondral lesions of the talus based on the MRI findings *(32)* (Table 2).

In 1999, based on a review of 430 hindfoot MR images, including 18 osteochondral lesions, Hepple and colleagues suggested a revised classification scheme to take into account the detail now available on MRI scans *(34)* (Table 3).

A modification of Cheng's arthroscopic scale *(35)*, adapted for MRI, was proposed by Mintz and colleagues *(24)* (Table 4).

It is believed that arthroscopy is the most accurate modality at determining the status of the cartilage overlying the lesion and the key to guiding subsequent treatment. Arthroscopic grading of the cartilage overlying the osteochondral lesion by visualizing and probing was described by Pritsch and coworkers *(10)* (Table 5).

Some authors *(24,36)* have used the Cheng-Ferkel arthroscopy-based staging system when comparing and analyzing their results *(35)* (Table 6).

With improving imaging modalities and understanding of the disease, the staging systems have become more detailed in an attempt to subclassify and prognosticate. Unfortunately, there is no one classification system that is universally accepted by clinicians, but Berndt and Harty's work *(15)* has remained the basis from which the other grading systems have evolved. The current gold standard for diagnosis and key to subsequent care is arthroscopy, but as MRI technology improves it may prove to be as useful, especially in lower-grade lesions for which surgery may not be indicated.

NONOPERATIVE TREATMENT

Traditionally, the indications for conservative treatment are stable lesions with intact cartilage, such as Berndt and Harty stage 1 and 2 lesions, as well as medial stage 3 lesions. Tol and colleagues performed a detailed analysis of articles published from 1966 to 1999 describing the results of treatment strategies for OCD of the talus. They concluded that because the articles were variable in nature and there were no randomized clinical trials, no definite conclusions could be made regarding the most superior treatment. They did mention, however, that ankles that received no treatment had a success rate of less than 45% *(37)*.

Table 2
Anderson et al. (32): MRI Classification of Osteochondral Lesions of the Talus

Stage 1	Subchondral trabecular bone compression respecting the chondral layer
Stage 2A	Appearance of local cystic lesion in the subchondral layer
Stage 2	Fragment in site of injury but incompletely separated from chondral joint surface
Stage 3	Undisplaced fragment is separated by synovial fluid from the bony crater
Stage 4	Displaced fragment in the joint space

Table 3
Hepple et al. (34): MRI Classification of Osteochondral Lesions of the Talus

Stage 1	Articular cartilage damage only
Stage 2a	Cartilage injury with underlying fracture and surrounding bony edema
Stage 2b	Stage 2a without surrounding bony edema
Stage 3	Detached but undisplaced fragment
Stage 4	Detached and displaced fragment
Stage 5	Subchondral cyst formation

Table 4
Mintz et al. (24): MRI Classification of Osteochondral Lesions of the Talus

Stage 0	Normal
Stage 1	Hyperintense but morphologically intact cartilage surface
Stage 2	Fibrillation or fissures not extending to bone
Stage 3	Flap present or bone exposed
Stage 4	Loose, undisplaced fragment
Stage 5	Displaced fragment

Table 5
Pritsch et al. (10): Arthroscopic Grading of Osteochondral Lesions of the Talus

Grade 1	Intact, firm, shiny cartilage
Grade 2	Intact but soft cartilage
Grade 3	Frayed cartilage

Table 6
Cheng and Ferkel (35): Arthroscopic Staging System for Classification of Osteochondral Lesions of the Talus

Stage	*Findings*	*Stability*
A	Smooth, intact, but soft or ballotable cartilage	Stable
B	Rough surface	Stable
C	Fibrillation or fissuring	Stable
D	Cartilage flap present or bone exposed	Unstable
E	Loose, undisplaced fragment	Unstable
F	Displaced fragment	Unstable

It has been noted that, even when lesions become asymptomatic, many do not appear to heal radiographically when treated nonoperatively *(6)*. Shearer and colleagues studied 35 ankles with what they called stage 5 osteochondral lesions, which were chronic cystic lesions in the talus. With nonsurgical management, they noted that most lesions remain radiographically stable and that there is poor correlation between changes in lesion size and clinical outcome. Their clinical results, however, also showed that only 54% have a good or excellent clinical result at an average of 38 mo after diagnosis and 88 mo after symptom onset, and that lateral lesions fared better than medial ones *(38)*.

The prescription for nonoperative treatment varies greatly, from allowing the patient activity with no restriction to non-weight bearing with cast immobilization on the affected extremity acutely. In general, patients with more chronic symptoms are discouraged from engaging in activities that cause considerable discomfort or symptoms.

OPERATIVE TREATMENT

Indications for operative therapy of osteochondral lesions of the talus include a displaced acute lesion (Berndt and Harty stage 4) or chronic lesions with considerable symptoms that have persisted for at least 3 mo. Surgical options depend on whether the cartilage injury is partial or full thickness and whether it is associated with underlying changes in the subchondral bone. The stability of the fragment and the condition of the articular cartilage also determine the algorithm to be pursued. The options in a symptomatic stable lesion with cartilage intact is limited to drilling, either antegrade or retrograde, as well as retrograde bone grafting to fill a bony defect under an intact cartilage layer. In unstable lesions, the options include excision of the fragment, stimulative treatments such as excision combined with curettage and drilling, osteochondral grafting, or autologous chondrocyte transplantation (ACT). Usually, the approach taken in treating talar dome defects is to pursue the least aggressive, simplest, and lowest-risk treatment with a good chance of success first. Small lesions, less than 8 mm, are almost always treated with arthroscopy and drilling as a primary procedure. The more aggressive and expensive treatment modalities, such as osteochondral autografting, ACT, and allograft replacement, are generally reserved for large lesions, revisions, and failures. This generalization should be modified if indicated by patient factors such as age or activity level or the lesion size and location.

Many of these strategies for treating cartilaginous defects in the talus have made use of techniques that have been tried with some success in other joints, such as the knee. Although early results of techniques such as mosaicplasty, large allografts, and ACT have shown promising results to varying degrees, it is important to remember that the ankle joint is very different from the knee, both mechanically and biologically. In the knee, increased success in using these techniques is related to offloading the injured part of the joint with corrective osteotomies. In the ankle, the etiology of osteochondral lesions is not known to be related to deviations in mechanical axes that can be corrected concurrently with the cartilage repair. As well, the properties of the cartilage in lower extremity joints are not equal, and the ankle cartilage is thinner *(39–41)*.

In 1986, Baker et al. were among the first to describe the use of arthroscopy for the diagnosis and treatment of talar osteochondral lesions *(12)*. Arthroscopy has replaced arthrotomy of the ankle as the diagnostic and therapeutic approach of choice. Arthroscopy, with modern techniques and noninvasive distraction devices, provides excellent visualization, minimal complications, and decreased morbidity *(42–44)*. Currently, some of the indications for ankle

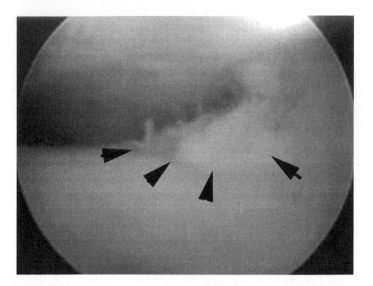

Fig. 4. Arthroscopic view of fibrillated unstable cartilage flap (large arrows) overlying OLT.

arthroscopy include osteochondral lesions of the talus, acute articular fractures, synovitis, loose bodies, degenerative joint disease, and soft tissue impingement.

Arthroscopic examination of the ankle permits complete examination of intra-articular structures and pathology. In the treatment of small defects and stable lesions, arthroscopic procedures such as debridement, synovectomy, and retrograde drilling have distinct advantages over open techniques. Andrews's group was among the first to document outcomes with ankle arthroscopy and demonstrated that the best results at a mean follow-up of 2 yr were achieved in patients with synovitis and transchondral defects of the talus *(45)*.

The technique for ankle arthroscopy has the patient supine with a thigh tourniquet and a padded thigh holder. After limb exsanguination, the tourniquet is inflated, and the landmarks of the ankle are palpated and marked. The ankle is placed in a noninvasive distractor device, and the joint is insufflated with saline solution via an anteromedial approach. An anteromedial portal is established first using a nick-and-spread technique. This portal is located just medial to the anterior tibial tendon and is usually made approximately half a centimeter below the joint line. A 2.7-mm 30° arthroscope is used, and an anterolateral portal is established just lateral to the extensor tendons, paying special attention to protect the superficial peroneal nerve. Most commonly, the arthroscope is placed in the anterior portal on the opposite side of the lesion, and the working instruments are placed through the anterior portal that is closest to the lesion. A posterolateral outflow is established just lateral to the Achilles tendon, in the space between the Achilles and peroneal tendons, and can be converted to a portal if required for visualization. A complete inspection of the joint is performed, and the cartilage surface of the talus and tibia is probed for softening, fissure, flaps, or defects (Fig. 4).

Excision

If an osteocartilaginous flap (Berndt and Harty stage 3) or loose body (stage 4) is encountered during diagnostic arthroscopy, then the decision must be taken whether it can be fixed to its base or whether it needs to be removed. Fixation of a displaced osteochondral fragment can be undertaken only if it can be reduced anatomically and the cartilaginous surface appears well preserved, which is unlikely in a chronic osteochondral lesion. As well, if the cartilage is detached from the bone, it must be excised. Many years ago, an acceptable treatment was the removal of the fragment, either arthroscopically or open, and either no treatment or simple curettage of the talar bony bed. Tol et al. have shown that, in the 14 results of studies describing the outcome of excision alone, good-to-excellent results were only seen in 38% of patients (37). Currently, the excision of the fragment in a large chronic lesion is usually accompanied by one of the cartilage repair techniques reviewed next.

Excision and Curettage

Tol and colleagues performed a review of literature from 1966 to 1998, which included 14 studies describing excision alone, 11 studies reporting on excision with curettage, and no randomized clinical trials. The best outcomes were in patients who underwent excision, curettage, and drilling of advanced osteochondral lesions, as 85% had good-to-excellent results. In contrast to that figure, only 78% had good results with excision and curettage, and 38% did well following excision alone (37). In most cases, the excision and curettage was performed by arthrotomy or mini-arthrotomy. The same group also published a meta-analysis of 39 studies published from 1966 to 2000 describing the results of treatment strategies for OCD of the talus. The success rates they presented for the various treatment modalities were unchanged from their earlier publication, and they concluded that excision, curettage, and drilling or excision and curettage alone could be recommended as treatment modalities, but excision alone was not recommended (46).

Frank et al. reported on 9 patients who underwent arthroscopic removal of the loose body and curettage of the necrotic bone. With a clinical follow-up of 10–24 mo, 6 patients with chronic OCD did well; one did poorly (47). The first long-term functional outcome of arthroscopic excision and curettage was published by Baker et al. Of their 12 patients, 10 were rated good or excellent, 1 was fair, and 1 had a poor rating at an average follow-up of 10 yr. Interestingly, radiographs showed minimal to no degenerative changes in the ankle and residual subchondral changes at the site of the lesion. Based on these findings, they argued that arthroscopic debridement and curettage yield successful results at 10 yr, with minimal morbidity (12,48). Others have also shown favorable long-term results with arthroscopic debridement and curettage or abrasion (49).

Kelberine et al. reported on 48 cases of arthroscopic surgery for osteochondral talar lesions, with an average follow-up of 5 yr. In 18 cases, there was an anterolateral loose fragment, which was merely excised in 16 cases and fixed in 2 cases. In contrast, of the 30 chronic lesions, 27 underwent excision of the necrotic area with curettage of the subchondral bone. These chronic cases did not fare as well as the acute osteochondral fractures, with only 20 of 30 having good or excellent results at follow-up. The authors emphasized that there is a significant prognostic distinction between osteochondral injuries in the anterolateral aspect of the talar dome, which are traumatic and recent in onset, and the more necrotic chronic medial lesions (50). Ogilvie-Harris and Sarrosa reported on 8 patients who underwent arthroscopic debridement and abrasion for persistent symptoms after failed open surgery for OCD. They found a statistically significant improvement in pain, swelling, limp, and activity level at a mean of 38 mo postarthroscopy (51).

Drilling/Microfracture

Prior to the universal use of arthroscopy in treating osteochondral lesions of the ankle, drilling and microfracture techniques were done open to stimulate healing by penetrating the subchondral bone. The removal of debris and penetration of the subchondral bone to induce bleeding has been shown to bring osteoprogenitor cells into the defect and stimulate the growth of fibrocartilage. Although the properties of fibrocartilage are inferior to hyaline cartilage *(52)*, there have been good clinical results to support this treatment.

Several authors presented results of open drilling or microfracture in treating defects of the talus. O'Farrell and Costello assessed the outcome of 24 patients at a mean of 47 mo after open removal of the osteochondritic fragment and drilling of some of the lesions. The authors concluded that drilling of the base improved the results, and that chronic lesions had less successful outcomes *(53)*. In Nash et al.'s study of 9 patients with traumatic-onset osteochondral lesions, 8 had good results at a mean of 15 mo after K-wire drilling *(54)*.

Flick and Gould also performed open curettage and drilling of the lesion base and described a technique that allowed access to posteromedial talar dome lesions without requiring a medial malleolar osteotomy. These lesions were approached through the tibialis anterior tendon sheath, with a grooving of the anteromedial distal tibia articular surface. Of the 19 patients in their study, 79% had good or excellent results at a mean follow-up of 24 mo *(14)*.

Loomer's group had similar clinical results, with 42% excellent and 32% good results, although they noted a discrepancy between the resolution of symptoms and the actual radiographic healing *(8)*. Alexander and Lichtman looked at the long-term results of open drilling performed between 1957 and 1977 on 25 patients, at an average of 65 mo postoperatively. Of the 25 patients, 22 had good or excellent results, and these positive results seemed to apply even when the procedure was performed for chronic lesions. They also noted that patients seemed to improve clinically for as long as 18 mo, and that the clinical benefits appeared to persist, with good long-term results *(55)*. Angermann and Jensen did note some deterioration in clinical results with long-term follow-up of 9–15 yr but would still recommend the procedure even in patients with long-standing symptoms *(56)*.

The ability to drill arthroscopically significantly reduces the morbidity associated with open procedures. Several techniques have been described to access the posteromedial talar lesions, including transmalleolar drilling, anteromedial grooving of the distal tibia, and the use of an anterior cruciate ligament guide for aiming precision. The drilling is usually performed with small Kirschner wires to perforate the subchondral bone and may be done in the bony talar bed after fragment excision and curettage or through intact cartilage in earlier stage osteochondral lesions (Fig 5).

Van Bueken and colleagues had 13 good-to-excellent results in 15 patients treated with arthroscopic drilling, with a mean follow-up of 26 mo *(42)*. In Schuman et al.'s group of 38 patients, good or excellent results were seen in 86% of patients undergoing a first procedure. Those undergoing a revision procedure had only slightly diminished success rates, with 75% having good or excellent results *(57)*.

Earlier stage lesions that have failed conservative therapy are also an indication for arthroscopic evaluation and drilling. In the past, this drilling was done antegrade through intact articular cartilage in an attempt to induce healing in the underlying necrotic bone. Kumai and colleagues looked at the functional results in 18 ankles at a mean of 4.6 yr postoperatively. All patients had intact articular cartilage overlying the lesion and underwent transmalleolar antegrade arthroscopic drilling with 1.2-mm Kirschner wires. All ankles had clinical improvement, with 13 rated as good and 5 as fair. They also noted that better results were seen in patients under 30 yr of age and in more acute lesions *(58)*.

A technique has been devised that allows drilling in a retrograde fashion through the talus so intact articular cartilage that covers a stable osteochondral lesion is not violated. This

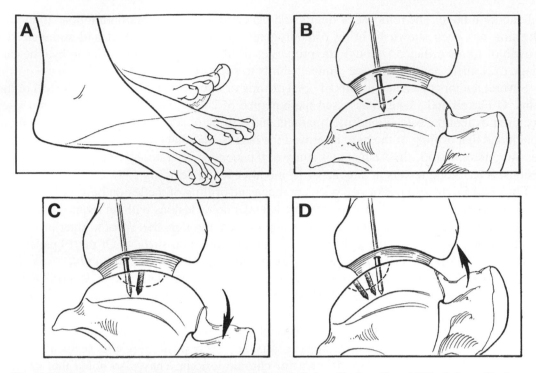

Fig. 5. Technique of antigrade drilling through the medial malleolus. One drill hole in malleolus can be used for multiple drill holes in the talus. (Reprinted from ref. *59* with permission from Elsevier.)

avoids iatrogenic cartilage injury and hemarthrosis and allows bone grafting to be performed through the drill holes. Described by Ferkel *(59)*, it uses a hinged small joint aiming device, such as the Micro Vector Drill Guide (Smith and Nephew, Andover, MA) to access posteromedial osteochondral lesions. The guide is placed through the anteromedial portal, with the tip on the lesion. The distal aiming arm and drill guide are positioned to enter inferolaterally through the sinus tarsi (Fig. 6). The articulated arm allows multiple drill holes to be placed with Kirschner wires and cannulated drills. An image intensifier can be used concomitantly to determine the depth of penetration of the Kirschner wires and drill *(60)*.

Conti's group reported on 16 patients who underwent medial talar dome percutaneous retrograde drilling through the sinus tarsi. The patients were assessed at an average of 2 yr postintervention using the American Orthopaedic Foot and Ankle Society (AOFAS) Ankle-Hindfoot Scale and improved from a mean of 53.9 of 100 points preoperatively to 82.6 points postoperatively. The authors concluded that their short-term results were comparable to the results reported with other techniques *(61)*.

Bone Grafting

Bone grafting can now be done in contained lesions with intact cartilage via a retrograde technique as described for drilling of osteochondral lesions of the talus. After drilling and curetting from the sinus tarsi up into the dome of the talus, bone graft can be tamped into the space left after evacuation of the necrotic bone (Fig. 7). To our knowledge, there are no studies that looked at this form of treatment specifically. Open anterograde autologous bone grafting was abandoned after earlier studies showed a high failure rate, with half of the patients requiring further surgery *(62)*.

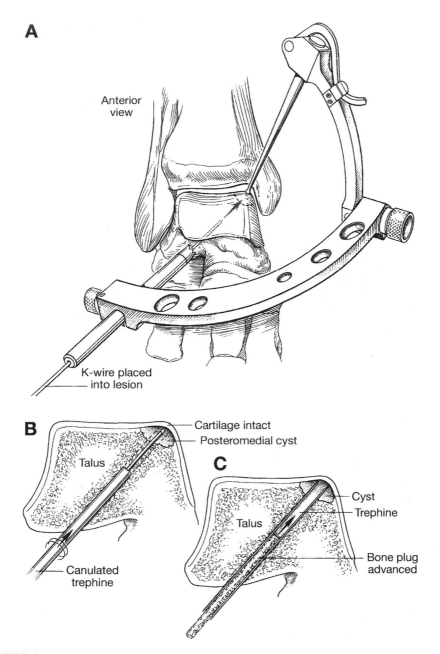

Fig. 6. With intact cartilage, retrograde drilling of the talus can be done in the following steps. **(A)** K-wire into the guide and fluroscan are used to localize the lesion with hinged drill over the wire. **(B)** Trephine or drill is advanced over the K-wire to remove necrotic bone but leave cartilage intact. **(C)** Bone graft can then be advanced into the lesion and a tamp used to pack the bone graft. (Reprinted from ref. *59* with permission from Elsevier.)

Fixation

Fixation of acute osteochondral lesions has been described, although few results are available in the literature. Under arthroscopic guidance, the fracture fragment and talar defect are identified. If the fracture fragment is devoid of bone, then it should be excised. If the fracture is truly osteochondral, then the edges should be debrided so that the cartilage edge is perpendicular.

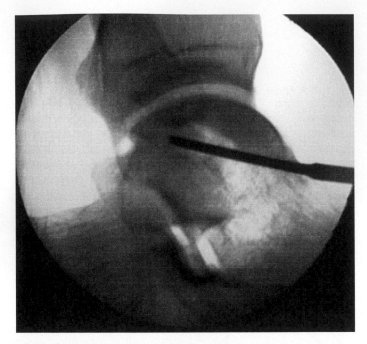

Fig. 7. Lateral radiograph of retrograde bone grafting of large osteochondral lesion.

The defect in the talus is debrided to a bleeding bony base and drilled with a 0.062-in. K-wire. The free piece is reduced into the defect; if the reduction is adequate, then it is held temporarily with Kirschner wires. Very large fragments can be kept reduced with countersunk or bioabsorbable screws; slightly smaller fragments can be fixed with bioabsorbable pins. Cannulated screw systems are especially useful in performing a percutaneous, arthroscopic-assisted fixation. Lateral lesions are usually instrumented most easily through the anterolateral portal. Medial lesions tend to be more posterior and can require a medial malleolar osteotomy for access if plantar flexing the foot does not suffice *(60)*.

Angermann and Riegels-Nieslsen reported on six osteochondral fractures of the talar dome fixed with fibrin sealant. They reported that all lesions healed with no adverse effects, and that 3 of 4 athletes had returned to sports by 1 yr *(63)*.

Allograft

Advantages of allograft use include decreased patient morbidity, shorter surgical time, smaller incisions, and the ability to resurface large lesions. Disadvantages of this technique include the risk of disease transmission, slower biological healing, potential for immune response, the question of survival of the implanted cartilage, as well as the logistics of graft procurement and storage *(64)*. The technique is usually reserved for focal arthritic areas in the ankle and large defects not amenable to mosaicplasty or cartilage cell transplantation. Meticulous technique in achieving host-donor fit and incorporation of the graft-host interface are keys to the success of fresh osteochondral allografts *(65)*.

The viability of chondrocytes depends in large part on the harvesting and preservation of the grafts. Viability of the cartilage and the survival of chondrocytes is key to successful clinical outcomes with osteochondral allograft transplantation. Ideally, allograft procurement is within 24 h of death and is transplanted by 72 h (no more than 7 d). Fresh frozen allografts have shown decreased cell viability compared to fresh allografts *(66,67)*. Cell survival as low as 20–30% has been published following cryopreservation, but this viability appears to be improved in cartilage stored by refrigeration *(68)*. In allografts implanted fresh, the donor screening must be extensive to decrease the risk of disease transmission. Although there is documented immunogenicity, there have been, to our knowledge, no reports of clinical problems from graft rejection as the chondrocytes seem to be immunoprivileged.

Technique of selection and implantation involves matching the donor to the host bone using radiography. Any mechanical axis deviation or ankle instability needs to be addressed and corrected. After arthrotomy, the defect is prepared and its size measured. The donor graft is harvested and trimmed to the appropriate size and lavaged, and repeated fittings are performed to ensure an anatomic fit. Tontz and colleagues have described using the cutting blocks from the Agility (Depuy, Warsaw, IN) ankle arthroplasty system to achieve reproducible cuts and match the host defect to the donor graft *(65)*. The graft is fixed using screws. Postoperatively, the patient is kept non-weight bearing for 6–12 wk until evidence of incorporation is seen. During that time, after wound healing, some range of motion exercises are encouraged.

Gross and colleagues reported on long-term outcomes of 9 patients who underwent fresh osteochondral allograft transplantation of the talus, 8 for OCD and 1 for traumatic open fracture of the talus. At a mean of 11 yr, ranging from 4 to 19 yr, 6 of the 9 grafts remained *in situ*. Three patients underwent ankle arthrodesis during that time for failure of the graft. Interestingly, the failures were not caused by progression of the original arthritic condition, but rather they were all secondary to graft failure with resorption and fragmentation of the graft *(69)*.

Tontz and colleagues presented the outcomes of 12 patients who underwent tibiotalar fresh allografting. At a mean follow-up of 21 mo, all grafts had healed at the host-donor interface, and the patients had a significant improvement in function and decrease in pain. Range of motion, however, did not consistently improve, and complications included intraoperative fracture in 1 patient and graft collapse requiring revision allografting in another *(65)*.

Mosaicplasty

Despite satisfactory clinical results in small lesions with other techniques such as arthroscopic debridement, chondral shaving, and drilling, these methods substitute fibrocartilagenous repair tissue for the damaged articular cartilage. In lesions larger than 1.0 cm^2, healing of the lesion with introduction of hyalinelike cartilage is ideal as it has better mechanical properties than fibrocartilage *(52)*. In principle, autogenous osteochondral transplantation fills these criteria.

Initially, one osteochondral plug was harvested from the knee and placed in modest defects of the talus because the harvest site morbidity limited the application of this technique to small lesions. A technique called mosaicplasty was then developed for use in the knee, where several small grafts were press-fit into a chondral defect, allowing more plugs to be harvested with minimal morbidity *(70)*. This was then soon extrapolated to the ankle to treat osteochondral lesions of the talus. Currently, this technique is indicated in lesions approx 8–30 mm^2 with frayed or absent cartilage and necrotic subchondral bone, failure of previous surgery, age less than 50 yr, and absence of arthritis or "kissing" lesions *(71)*.

Prior to performing mosaicplasty, ankle arthroscopy is undertaken to evaluate the size and location of the lesion and to assess for other intra-articular pathology. This can be performed in a staged fashion but is usually done at the same sitting. Advantages of mosaicplasty include proven good incorporation, no risk of disease transmission with autograft plugs, and performance as

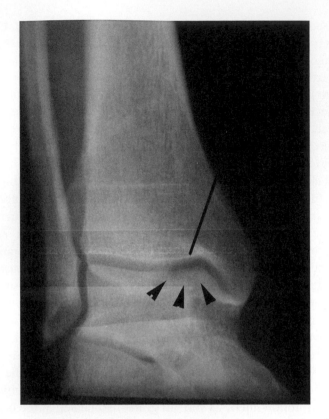

Fig. 8. Medial osteochondral lesion (large arrows) with proposed medial malleolar osteotomy for perpendicular access to lesion for osteochondral allograft plug.

a single-setting procedure. There are, however, limitations to the technique, which include the added morbidity of the knee harvest site, size limitations, and the challenge to achieve symmetry and surface congruity with multiple grafts. In addition, the space between the grafts fills with fibrocartilage, creating a repair that is not perfectly uniform.

When performing osteochondral autografts, perpendicular access to the lesion is required to achieve proper resurfacing and seat the grafts. Especially when the talar lesion is medial, a medial malleolar osteotomy is most often required to achieve adequate exposure. Under image intensifier guidance, the position for the proposed osteotomy is determined that will allow perpendicular access to the lesion. A medial skin incision overlying the medial malleolus is performed, and the malleolus is predrilled and tapped to allow for easier reduction and fixation once the grafting is completed. An oblique osteotomy is commonly performed with the oscillating saw and is finished by breaking through the articular tibial cartilage with the osteotome (Fig. 8). The malleolar osteotomy is eventually reduced anatomically and fixed with two 4.0-mm malleolar screws. Sammarco and Makwana described access to the talus through a replaceable bone block removed from the anterior tibial plafond *(72)*. Rarely, if access on the lateral side is limited, an oblique osteotomy of the fibula and the bony tibial site of attachment of the anterior tibiofibular syndesmosis is performed. Alternatively, the anterior talofibular ligament can be sectioned; the fibula is left attached to its posterior soft tissue attachments and is hinged posteriorly to allow access to the joint. Eventually, the fibula is repaired with a six-hole plate and possibly a lag screw *(73,74)*.

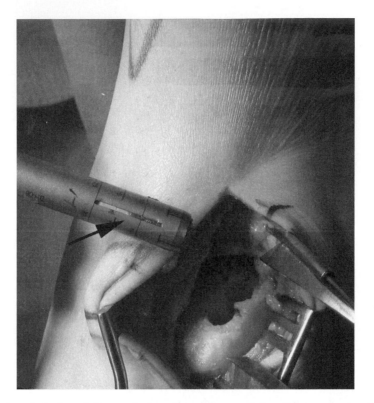

Fig. 9. Osteochondral plug delivery device slotted for precision (large arrow) with plug ready to be inserted into drilled recipient sites.

Once access is ensured, the osteochondral lesion is debrided to a stable base of healthy bone, and any unstable cartilaginous flaps are excised. A healthy vertical rim of cartilage is necessary. The lesion is then sized to determine the approximate number and size of the osteochondral plugs to be harvested and used. Grafts measuring from 3.5 to 10 mm can be used in combination to allow for contouring and as precise a fill as possible. These osteochondral grafts are usually harvested from the ipsilateral knee joint, from the periphery of the medial or lateral femoral condyles, either arthroscopically assisted or via mini-arthrotomy. The plugs are removed from the femur with a tubular double-edge chisel, and there is a 0.1- to 0.2-mm expansion in their diameter on removal, which ultimately allows for a press-fit in a drill hole of the same size.

The grafts are then sequentially inserted using a windowed delivery tube and are gently tamped (Fig. 9). Care is taken to leave the cartilage flush with the healthy surface, avoiding a step deformity; once all the plugs are seated, the ankle is irrigated to remove loose bodies, and the grafts are observed through a range of motion to ensure congruency *(73)* (Fig. 10). Postoperatively, the patient is kept nonweight bearing for 4–6 wk, but usually motion is allowed after wound healing. Some surgeons, however, prefer to immobilize their patients for 4–6 wk to ensure that the malleolar osteotomy site heals adequately.

A few authors prefer to harvest the plugs from areas of the talus that are not critically involved in weight bearing, such as the medial or lateral talar articular facet on the same side as the lesion *(72)*. The rationale behind this is that knee and ankle cartilage are qualitatively different in thickness and function *(75)*, and that talar cartilage is best replaced by the same

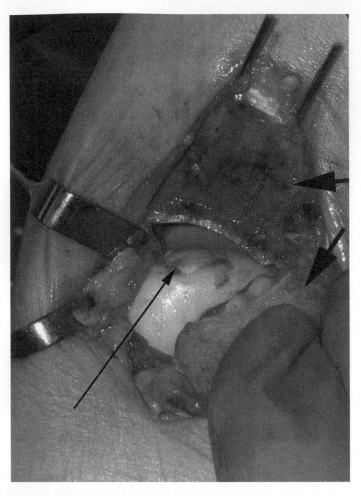

Fig. 10. Osteochondral allograft plug placed into drilled defect in talus (thin arrow), accessed via medial malleolar osteotomy (large arrows).

type of articular cartilage. Their clinical results in 12 patients were excellent, with significant improvements from preoperative functional scores. This particular technique is limited to 8-mm lesions and smaller given the limited area of the donor site.

Choung and Christensen performed cadaveric loading experiments to assess the best size of grafts that would restore the contact pressures to a normal level. They created an 8×12 mm ovoid chondral defect in a cadaveric talus, which was then filled with grafts, and axially loaded it to assess contact pressures and total contact area. When filled with 6-mm grafts, there was less-optimal restoration of normal parameters; the 4-mm plugs nearly restored the joint contact area and pressure to normal, intact levels. They concluded that focal talar dome defects should be repaired with multiple small osteochondral cylindrical grafts, which could be of talar origin *(76)*.

Several authors have reported results with the osteochondral autograft mosaicplasty technique. Hangody's group was the first to popularize this technique and have published their experiences since 1997. In 1997, their preliminary results of mosaicplasty for OCD lesions of the talus in 11 patients were released. They used tubular chisels via arthrotomy to harvest cylindrical grafts from minimally weight-bearing areas of the ipsilateral knee. These grafts were then implanted into the talar defects, which had been drilled to accommodate the grafts. At a mean follow-up of 16 mo, all patients had excellent results (Hannover scale) and had returned to activities *(77)*. They have followed up this report with one reporting clinical outcomes of 36 patients at a mean of 4.2 (2–7) yr postoperatively. The patients had 94% good-to-excellent results by the Hannover scoring system for ankle function, with no donor site morbidity at the knee. Eight patients underwent second-look arthroscopy, which showed normal-looking cartilage, and biopsies in 4 ankles revealed a predominance of Type 2 collagen in the cartilage *(73)*. Some comparative studies have shown improved results with osteochondral autografting compared with traditional treatments such as debridement, curettage, and drilling *(78,79)*. Prospective studies have confirmed the good intermediate-term results and durability of this technique *(80–83)*.

Al-Shaikh et al. reported on 19 patients with osteochondral lesions of the talus who were treated with autologous osteochondral grafting taken from the ipsilateral femoral condyle. The group included 13 who had failed prior excision, curettage, and drilling. The average size of the lesion was 12 × 10 mm. Ankle exposure was obtained by medial malleolar osteotomy in 13 patients, arthrotomy in 5, and lateral malleolar osteotomy in 1. At a mean follow-up of 16 mo, the average postoperative AOFAS Ankle-Hindfoot score was 88 (of 100) points, with excellent function and minimal morbidity at the knee. It also proved to be an effective salvage following previous failed procedures *(84)*.

Lee and colleagues reported on outcomes of 18 symptomatic Berndt and Harty stage 3 and 4 osteochondral lesions of the talus treated with mosaicplasty. The mean size of the defect was 13.6 × 7.2 mm and was filled with two or three 6- or 7-mm osteochondral grafts harvested from the superomedial margin of the ipsilateral knee. At a mean follow-up of 36 mo, 16 of 18 ankles had excellent results; 2 had good results. Second-look arthroscopy in 16 ankles revealed congruity between the grafts and native cartilage in 14, with some fissuring of the grafts in 2 *(85)*.

Autologous Chondrocyte Transplantation

As with mosaicplasty, the approach to larger osteochondral lesions is to replace the damaged articulating surface with hyaline cartilage to obtain satisfactory and durable clinical outcomes. In clinical and animal experiments *(86,87)*, investigators have repaired these lesions by injecting cultured autologous chondrocytes into the defect under a periosteal flap. ACT has shown that it provides coverage of the defect with hyaline-type cartilage *(88,89)*. Although initially described in humans for treatment of osteochondral lesions of the knee with excellent intermediate results *(88,90–92)*, the technique has now been applied to lesions of the talus *(93)*.

Although the joints are biomechanically very different, the same procedure was essayed in the ankle for repair of large osteochondral lesions of the talus. The procedure is staged and involves a harvesting phase as well as an implantation phase. In the first phase, diagnostic ankle arthroscopy is performed. After inspecting and probing the joint for pathology, first-line treatments such as debridement and drilling of the subchondral bone are performed to stimulate healing in the observed osteochondral defect. Ipsilateral knee arthroscopy should then be performed using a sharp curette to obtain an articular cartilage biopsy for culture. The preferred knee donor site is the lateral margin of the intercondylar notch, but the superior lateral and medial edges of the notch are acceptable as well. These cartilage biopsies should be full thickness and measure 3–4 mm in width and 10 mm in length *(94)*. This cartilage for ACT is not harvested from the ankle as loss of even this small amount of cartilage could be additionally detrimental to the mechanics of the ankle joint *(95)*. Taking cartilage for cell expansion from the talar lesion itself, however, has been described *(96)*. The samples are expediently sent to a laboratory specializing in cell expansion for processing and cell culturing, which is done under sterile conditions to avoid microbial contamination.

The second phase, consisting of the reimplantation of the chondrocytes, can be planned as early as 14 d after starting the cell culturing. An arthrotomy is performed, with a malleolar osteotomy if necessary. The lesion is thoroughly debrided to remove all fibrous tissue, although the subchondral bone is left intact to avoid bleeding at the base. The lesion should be contained and surrounded by a vertical rim of healthy cartilage. The lesion is sized with a template cut to size, and a periosteal patch is then harvested with those dimensions from the distal tibia. The periosteum is cut sharply 2–3 mm wider than the template with the 15 blade, and then a periosteal elevator is used to remove the graft, which is kept moistened in saline. Marking the outer layer with the sterile surgical pen will help differentiate the outer and cambium layers once it is freed from the tibia.

The periosteal graft is then placed over the defect with the cambium layer facing into the lesion and trimmed to provide an exact fit without any overhang. To anchor the graft, the four corners are sutured to the adjacent articular cartilage with 6-0 vicryl suture, and then subsequent sutures are placed at 2- to 3-mm intervals. The periphery is augmented with Tisseel fibrin sealant (Baxter Healthcare Corp., Deerfield, IL) to provide a watertight seal. This is tested for leaks by injecting saline under the periosteal graft pouch. The saline is withdrawn, and the autologous chondrocytes are injected under the periosteum with a blunt-tipped, plastic, 18-gage angiocatheter. The last opening is sutured with the 6-0 vicryl and sealed with Tisseel *(94)*.

Postoperatively, patients receive antibiotics for 24 h, and they wear thromboembolic stockings and a hinged ankle brace limiting motion to between 10° of dorsiflexion and 10° of plantar flexion. They begin continuous passive motion at 8 h after surgery, which continues for two weeks.

Mosaicplasty and ACT have similar therapeutic indications, and are both capable of reconstructing hyaline cartilage with similar clinical results. The advantage ACT has over mosaicplasty is the smooth contour of cartilage that results. Curettage and drilling have had good clinical results, but are histologically inferior without the ability to restore hyaline cartilage *(97)*. Disadvantages of the ACT technique are the necessity to stage the procedure, the costs involved in the process, and the long duration of recovery. As well, for lesions with significant bony defects, which are common in the talus, bone grafting with a double-layer periosteal patch is required.

Giannini and colleagues reported their results on 8 patients who underwent ACT for large osteochondral defects of the talus since 1997. At a mean follow-up of 24 mo, patients had excellent results, with an average of 91 of 100 points on the AOFAS ankle scale postoperatively. Furthermore, histology confirms the presence of chondrocytes and type II collagen, which are typical of hyaline cartilage *(93)*. Koulalis et al. reviewed their results for 8 patients after ACT for medial talar osteochondral lesions. All clinical results were excellent to good at a mean of 17 mo postoperatively, with no complications. The 3 patients who underwent a second-look arthroscopy at 6 mo had complete coverage of the defect with cartilaginous-appearing tissue *(98)*.

Mandelbaum et al. summarized the results of autologous chondrocyte grafting for osteochondral lesions of the talus in 14 patients of Brittberg and Peterson's. This represents the largest group with the longest follow-up to date. At a mean follow-up of 32 mo, Finsen ankle scores showed significant improvements in walking ability, pain relief, and activity levels in 79% of patients. It was noted, however, that 21% did poorly, and that half of the patients required a subsequent arthroscopy to debride overgrowth of the periosteal cover *(94)*.

PERSONAL EXPERIENCE

In treating symptomatic osteochondral lesions of the talus, the size of the lesion dictates the first line of treatment. For small defects (< 8 mm in diameter), the preference of the senior author (J. T. D.) is to drill the lesion arthroscopically. In large cystic lesions with minimal cartilage damage, we have found retrograde drilling and bone grafting to be quite helpful. In our experience, it is not likely that large lesions, especially those over 10 mm in diameter, will do well with drilling. For these larger lesions, we have used mosaicplasty with a success rate of approx 80% based on the resolution of pain. The biggest challenge continues to be the treatment of very large lesions, especially those with diameters over 20 mm and a large amount of bony involvement. For mosaicplasty to work well, both a good bony bed and careful fitting and contouring are extremely important. Our personal preference is to use fewer plugs of a larger size to decrease the gap space and maximize donor-to-recipient bone contact rather than donor plug-to-donor plug contact. Patients who have fared the best are those with lesions that required only one or two osteochondral plugs and in whom a near-perfect fit of the plug was achieved. Donor site morbidity at the knee has been minimal so far.

To further avoid donor site morbidity, ACT is an attractive option, but restoring a good subchondral bone surface, which is frequently disrupted in ankle cartilage lesions, is more problematic. We have therefore not used ACT and cannot provide personal experience or results (Fig. 11).

FUTURE DIRECTIONS

The future for treating cartilage defects in the ankle lies with the field of articular cartilage engineering, looking for a combination of donor cells, scaffolding, and induction substances that will allow for cartilage regrowth in vivo. Animal studies have focused on polymer matrices that can be used as vehicles for implantation of the chondrocytes into the defects *(99–102)*. As well, a focus has been placed on an in vitro manipulation of cells and scaffolding matrices to produce mature biosynthetic grafts that are ready to be implanted *(103–105)*. There have been promising results with these technologies *(99,105,106)*.

Giannini and colleagues have been experimenting with the use of these cell-laden adhesive patches, which would decrease the morbidity of the ACT by performing less-invasive surgery and obviating the need for the periosteal patch *(97)*. Agung and colleagues' technique of transplanting tissue-engineered cartilage, by which a cartilagelike tissue is made in vitro by culturing chondrocytes in a three-dimensional atelocollagen gel matrix, has been attempted with success in the talus *(107)*. Although the long-term results are not yet available with respect to the durability of those tissues, these exciting advances may play a role in the future of cartilage repair.

CONCLUSION

Osteochondral lesions of the talus represent a significant source of disability to those affected. The approach to treatment depends on a number of patient factors, such as age,

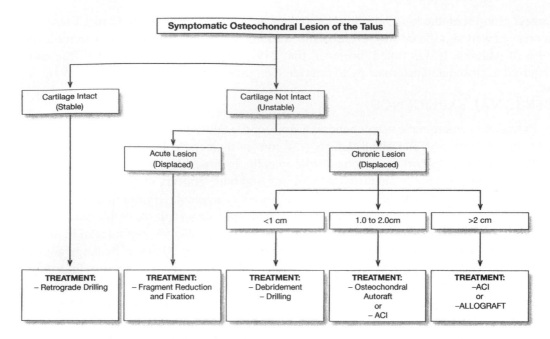

Fig. 11. Our treatment algorithm for osteochondral lesions of the talus.

activity level, and duration of symptoms, as well as factors pertaining to the lesion itself, such as location, size, cartilage status, and presence of diffuse degenerative changes. Nonoperative treatment of osteochondral lesions of the talus has been shown to provide a successful clinical outcome in less that half of the cases; good-to-excellent short-term results have been published for over 80% of those who are operatively treated. Operative options must be individualized, but the most popular techniques include arthroscopic debridement and drilling, osteochondral mosaicplasty, and ACT. These procedures all have their advantages and disadvantages, and there remains no consensus regarding a gold standard treatment. The future for treating cartilage defects in the ankle is likely to involve implants that allow cartilage regrowth and are positioned by minimally invasive surgical techniques.

REFERENCES

1. Navid DO, Myerson MS. Approach alternatives for treatment of osteochondral lesions of the talus. Foot Ankle Clin 2002;7:635–649.
2. Pare A. Oeuvres Completes. Vol. 3. Paris: Balliere; 1840–1841:32.
3. Konig F. Ueber freie Korper in den Gelenken. Deutsche Zeitschr Chir 1888;27:90–109.
4. Kappis M. Weitere Beitrage zur traumatisch-mechanischen Enstehung der "spontanen" Knorpelablosungen (sog. Osteochondritis dissecans). Deutsche Zeitschr Chir 1922;171:13–29.
5. Guhl J, Kohn H, Zoltan D. Ankle arthroscopy. Surg Rounds Orthop 1989:51–62.
6. Canale ST, Belding RH. Osteochondral lesions of the talus. J Bone Joint Surg Am 1980;62: 97–102.
7. Taga I, Shino K, Inoue M, Nakata K, Maeda A. Articular cartilage lesions in ankles with lateral ligament injury. An arthroscopic study. Am J Sports Med 1993;21:120–126; discussion 126–127.
8. Loomer R, Fisher C, Lloyd-Smith R, Sisler J, Cooney T. Osteochondral lesions of the talus. Am J Sports Med 1993;21:13–19.
9. Thompson JP, Loomer RL. Osteochondral lesions of the talus in a sports medicine clinic. A new radiographic technique and surgical approach. Am J Sports Med 1984;12:460–463.

10. Pritsch M, Horoshovski H, Farine I. Arthroscopic treatment of osteochondral lesions of the talus. J Bone Joint Surg Am 1986;68:862–865.
11. Parisien JS. Arthroscopic treatment of osteochondral lesions of the talus. Am J Sports Med 1986;14:211–217.
12. Baker CL, Andrews JR, Ryan JB. Arthroscopic treatment of transchondral talar dome fractures. Arthroscopy 1986;2:82–87.
13. Schafer DB. Cartilage repair of the talus. Foot Ankle Clin 2003;8:739–749.
14. Flick AB, Gould N. Osteochondritis dissecans of the talus (transchondral fractures of the talus): review of the literature and new surgical approach for medial dome lesions. Foot Ankle 1985; 5:165–185.
15. Berndt AL, Harty M. Transchondral fractures (osteochondritis dissecans) of the talus. Am J Orthop 1959;41-A:988–1020.
16. Yao J, Weis E. Osteochondritis dissecans. Orthop Rev 1985;14:190–204.
17. Hintermann B, Boss A, Schafer D. Arthroscopic findings in patients with chronic ankle instability. Am J Sports Med 2002;30:402–409.
18. Loren GJ, Ferkel RD. Arthroscopic assessment of occult intra-articular injury in acute ankle fractures. Arthroscopy 2002;18:412–421.
19. Hintermann B, Regazzoni P, Lampert C, Stutz G, Gachter A. Arthroscopic findings in acute fractures of the ankle. J Bone Joint Surg Br 2000;82:345–351.
20. Komenda GA, Ferkel RD. Arthroscopic findings associated with the unstable ankle. Foot Ankle Int 1999;20:708–713.
21. Canosa J. Mirror image osteochondral defects of the talus and distal tibia. Int Orthop 1994; 18:395–396.
22. Frey C. Foot and ankle arthroscopy and endoscopy. In: Myerson M, ed. Foot and Ankle Disorders. Vol. 2. Philadelphia: Saunders; 2000:1477–1511.
23. Urman M, Ammann W, Sisler J, et al. The role of bone scintigraphy in the evaluation of talar dome fractures. J Nucl Med 1991;32:2241–2244.
24. Mintz DN, Tashjian GS, Connell DA, Deland JT, O'Malley M, Potter HG. Osteochondral lesions of the talus: a new magnetic resonance grading system with arthroscopic correlation. Arthroscopy 2003;19:353–359.
25. De Smet AA, Fisher DR, Burnstein MI, Graf BK, Lange RH. Value of MR imaging in staging osteochondral lesions of the talus (osteochondritis dissecans): results in 14 patients. AJR Am J Roentgenol 1990;154:555–558.
26. Dipaola JD, Nelson DW, Colville MR. Characterizing osteochondral lesions by magnetic resonance imaging. Arthroscopy 1991;7:101–104.
27. Yulish BS, Mulopulos GP, Goodfellow DB, Bryan PJ, Modic MT, Dollinger BM. MR imaging of osteochondral lesions of talus. J Comput Assist Tomogr 1987;11:296–301.
28. McCauley TR, Disler DG. Magnetic resonance imaging of articular cartilage of the knee. J Am Acad Orthop Surg 2001;9:2–8.
29. Potter HG, Linklater JM, Allen AA, Hannafin JA, Haas SB. Magnetic resonance imaging of articular cartilage in the knee. An evaluation with use of fast-spin-echo imaging. J Bone Joint Surg Am 1998;80:1276–1284.
30. Recht M, White LM, Winalski CS, Miniaci A, Minas T, Parker RD. MR imaging of cartilage repair procedures. Skeletal Radiol 2003;32:185–200.
31. Higashiyama I, Kumai T, Takakura Y, Tamail S. Follow-up study of MRI for osteochondral lesion of the talus. Foot Ankle Int 2000;21:127–133.
32. Anderson IF, Crichton KJ, Grattan-Smith T, Cooper RA, Brazier D. Osteochondral fractures of the dome of the talus. J Bone Joint Surg Am 1989;71:1143–1152.
33. Nelson DW, DiPaola J, Colville M, Schmidgall J. Osteochondritis dissecans of the talus and knee: prospective comparison of MR and arthroscopic classifications. J Comput Assist Tomogr 1990;14:804–808.
34. Hepple S, Winson IG, Glew D. Osteochondral lesions of the talus: a revised classification. Foot Ankle Int 1999;20:789–793.

35. Cheng MS, Ferkel RD, Applegate GR. Osteochondral lesions of the talus: a radiologic and surgical comparison. Paper presented at: AAOS Annual Meeting; February 1995; New Orleans.

36. Assenmacher JA, Kelikian AS, Gottlob C, Kodros S. Arthroscopically assisted autologous osteochondral transplantation for osteochondral lesions of the talar dome: an MRI and clinical follow-up study. Foot Ankle Int 2001;22:544–551.

37. Tol JL, Struijs PA, Bossuyt PM, Verhagen RA, van Dijk CN. Treatment strategies in osteochondral defects of the talar dome: a systematic review. Foot Ankle Int 2000;21:119–126.

38. Shearer C, Loomer R, Clement D. Nonoperatively managed stage 5 osteochondral talar lesions. Foot Ankle Int 2002;23:651–654.

39. Al-Ali D, Graichen H, Faber S, Englmeier KH, Reiser M, Eckstein F. Quantitative cartilage imaging of the human hind foot: precision and inter-subject variability. J Orthop Res 2002;20:249–256.

40. Kempson GE. Relationship between the tensile properties of articular cartilage from the human knee and age. Ann Rheum Dis 1982;41:508–511.

41. Kempson GE. Age-related changes in the tensile properties of human articular cartilage: a comparative study between the femoral head of the hip joint and the talus of the ankle joint. Biochim Biophys Acta 1991;1075:223–230.

42. Van Buecken K, Barrack RL, Alexander AH, Ertl JP. Arthroscopic treatment of transchondral talar dome fractures. Am J Sports Med 1989;17:350–355;discussion 355–356.

43. Ewing JW. Arthroscopic management of transchondral talar-dome fractures (osteochondritis dissecans) and anterior impingement lesions of the ankle joint. Clin Sports Med 1991;10:677–687.

44. Amendola A, Petrik J, Webster-Bogaert S. Ankle arthroscopy: outcome in 79 consecutive patients. Arthroscopy 1996;12:565–573.

45. Martin DF, Baker CL, Curl WW, Andrews JR, Robie DB, Haas AF. Operative ankle arthroscopy. Long-term followup. Am J Sports Med 1989;17:16–23; discussion 23.

46. Verhagen RA, Struijs PA, Bossuyt PM, van Dijk CN. Systematic review of treatment strategies for osteochondral defects of the talar dome. Foot Ankle Clin 2003;8:233–242, viii–ix.

47. Frank A, Cohen P, Beaufils P, Lamare J. Arthroscopic treatment of osteochondral lesions of the talar dome. Arthroscopy 1989;5:57–61.

48. Baker CL Jr, Morales RW. Arthroscopic treatment of transchondral talar dome fractures: a long-term follow-up study. Arthroscopy 1999;15:197–202.

49. Ogilvie-Harris DJ, Sarrosa EA. Arthroscopic treatment of osteochondritis dissecans of the talus. Arthroscopy 1999;15:805–808.

50. Kelberine F, Frank A. Arthroscopic treatment of osteochondral lesions of the talar dome: a retrospective study of 48 cases. Arthroscopy 1999;15:77–84.

51. Ogilvie-Harris DJ, Sarrosa EA. Arthroscopic treatment after previous failed open surgery for osteochondritis dissecans of the talus. Arthroscopy 1999;15:809–812.

52. Buckwalter JA, Mow VC, Ratcliffe A. Restoration of Injured or Degenerated Articular Cartilage. J Am Acad Orthop Surg 1994;2:192–201.

53. O'Farrell TA, Costello BG. Osteochondritis dissecans of the talus. The late results of surgical treatment. J Bone Joint Surg Br 1982;64:494–497.

54. Nash WC, Baker CL, Jr. Transchondral talar dome fractures: not just a sprained ankle. South Med J 1984;77:560–564.

55. Alexander AH, Lichtman DM. Surgical treatment of transchondral talar-dome fractures (osteochondritis dissecans). Long-term follow-up. J Bone Joint Surg Am 1980;62:646–652.

56. Angermann P, Jensen P. Osteochondritis dissecans of the talus: long-term results of surgical treatment. Foot Ankle 1989;10:161–163.

57. Schuman L, Struijs PA, van Dijk CN. Arthroscopic treatment for osteochondral defects of the talus. Results at follow-up at 2 to 11 yr. J Bone Joint Surg Br 2002;84:364–368.

58. Kumai T, Takakura Y, Higashiyama I, Tamai S. Arthroscopic drilling for the treatment of osteochondral lesions of the talus. J Bone Joint Surg Am 1999;81:1229–1235.

59. Barnes CJ, Ferkel RD. Arthroscopic debridement and drilling of osteochondral lesions of the talus. Foot Ankle Clin 2003;8:243–257.

60. Tucker TJ, Ferkel RD. Arthroscopic-assisted management of ankle fractures. In: McGinty JB, ed. Operative Arthroscopy. Philadelphia: Lippincott Williams and Wilkins; 2003:908–923.
61. Taranow WS, Bisignani GA, Towers JD, Conti SF. Retrograde drilling of osteochondral lesions of the medial talar dome. Foot Ankle Int 1999;20:474–480.
62. Kolker D, Murray M, Wilson M. Osteochondral defects of the talus treated with autologous bone grafting. J Bone Joint Surg Br 2004;86:521–526.
63. Angermann P, Riegels-Nielsen P. Fibrin fixation of osteochondral talar fracture. Acta Orthop Scand 1990;61:551–553.
64. Tasto JP, Ostrander R, Bugbee W, Brage M. The diagnosis and management of osteochondral lesions of the talus: osteochondral allograft update. Paper presented at: Arthroscopy Association of North America; Feb., 2004; Orlando, Florida.
65. Tontz WL Jr, Bugbee WD, Brage ME. Use of allografts in the management of ankle arthritis. Foot Ankle Clin 2003;8:361–373, xi.
66. Rodrigo JJ, Thompson E, Travis C. Deep-freezing vs 4° preservation of avascular osteocartilaginous shell allografts in rats. Clin Orthop 1987:268–275.
67. Stevenson S, Dannucci GA, Sharkey NA, Pool RR. The fate of articular cartilage after transplantation of fresh and cryopreserved tissue-antigen-matched and mismatched osteochondral allografts in dogs. J Bone Joint Surg Am 1989;71:1297–1307.
68. Csonge L, Bravo D, Newman-Gage H, et al. Banking of osteochondral allografts, part II. Preservation of chondrocyte viability during long-term storage. Cell Tissue Bank 2002;3:161–168.
69. Gross AE, Agnidis Z, Hutchison CR. Osteochondral defects of the talus treated with fresh osteochondral allograft transplantation. Foot Ankle Int 2001;22:385–391.
70. Matsusue Y, Yamamuro T, Hama H. Arthroscopic multiple osteochondral transplantation to the chondral defect in the knee associated with anterior cruciate ligament disruption. Arthroscopy 1993;9:318–321.
71. Giannini S, Vannini F. Operative treatment of osteochondral lesions of the talar dome: current concepts review. Foot Ankle Int 2004;25:168–175.
72. Sammarco GJ, Makwana NK. Treatment of talar osteochondral lesions using local osteochondral graft. Foot Ankle Int 2002;23:693–698.
73. Hangody L, Kish G, Modis L, et al. Mosaicplasty for the treatment of osteochondritis dissecans of the talus: 2- to 7-yr results in 36 patients. Foot Ankle Int 2001;22:552–558.
74. Gautier E, Kolker D, Jakob RP. Treatment of cartilage defects of the talus by autologous osteochondral grafts. J Bone Joint Surg Br 2002;84:237–244.
75. Treppo S, Koepp H, Quan EC, Cole AA, Kuettner KE, Grodzinsky AJ. Comparison of biomechanical and biochemical properties of cartilage from human knee and ankle pairs. J Orthop Res 2000;18:739–748.
76. Choung D, Christensen JC. Mosaicplasty of the talus: a joint contact analysis in a cadaver model. J Foot Ankle Surg 2002;41:65–75.
77. Hangody L, Kish G, Karpati Z, Szerb I, Eberhardt R. Treatment of osteochondritis dissecans of the talus: use of the mosaicplasty technique—a preliminary report. Foot Ankle Int 1997;18:628–634.
78. Greenspoon J, Rosman M. Medial osteochondritis of the talus in children: review and new surgical management. J Pediatr Orthop 1987;7:705–708.
79. Draper SD, Fallat LM. Autogenous bone grafting for the treatment of talar dome lesions. J Foot Ankle Surg 2000;39:15–23.
80. Hangody L, Feczko P, Bartha L, Bodo G, Kish G. Mosaicplasty for the treatment of articular defects of the knee and ankle. Clin Orthop 2001:S328–S336.
81. Hangody L, Fules P. Autologous osteochondral mosaicplasty for the treatment of full-thickness defects of weight-bearing joints: 10 yr of experimental and clinical experience. J Bone Joint Surg Am 2003;85-A(suppl 2):25–32.
82. Hangody L. The mosaicplasty technique for osteochondral lesions of the talus. Foot Ankle Clin 2003;8:259–273.

83. Scranton PE Jr, McDermott JE. Treatment of type V osteochondral lesions of the talus with ipsilateral knee osteochondral autografts. Foot Ankle Int 2001;22:380–384.

84. Al-Shaikh RA, Chou LB, Mann JA, Dreeben SM, Prieskorn D. Autologous osteochondral grafting for talar cartilage defects. Foot Ankle Int 2002;23:381–389.

85. Lee CH, Chao KH, Huang GS, Wu SS. Osteochondral autografts for osteochondritis dissecans of the talus. Foot Ankle Int 2003;24:815–822.

86. Grande DA, Pitman MI, Peterson L, Menche D, Klein M. The repair of experimentally produced defects in rabbit articular cartilage by autologous chondrocyte transplantation. J Orthop Res 1989;7:208–218.

87. Breinan HA, Minas T, Hsu HP, Nehrer S, Sledge CB, Spector M. Effect of cultured autologous chondrocytes on repair of chondral defects in a canine model. J Bone Joint Surg Am 1997;79: 1439–1451.

88. Minas T, Peterson L. Advanced techniques in autologous chondrocyte transplantation. Clin Sports Med 1999;18:13–44, v–vi.

89. Brittberg M, Lindahl A, Nilsson A, Ohlsson C, Isaksson O, Peterson L. Treatment of deep cartilage defects in the knee with autologous chondrocyte transplantation. N Engl J Med 1994;331: 889–895.

90. Minas T, Chiu R. Autologous chondrocyte implantation. Am J Knee Surg 2000;13:41–50.

91. Minas T. Autologous chondrocyte implantation for focal chondral defects of the knee. Clin Orthop 2001:S349–S361.

92. Peterson L, Minas T, Brittberg M, Lindahl A. Treatment of osteochondritis dissecans of the knee with autologous chondrocyte transplantation: results at 2 to 10 yr. J Bone Joint Surg Am 2003;85-A(suppl 2):17–24.

93. Giannini S, Buda R, Grigolo B, Vannini F. Autologous chondrocyte transplantation in osteochondral lesions of the ankle joint. Foot Ankle Int 2001;22:513–517.

94. Mandelbaum BR, Gerhardt MB, Peterson L. Autologous chondrocyte implantation of the talus. Arthroscopy 2003;19(suppl 1):129–137.

95. Sammarco GJ, Burstein AH, Frankel VH. Biomechanics of the ankle: a kinematic study. Orthop Clin North Am 1973;4:75–96.

96. Giannini S, Buda R, Faldini C, et al. Surgical treatment of the osteochondral lesions of the talus (OLT) in young active patients. Paper presented at: American Academy of Orthopaedic Surgeons 72nd Annual Meeting; 2005; Washington, DC.

97. Giannini S, Vannini F, Buda R. Osteoarticular grafts in the treatment of OCD of the talus: mosaicplasty vs autologous chondrocyte transplantation. Foot Ankle Clin 2002;7:621–633.

98. Koulalis D, Schultz W, Heyden M. Autologous chondrocyte transplantation for osteochondritis dissecans of the talus. Clin Orthop 2002:186–192.

99. Frenkel SR, Toolan B, Menche D, Pitman MI, Pachence JM. Chondrocyte transplantation using a collagen bilayer matrix for cartilage repair. J Bone Joint Surg Br 1997;79:831–836.

100. Nehrer S, Breinan HA, Ramappa A, et al. Canine chondrocytes seeded in type I and type II collagen implants investigated in vitro. J Biomed Mater Res 1997;38:95–104.

101. Nehrer S, Breinan HA, Ramappa A, et al. Chondrocyte-seeded collagen matrices implanted in a chondral defect in a canine model. Biomaterials 1998;19:2313–2328.

102. Niederauer GG, Slivka MA, Leatherbury NC, et al. Evaluation of multiphase implants for repair of focal osteochondral defects in goats. Biomaterials 2000;21:2561–2574.

103. Minas T, Nehrer S. Current concepts in the treatment of articular cartilage defects. Orthopedics 1997;20:525–538.

104. Ochi M, Uchio Y, Tobita M, Kuriwaka M. Current concepts in tissue engineering technique for repair of cartilage defect. Artif Organs 2001;25:172–179.

105. Ochi M, Uchio Y, Kawasaki K, Wakitani S, Iwasa J. Transplantation of cartilage-like tissue made by tissue engineering in the treatment of cartilage defects of the knee. J Bone Joint Surg Br 2002;84:571–578.
106. Schreiber RE, Ilten-Kirby BM, Dunkelman NS, et al. Repair of osteochondral defects with allogeneic tissue engineered cartilage implants. Clin Orthop 1999:S382–S395.
107. Agung M, Ochi M, Adachi N, Uchio Y, Takao M, Kawasaki K. Osteochondritis dissecans of the talus treated by the transplantation of tissue-engineered cartilage. Arthroscopy 2004;20:1075–1080.

19

Management of Cartilage Injuries in the Hip

Bryan T. Kelly, MD, Patrick P. Sussmann, MD, and Robert L. Buly, MD

Summary

Within the discipline of sports medicine, articular cartilage injuries in the hip have received considerably less attention than other joints, largely due to the difficulty that practitioners have had with accurate assessment. Non-arthritic cartilage injuries in the hip refer to focal chondral defects on either the femoral or acetabular side of the joint. Focal chondral defects on the femoral side are relatively uncommon, however, and may result from axial loading or shear injury of the head within the socket. Subluxation events of the femoral head seen in high-energy contact sports may result in these types of focal chondral injuries. Cartilage injuries on the acetabular side are more common and typically present as localized cartilage delamination in the anterior-superior weight-bearing zone of the acetabular rim. The most common underlying condition resulting in these types of cartilage defects is femoroacetabular impingement. This chapter discusses current surgical indications and techniques appropriate for management of these injuries as well as clinical and radiographic methods to detect focal cartilage lesions in the hip joint.

Key Words: Hip; cartilage injury; femoro-acetabular impingement.

INTRODUCTION

Articular cartilage injuries are some of the most challenging orthopedic injuries to treat. Within the discipline of sports medicine, articular cartilage injuries in the hip have received considerably less attention compared to other joints, largely because of the inherent difficulties that practitioners have had with accurately assessing pathological conditions in this area. Prior to the advent of highly specific magnetic resonance imaging (MRI) techniques, hip pain in the young was typically earmarked as "early arthritis"; little consideration for soft tissue anatomy and injury in and around the joint was given.

In the young patient, hip pain is often characterized by nonspecific symptoms, normal radiographs, and vague clinical findings. Common causes of hip and groin pain in young patients include adductor muscle pathology, hip flexor tendonitis, osteitis pubis, and trochanteric bursitis. Other less-common clinical entities include psoas strain, psoas bursitis, stress fractures, nerve entrapment syndromes, hip synovitis, hip joint osteoarthritis, and referred pain (1–3). However, intra-articular nonarthritic pathology of the hip joint has gained attention. Disorders of the labrum, ligamentum teres, iliofemoral ligament, and chondral surfaces of the femoral head and acetabulum are now recognized as potential sources of hip and groin pain in the younger patient (4–5). A careful history and physical examination aids the diagnosis of an intra-articular, extra-articular, or referred source of pain. Without proper

From: *Cartilage Repair Strategies*
Edited by: Riley J. Williams © Humana Press Inc., Totowa, NJ

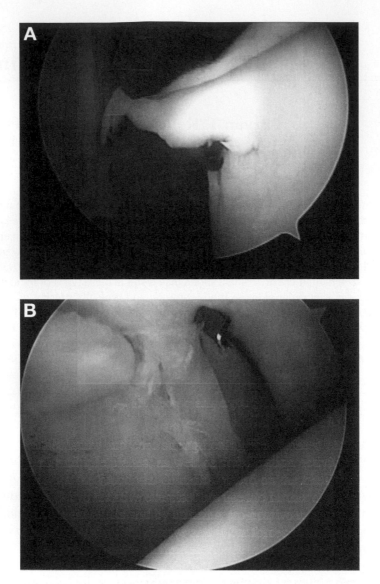

Fig. 1. Chondral injuries in the hip joint can occur as (**A**) focal injuries on the femoral head or (**B**) delamination injuries along the rim of the acetabulum. These delamination lesions are typically secondary to femoroacetabular impingement and occur most commonly in the anterior-superior weight-bearing zone of the acetabulum.

visualization of the articular surface using MRI or arthroscopy, the diagnosis of an articular lesion of the hip remains difficult.

Nonarthritic cartilage injuries in the hip refer to focal chondral defects on either the femoral or acetabular side of the joint (Fig. 1A,B). Focal chondral defects on the femoral head (Fig. 1A) are relatively uncommon and may result from axial loading or shear injury of the head within the socket *(6)*. Subluxation events of the femoral head, as seen in high-energy contact sports, may result in these types of focal chondral injuries *(7,8)*. Cartilage injuries on the acetabulum are common. These injuries typically present as localized cartilage delamination defects in the anterior-superior weight-bearing zone of the acetabular rim (Fig. 1B). The most common underlying condition resulting in these types of cartilage defects is femoroacetabular impingement (FAI) *(9–12)*. This chapter discusses current surgical indications and techniques appropriate for management of these injuries as well as clinical and imaging methods that are used to detect focal cartilage lesions in the hip joint.

ETIOLOGY OF CHONDRAL LESIONS OF THE FEMORAL HEAD

Chondral damage in the hip has traditionally been associated with progressive generalized joint deterioration (osteoarthritis, rheumatoid arthritis). However, there are several other mechanisms that can result in focal chondral lesions of the femoral head; these mechanisms include trauma, osteonecrosis, underlying bony deformity, and dysplastic conditions. Femoral head chondral lesions that are detectable by conventional radiography are usually degenerative. However, advancements in MRI and hip arthroscopy have facilitated greater appreciation of the spectrum of cartilage lesions that can affect the hip joint.

The articular cartilage of the femoral head is thickest on the medial and central surfaces; this observed cartilage thickness is adapted to the loading pattern of the hip joint *(13)*. The normal thickness of articular cartilage correlates with the surface pressure within the joint. The higher the peak joint reactive forces, the thicker the articular cartilage is. Approximately 70% of the femoral head chondral surface is involved in load transfer across the joint *(14)*; as such, the majority of the femoral head cartilage may be subject to injury in circumstances of unusually high load transfer across the hip joint. The grade and character of cartilage lesions depend on the mechanism of injury and the stage at which the lesion is detected. The characteristics of early-stage lesions often give important information regarding the mechanism of injury. Lesions can present as shear injuries, delamination, chondral flaps, fissuring, fractures, and punch or impaction injuries. After progression to an advanced stage degenerative condition, these lesions often lose these specific characteristics.

Acute isolated traumatic articular surface injuries most commonly occur from impact loading across the hip joint *(6,15)*. These traumatic injuries may involve articular cartilage alone or result in osteochondral fractures. There appears to be a particular propensity for this injury pattern in young, physically fit adult males who suffer impact loading at the greater trochanter in association with a high-energy activity (sports, trauma). The so-called lateral impact injury occurs following a blow to the greater trochanter; the subcutaneous location of the greater trochanter limits its ability to absorb large forces *(6)*. The high bone density of this region allows impact on this area to transfer energy and load to the hip joint surface, resulting in chondral lesions of the femoral head or acetabulum without associated osseous injury. Arthroscopic findings in this clinical scenario will commonly support this lateral impact mechanism *(6)*.

The type and degree of injury vary depending on the amount and direction of the impact load. The spectrum of resulting injuries can vary from a subchondral contusion, to a shear injury of the articular cartilage, to a complete fracture of the femoral head. During posterior-directed loading, the femoral head is forced against the labrum and the rim of the posterior wall. This can lead to shear injuries at the level of the articular cartilage as well as associated fractures of the subchondral bone. With less axial loading and incomplete subluxation of the femoral head, injuries can be limited to the articular cartilage and capsulolabral complex *(6)*. Cartilage injury may occur even with minor trauma, as chondrocyte death has been reported to occur at 20–30% of strain of articular cartilage specimens *(16)*. Injured cartilage that loses

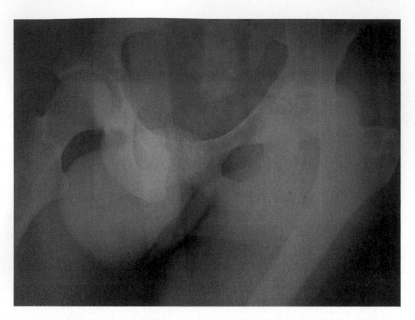

Fig. 2. AP pelvis x-ray demonstrating a posterior fracture dislocation of the hip.

its congruity by a crush injury, indentation, or fragmentation results in loss of joint function and results in progressive joint degeneration *(15)*.

More violent injuries that result in hip dislocations will often lead to indentation fractures of the femoral head in addition to fractures of the acetabulum (Fig. 2). As a result of the typical position of the extremity in relationship to the body (flexed hip with posterior-directed force), axial impact load in these cases is most commonly transferred posteriorly *(17,18)*. Although these injuries are most often the result of high-energy trauma, they do occur in high-impact collision sports and subject the patient to an increased risk for the development of avascular necrosis (AVN) of the femoral head *(7,8)*. Brumback et al. recognized indentation or crush injuries to the femoral head associated with anterior dislocation *(19)*.

The incidence of femoral head fractures with hip dislocations has been reported to be as high as 7% *(17,18,20)* (Fig. 3A,B). This number does not include chondral or soft tissue injuries, which we believe have a higher incidence. To our knowledge, there is no study that has reported the incidence of cartilage injury after hip dislocation or subluxation. Avulsion fractures of the femoral head in conjunction with ligamentum teres disruption are reported to be one of the most common fractures and involve the displacement of a variable-size fragment of bone from the fovea of the femoral head *(21)*. Brumback et al. and Epstein et al. described most of their femoral head fractures as shear- or cleavage-type fractures *(18–20)*.

Avascular necrosis is another cause of focal chondral injury to the femoral head. In AVN, the femoral head articular cartilage injury is secondary to the loss of structural integrity of the subchondral bone; collapse of bone is common. The extent of chondral pathology depends on the degree of collapse of the underlying subchondral bone. A wide spectrum of cartilaginous lesions is associated with AVN, ranging from mild chondromalacia to severe chondral fractures with complete collapse.

Avascular necrosis of the femoral head has a large variety of etiologies *(22,23)*. Many of the pathological mechanisms of nontraumatic AVN include excessive alcohol intake,

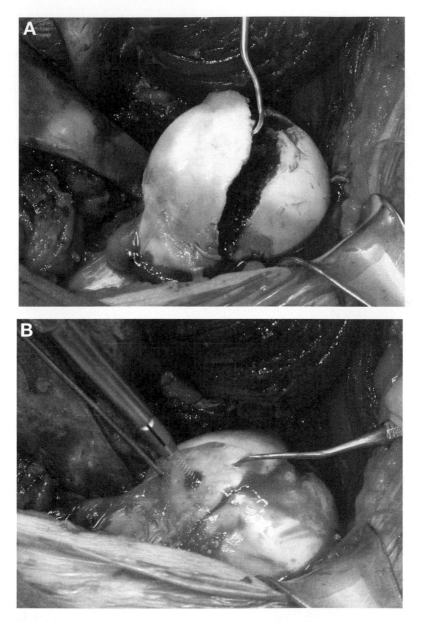

Fig. 3. Anterior Pipkin fracture of the left femoral head after hip dislocation in a skiing accident. (**A**) A surgical dislocation has been performed for exposure. (**B**) Repair of the major fragment with absorbable screws.

corticosteroid use, hemoglobinopathies, and slipped capital femoral epiphysis *(22)*. Although less common, AVN of the femoral head has been reported in sport injuries resulting from subluxation or dislocation of the hip. Nonspecific groin pain can be the only clinical presentation in these patients, which makes a high suspicion and critical evaluation for predisposing factors important in establishing the diagnosis *(7,8)*. With radiographic changes visible as late as 3 mo after the injury, MRI has become a sensitive and specific test for detecting AVN. The treatment of articular cartilage lesions in the hip secondary to AVN is dependent on the stage of the disease (24–26).

Cartilage lesions of the femoral head can also result from anatomic abnormalities, such as congenital hip disease (dysplasia, Legg Perthes disease) and slipped capital femoral epiphysis. There have been several reports of the incidence of acute chondrolysis following slipped capital femoral epiphysis (27) Narrowing of the joint space has been reported as early as 1 yr after the acute slip injury. Surgical treatment in early stages of this disease has not been recommended, however; surgery has been reserved for later stages and includes osteotomy, arthrodesis, and arthroplasty. Advancements in surgical techniques that facilitate access to the hip joint have allowed an earlier approach to early-stage degenerative disease. Specifically, hip arthroscopy may be used to address early-stage chondral lesions to preserve maximal function.

DISEASE PROGRESSION AND CONSERVATIVE TREATMENT

Although the natural history of the focal hip chondral lesion has not been well documented, clinical observations indicate that these chondral lesions will frequently result in pain and functional impairment. When large, these lesions tend to progress in size, possibly to osteoarthritis within a relatively short period (28–32). Animal models suggest that large full-thickness osteochondral defects will undergo degenerative change that occurs around the rim of the defect and, in as little as 1 yr, progress to global joint degradation (33). This progression has been similarly predicted in finite-element models of osteochondral damage. These models have shown that compressive strains reach maximum values around the rim of a defect, and that as defects become larger, the compressive strain values increase concomitantly (34).

Despite this grim prognosis, patients presenting with the symptoms and radiographic evidence of chondral injury are initially managed with nonsurgical treatment, including activity modification, weight reduction, physical therapy, bracing, and medications. Medications such as nonsteroidal anti-inflammatory drugs have not been shown to be any more effective than simple analgesics such as acetaminophen in the treatment of symptomatic cartilage lesions (35). The use of MRI to document chondral lesion progression and to predict outcomes for conservative treatment has been reported.

In a small series, De Smet et al. documented lesion size and reported that 10 of 12 conservatively treated patients who had hip cartilage lesions larger than 160 mm^2 had poor clinical outcomes. Furthermore, 6 of 6 patients who had cartilage fractures or surface defects detected by MRI had poor results with conservative management. The authors concluded that, based on their clinical experience and this study, cartilage defects or fractures that are detected by MRI will result in chronic pain and disability unless surgically treated (36,37).

EXISTING SURGICAL TREATMENTS AND PATIENT SELECTION

Because little is known about the natural history of chondral defects, it is often difficult to decide when, or if, to treat these defects surgically (38). Nonetheless, as in other joints, the long-term consequences of chondral lesions in the hip are concerning, and surgical treatment is preferred when symptoms persist and create unacceptable levels of pain and dysfunction. As in the knee, full-thickness defects of the femoral head articular cartilage have a poor capacity for repair because of the lack of blood supply. These lesions rarely heal spontaneously regardless of their etiology (39–44). As such, there is little expectation that these lesions will ultimately cease causing symptoms. The difficulty in diagnosing these lesions as well as the inability to improve symptoms with conservative management provide a reasonable rationale for the use of hip surgery in the treatment of these injuries. Moreover, the use of arthroscopy is a particularly attractive option in these cases because of the minimally invasive nature of the approach. In the presence of persistent symptoms, hip arthroscopy is useful for the evaluation of chondral injury, the debridement of chondral flaps, and the removal of free cartilage fragments.

Relevant surgical techniques that have been applied in treatment of chondral lesions in other joints are now becoming increasingly utilized in the hip joint. Such procedures include lavage, debridement, abrasion arthroplasty, microfracture, drilling, osteochondral autograft transfer, allograft transplant, autogenous cell implantation, and partial resurfacing procedures *(35,39,40,42–48)*. In addition, a variety of different osteotomy procedures has been utilized within the hip joint as a means of rotating areas of focal chondral injury away from the weight-bearing zones of the femoral head. Although symptomatic improvement from arthroscopic debridement of unstable cartilage flaps is encouraging, future advancement in surgical techniques will focus on more predictable cartilage resurfacing procedures similar to those that are employed in the knee and the shoulder. Improvements in these techniques will allow surgeons not only to alleviate mechanical symptoms, but also to promote the long-term overall health of the hip joint *(5,6)*.

Debridement

The goal of debridement is to remove the mechanical irritation of incongruent cartilaginous flaps and loose bodies that typically characterize a full-thickness chondral defect. Debridement, along with arthroscopic lavage, is believed to bring relief by alleviating mechanical symptoms and reducing levels of synovial fluid metalloproteinases and other inflammatory enzymes in the joint space *(49)*.

Marrow Stimulation Techniques (Microfracture, Abrasion, Drilling)

Marrow stimulation techniques are dedicated to the enhancement of intrinsic cartilage repair mechanisms at the articular surface. Such methods, including the microfracture technique, have been performed for years using arthroscopic access, especially in the knee joint. Microfracture of small- and medium-size cartilage defects has been performed in many patients with full-thickness lesions of the femoral head (Fig. 4A,B).

Richard Steadman originally developed the microfracture technique approximately 20 years ago for the knee. The procedure attempts to enhance chondral resurfacing by creating vascular access channels to the underlying bone marrow within a symptomatic cartilage defect; the creation of these channels supports the creation of an enriched environment for tissue regeneration through the use of the body's natural vascular response to injury *(39,40,42–45)*. The microfracture technique allows blood to fill within the full-thickness chondral defects and organize into a fibrin clot. Marrow elements, including mesenchymal stem cells, growth factors, fibrin, and platelets, become trapped within the clot and defect. These cells undergo metaplasia to produce a reparative granulation tissue within the defect *(41,43,50)*. Gradual fibrosis of the reparative tissue occurs over the ensuing days after surgery, and the fibrous tissue undergoes progressive hyalinization and chondrification ultimately to produce a fibrocartilaginous mass that "heals" the defect. Steadman et al. *(43,50)* performed this procedure on over 1800 patients and reported predictably good results, with slow improvement in patient function over a period of 2 yr.

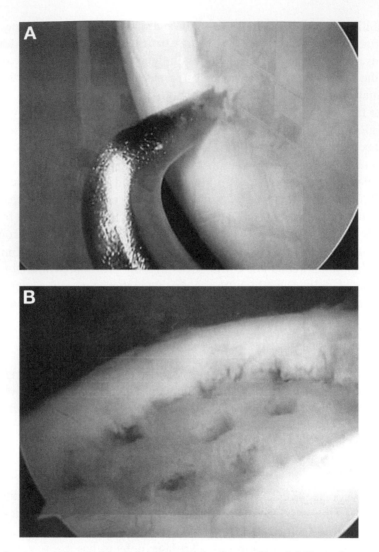

Fig. 4. Microfracture of focal chondral defects in the femoral head follows the same principles utilized in other joints. (**A**) After the calcified cartilage layer is removed, the subchondral bone is then penetrated by an awl with a 3–4 mm spacing of the holes to allow a superclot to fill the defect and adhere to the base of the defect. (**B**) Confirmation of bleeding from these microfracture holes should be made by evacuating the joint of all arthroscopy fluid.

The key to the success of the microfracture technique within the hip depends on the establishment of an optimal environment for the differentiation of pluripotential mesenchymal stem cells. This environment includes a source of marrow cells, provision of a matrix, removal of stress concentration, an intact subchondral plate, and some mechanical stimulation. Several factors affect the quality of the cartilaginous repair tissue in a full-thickness chondral defect treated by microfracture. First, the lesion must be debrided back to a stable rim; this enhances clot stability within the defect. Second, the calcified cartilage layer must be removed without violating the underlying subchondral bone. Third, the subchondral bone must be penetrated using an awl with a 3- to 4-mm spacing of the holes to allow the superclot to fill the defect and adhere to the base of the defect. Fourth, a strict postoperative rehabilitation regimen must be adhered to including immediate continuous passive motion (CPM) and protected weight bearing. Finally, abnormal mechanical axes should be corrected at the time of the microfracture procedure by hip osteotomy. If these basic principles are followed, then there is good potential for the formation of fibrocartilaginous tissue and ultimately significant improvement in patients' subjective and functional complaints. In our experience, the microfracture technique is more predictably good when performed for lesions of the acetabulum compared to the femur.

Chondral Transplant Procedures

Larger cartilage defects may be amenable to cartilage resurfacing procedures such as autogenous osteochondral transfer; these methods have been applied in the knee with success (Fig. 5A). There is limited experience with autologous osteochondral transplantation from the knee to the hip. Such procedures have been executed and have been technically successful; the early follow-up has been encouraging. Donor sites for these procedures can be from the ipsilateral knee or from the nonweight-bearing aspects of the femoral head-neck junction. Single or multiple cylindrical core grafts of articular cartilage and subchondral bone are taken from other articular areas within the knee or non-weight-bearing region of the hip (donor site) and transplanted into holes prepared within the defect (recipient site). The core grafts are then press-fit into the prepared holes so that the articular cartilage surface of the graft aligns to the natural remaining cartilage surface. This treatment is technically challenging, particularly in large defects *(51–53)*. With the current instrumentation available, these surgeries typically require surgical dislocation of the hip to expose the area of the femoral head in need of cartilage transplantation (Fig. 5A,B; *see* Color Plate 5, following p. 206). No long-term results or case series are available on these procedures.

Fresh or fresh-frozen allograft femoral head transplants can also be used for large symptomatic lesions employing techniques similar to the autograft procedure. In these cases, a single large allograft is used rather than multiple smaller plugs. Graft availability and the possible risk of disease transmission are issues that are relevant in the use of this treatment strategy. Again, this is a technically challenging surgical procedure, particularly when matching contours from allograft tissue to patient joint surfaces; an open surgical dislocation is necessary in the majority of cases *(51–55)*.

Autologous chondrocyte implantation (ACI) has been used in the knee joint with clinical success. The ACI method is a cell-based repair that relies on the creation of cartilage ground substance (collagen, proteoglycan) within a defect by chondrocytes that are surgically placed within the affected area. Autograft biopsies are taken in a first surgical procedure, expanded through laboratory techniques to increase the resident cell population of chondrocytes, and delivered back to the defect site in a second surgical procedure. This is a challenging surgical technique that requires the harvest and suture of a periosteal patch as a cover over the defect site. Sutures are placed through the surrounding hyaline articular cartilage surface. The expanded cell suspension is injected under the sutured patch, which must be sealed with fibrin sealants to maintain a watertight compartment *(56–61)*. Although the ACI procedure remains an option for the treatment of cartilage defects in the hip, the practical machinations of the approach and technical factors of the procedure itself make this method, in the case of hip cartilage lesions, a difficult undertaking. There is no study describing the results of ACI procedures in the hip.

Replacement and Resurfacing Procedures

Conventional joint replacements have a long history of achieving dramatic pain relief and restoration of function in arthritic patients. Ideally, these procedures are usually performed on

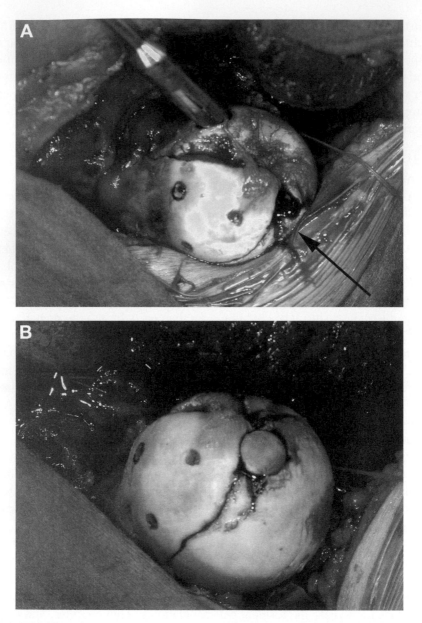

Fig. 5. (A) Surgical dislocation of the hip for exposure of an osteochondral defect at the apex of the femoral head (arrow). An osteochondral plug is harvested from the inferior pole of the femoral head. (**B**, *see* Color Plate 5, following p. 206.) View of the femoral head following fixation of the major fragment and delivery of the osteochondral plug.

elderly patients (age 65 and older) to minimize the likelihood of revision total joint arthroplasty. Primary total hip arthroplasty procedures have high rates of failure in young (less than 40 yr) and early-middle-aged (40–60 yr) patients *(62–65)*. Attempts have been made to preserve bone stock with partial resurfacing procedures that require only a minimum of bony removal *(66–72)*. Devices are now available that need only the removal of the area of cartilage loss; the remaining unaffected cartilage surfaces are untouched, and the natural radius of curvature of the femoral head is maintained (Fig. 6; *see* Color Plate 6, following p. 206.). Although these treatments have

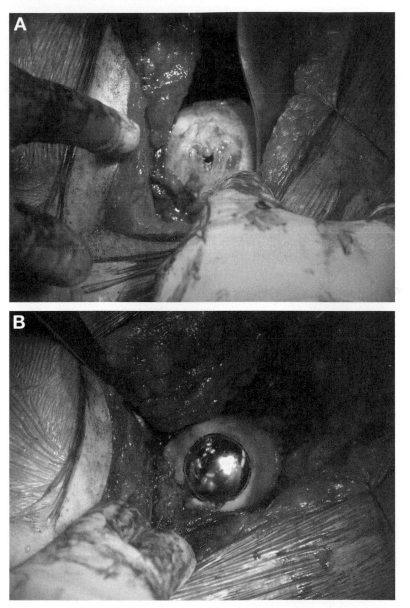

Fig. 6. *(Continued)*

been used clinically for more than 5 yr, there is a notable absence of comparative studies and long-term outcome information. Thus, these implants should be used with caution.

Osteotomies

The goal of osteotomy is to cause an alteration in joint reactive forces that results in an unloading of an area of the joint that is damaged or injured. A variety of osteotomy procedures have been applied to the hip; the procedures are performed to move areas of chondral injury or osteonecrosis out of the primary weight-bearing area of the hip joint. Hip osteotomies are morbid procedures as they typically require either a transverse cut across the proximal femur or multiple cuts through the pelvis with fixation of the segments *(48,73–77)*. The need for an osteotomy should be strongly considered in all cases for which a cartilage

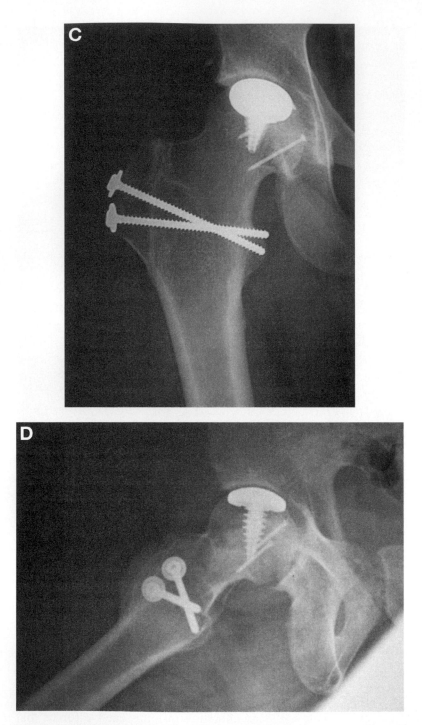

Fig. 6. (A) Partial resurfacing of a focal chondral defect of the femoral head with maintenance of the normal radius of curvature. **(B**, Color Plate 6, following p. 206.) Plain radiograph of the partial resurfacing implant. **(C)** AP and **(D)** lateral views of the hip after placement of a partial resurfacing prosthesis for an area of focal chondral depression secondary to a Pipkin fracture dislocation. The prosthesis was placed via a surgical dislocation of the hip for complete visualization of the entire femoral head.

resurfacing procedure is performed. Performing a cartilage repair procedure in a malaligned limb may result in early failure of the repair.

A careful examination of the published reports on the use of cartilage treatments in the hip joint illustrates that there is actually little overlap in the different treatment methods and the appropriate patient for each treatment. It is our belief that each of the existing cartilage repair methods is the most suitable for a specific patient profile. Therefore, there is limited opportunity to perform a comparative analysis between the different treatment methods. The critical determinants when establishing the appropriate treatment method for the affected patient are defect type, defect size, age, symptom severity, activity level, ability to complete postoperative protocol, and the presence of diseased joints elsewhere.

ETIOLOGY OF ACETABULAR CARTILAGE LESIONS: FEMOROACETABULAR IMPINGEMENT (FAI)

Cartilage injuries of the acetabulum are most common and typically present as localized cartilage delamination in the anterior-superior weight-bearing zone of the acetabular rim (Fig. 1B). The most common underlying condition resulting in these types of cartilage defects is femoroactabular impingement (FAI) *(9–12,78).* A high incidence of these chondral lesions has been reported in association with hip labral tears. In contrast, posterior acetabular cartilage lesions are more commonly associated with posterior-directed trauma from posterior subluxation or dislocation of the femoral head. As described, these traumatic events can be very subtle through repetitive posterior loading of the posterior rim of the acetabulum or by axial impact in high-energy contact sports.

Schmid et al. reported on 42 hips in 40 patients with a clinical diagnosis of FAI who were noted to have cartilage defects on the acetabulum based on magnetic resonance arthrogram. Cartilage lesions were subsequently confirmed at the time of open hip surgery, during which the entire cartilage surfaces were inspected. At the time of surgery, cartilage defects were identified in the anterosuperior part of the acetabulum in the majority of cases (37 of 42, 88%). Lesions were also found in the posterosuperior acetabulum (23 or 55%), anteroinferior acetabulum (12 or 29%), posteroinferior acetabulum (10 or 24%), and femoral head (10 or 24%) *(79).* They concluded that cartilage lesions are common in young and middle-aged patients with FAI and are most frequently found in the anterosuperior part of the acetabulum.

McCarthy et al. looked at 457 hip arthroscopies during a 6-yr period *(80,81).* They found that chondral injuries occurred in the anterior acetabulum in 269 cases (59%), the superior acetabulum in 110 cases (24%), and the posterior acetabulum in 114 cases (25%). In this study, these lesions were frequently associated with a labral tear and were often described as unstable flaps with a significant proportion of full-thickness cartilage loss. According to these authors, 70% of the anterior, 27% of the superior, and 36% of the posterior chondral injuries were Outerbridge grade III or IV. In addition, a clear decrement in outcome of patients with labral tears was observed in association with chondral acetabular lesions greater than 1 cm *(80,81).*

Acetabular rim wear in association with labral pathology is frequently the result of impingement of the femoral head against the anterior-superior acetabular rim during flexion of the hip. In these cases of impingement, it is necessary not only to address the areas of exposed cartilage with the types of techniques described for the femoral head, but also to address the underlying impingement lesion at the head-neck junction. This concept of FAI as a source of anterosuperior labral and chondral damage was introduced by Ganz et al. *(9–11,82).* These authors described a reproducible pattern of anterosuperior labral and chondral injury that resulted from abnormal contact between the femoral head-neck junction and the anterior acetabulum during

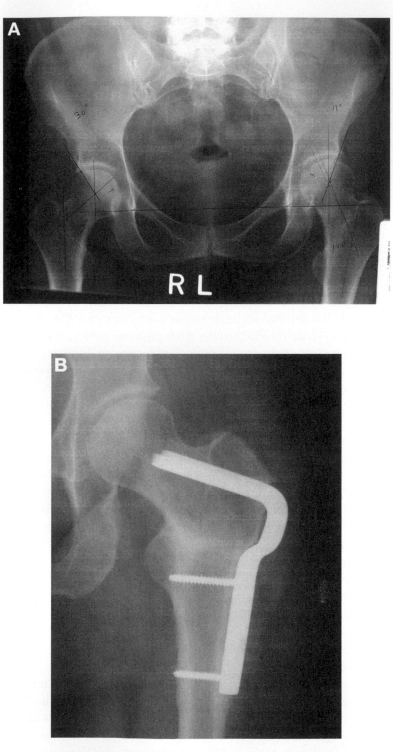

Fig. 7. (**A**) An excessively valgus orientation of the femoral neck (**A**) can be corrected with a femoral-sided vavus producing osteotomy (**B**).

terminal hip flexion (Fig. 7A–C). They directly observed this phenomenon after performing over 600 surgical hip dislocations for various hip conditions *(10,83)*. They described anatomic abnormalities of the proximal femur as well as the anterior acetabulum to explain the abnormal contact. Based on anatomic features and patterns of labral and chondral injuries, they classified FAI into two distinct entities: cam impingement and pincer impingement.

Cam impingement results from pathological contact of an abnormally shaped femoral head and neck with a morphologically normal acetabulum. This pattern of impingement is characterized by a femoral head-neck junction that is not spherical anteriorly and has increased radius of curvature (Fig. 8) *(84)*. As the hip flexes, this abnormal region engages the anterior acetabulum. The resultant shear forces that result from this contact produce the characteristic anterosuperior chondral injury and associated labral tear *(11,83,84)*.

The second type of FAI, pincer impingement, is the result of contact between an abnormal acetabular rim and a normal femoral head-neck junction. This pathological contact is the result of abnormal anterior acetabular "overcoverage." This can be the consequence of various different anatomic variants, including coxa profunda (protrusio), acetabular retroversion *(85)*, or deformity following trauma or periacetabular osteotomies *(10,82,86)*. This results in decreased joint clearance and repetitive contact between the femoral neck and acetabulum. Ultimately, this repetitive contact causes degeneration of the anterosuperior labrum much like in cam impingement. The injured labrum subsequently may become calcified, further worsening the anterior overcoverage. In addition, because the anatomic constraint in the native hip is so great, the contact can cause leverage of the head out of the acetabulum posteriorly, contributing to a *contre-coup* injury to the posteroinferior acetabulum *(87)*.

DISEASE PROGRESSION AND CONSERVATIVE TREATMENT

Femoroacetabular impingement is typically a disease of young active adults, who develop the insidious onset of hip and groin pain. However, older, more sedentary individuals may develop symptoms of FAI as well *(11)*. Generally, cam impingement is noted more frequently in the young, active patients; pincer impingement is seen more frequently in middle-aged women. Initial treatment of FAI begins with a trial of conservative management. Typically, this involves activity modification and anti-inflammatory medication. Failures of conservative management or the presence of labral or chondral injury noted by MRI are indications for surgery *(11)*.

In addition to its cause of disability and pain in a young athlete, FAI is suspected as an etiological factor in osteoarthritis. Ganz et al. *(10)* examined degenerative changes of the hip in elderly cadaveric specimens and in elderly patients undergoing hemiarthroplasty for fracture. The study demonstrated that the degenerative process appears to begin in the anterosuperior periphery of the acetabulum and not in the central weight-bearing zone. The findings in their study implicated FAI as the initiating event in degeneration of the hip associated with age.

In addition, Wagner et al. *(88)* examined the pathology of surgically excised impingement lesions at the time of open dislocation and debridement. The excised specimens demonstrated histological and biochemical changes consistent with osteoarthritic cartilage *(88)*. Support for a causal relationship between FAI and osteoarthritis has been further strengthened by studies that have demonstrated a link between mild hip deformities and osteoarthritic degeneration *(89)*. It is the belief of Ganz et al. *(10)* that FAI causes articular lesions that are precursors for what has traditionally been called idiopathic osteoarthritis of the hip.

Cam and pincer impingement differ in mechanism, epidemiology, and pathoanatomy; moreover, each diagnosis is treated differently by surgical management. Cam impingement

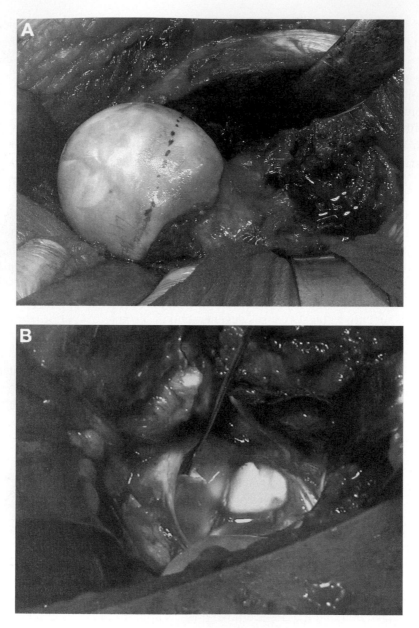

Fig. 8. *(Continued)*

is reported to occur with increasing frequency in young, athletic males. The chondral lesions are deep, and the labral tears are often extensive *(10,12,87)*. This is in contrast to pincer impingement, which is reported to occur more commonly in active middle-aged women *(10,85,90)*. The chondral lesions in the pincer type of impingement are typically smaller and more benign than those seen in cam impingement. It is not uncommon to see both of these lesions coexisting in a patient with FAI.

SURGICAL TREATMENTS AND PATIENT SELECTION

The goal of surgical intervention is to relieve the impingement by increasing hip clearance in flexion as well as addressing the associated labral and chondral pathology. Surgery

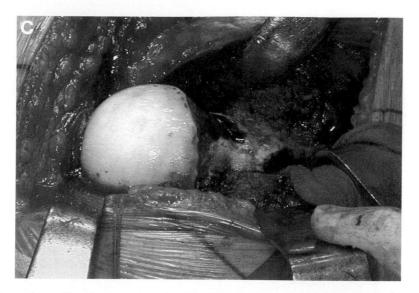

Fig. 8. Open view of impinging osteophyte in FAI at the anterior-lateral head-neck junction (**A**). Associated delamination lesion at the anterior-superior weight-bearing rim of the acetabulum (**B**). View of the head-neck junction after the osteophyte is removed (**C**).

is tailored to the underlying anatomic abnormality. Cam-type impingement, with prominence of the femoral head-neck region, is addressed on the femoral side with femoral neck osteochondroplasty. The goal of femoral neck osteochondroplasty is to re-create the anatomic spherical shape of the femoral head and to reduce the prominence of the femoral neck, which abuts the anterior labrum and acetabulum. Conversely, pincer impingement lesions often require resection osteoplasty of the acetabular rim with repair of the labrum to its proper anatomic position. When these lesions coexist, osteoplasty of both the femoral head-neck junction and the acetabular rim is required.

Classically, the surgical approach to these lesions has been a formal open surgical dislocation, including trochanteric osteotomy. This approach was espoused by Ganz et al. *(19,11,83)* for its ability to give a full view of the femoral head and acetabulum. Arthroscopic management of these lesions has been described but traditionally has focused on the labral tear and not on the underlying anatomic cause of the tear. Some authors have suggested that it is exceedingly difficult, if not impossible, to address these lesions arthroscopically *(11)*.

It is our contention that arthroscopic management of FAI provides excellent visualization and results in a shorter period of rehabilitation and fewer complications. Ongoing studies and clinical follow-up will help to answer the question regarding the clinical efficacy of the arthroscopic procedure and whether it produces equivalent clinical outcomes when compared to the open surgical approach. Hip arthroscopy can be performed in both the supine and lateral positions, depending on surgeon preference; all of the intra-articular structures in the hip joint can be seen through the combined use of 70° and 30° arthroscopes as well as the interchange of portals *(5)*.

As noted, the goal of surgical intervention is to relieve the symptomatic impingement and address any associated labral and chondral pathology. The classic open approach has been advocated because it provides excellent visualization of both the femoral head and acetabulum

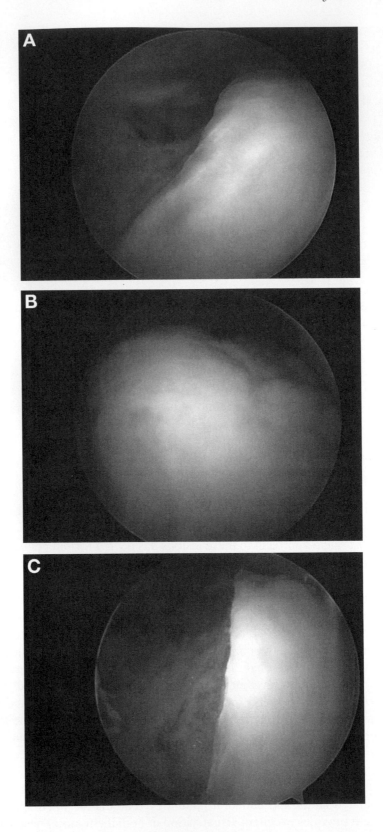

(9,11,83). However, open surgical dislocation is not without risk. Heterotopic ossification, postoperative joint stiffness, sciatic nerve injury, and trochanteric nonunion have been reported with this approach *(83)*. In addition, long-term rehabilitation requirements and time to return to sporting activity following open dislocation have not been fully reported. Moreover, the published midterm results of this technique are promising, but certainly not excellent. Of the first 19 patients reported at an average 4.7 yr of follow-up, 5 had already been converted to total hip arthroplasty *(9)*. Devising a technique that can minimize surgical trauma, enhance recovery, and optimize clinical results would be ideal.

Arthroscopic management of these lesions has been described recently *(91)*. These reports place more emphasis on how to most adequately address the source of FAI *(91)*. Traditionally, arthroscopic techniques have not addressed the underlying bony abnormalities but only the resultant injury to the labrum and the cartilage *(92)*. In fact, Lavigne et al. *(11)* reported that "the constrained hip renders access to the underlying cause of impingement technically challenging, if not impossible." We agree with Lavigne et al *(11)*. that to address the labral and chondral lesions associated with FAI adequately, the underlying anatomic deformity must be addressed. Standard hip arthroscopy portals and techniques are adequate for visualizing and debriding a diseased labrum but are incapable of addressing either the cam or pincer impingement lesions. Improved arthroscopic techniques utilizing additional accessory portals give direct access to both cam and pincer impingement lesions and provide excellent visualization (Fig. 9A–C). In addition, supplementary procedures such as microfracture, labral repair, and capsulorraphy can be performed concomitantly using arthroscopic techniques.

In summary, FAI is a source of many anterosuperior labral and chondral injuries on the acetabular side of the hip. Although management of this disorder has typically been addressed using open methods, the role of arthroscopy for the treatment of this disorder is evolving. Technological advancements in hip arthroscopy have allowed direct access to the source of the pathology without the need for hip dislocation. Additional studies are needed to define the long-term clinical impact of arthroscopic management on the natural history of FAI and how it compares with open approaches.

CLINICAL EXAM AND WORKUP

In most cases of traumatic chondral injuries in the femoral head, symptom onset is immediate. However, in some cases the injury will appear innocuous and have variable levels of dysfunction. Persistent symptoms such as intermittent catching or pain elicited by provocative maneuvers should prompt a more extensive diagnostic work-up. Groin pain associated with acetabular cartilage delamination and FAI is typically insidious in onset. The patient will often report months to years of gradually worsening hip pain. There is little guidance in the present literature on the sensitivity or specificity of physical examination to detect nonarthritic intra-articular pathology of the hip joint reliably.

A comprehensive patient history should be performed to assess the qualitative nature of the discomfort (pain, clicking, catching, instability, stiffness, weakness, or decreased performance). Other factors, including the specific location of the discomfort, the timing of symptoms, and the

---

Fig. 9. *(Opposite page)* View of the peripheral compartment and the anterior head-neck junction through the distal lateral portal with CAM impingement **(A,B)**. After arthroscopic osteochondroplasty, the head-neck offset is re-established **(C)**.

precipitating causes of symptoms and an assessment of any referred or systemic causes of hip pain should be included in the workup *(3,4,93)*. An intra-articular cause of intractable hip pain in the adult can present in a variety of ways. Patients may have pain in the anterior groin, anterior thigh, buttock, greater trochanter, or medial knee. Other symptoms include persistent clicking, catching, locking, giving way, or restricted range of motion. Symptoms may be preceded by a traumatic event, either a fall or twisting injury; however, insidious onset of hip pain may also be reported. Symptoms are typically exacerbated with activity and improved with rest.

Physical examination begins with an assessment of the patient's gait and posture and is best performed when the patient is unaware that of being watched. Antalgic gait patterns result in shortening of the stance phase, as well as shortening of the length of the step on the affected side secondary to pain. During a Trendelenburg gait, functionally or physiologically weakened gluteus medius forces shift the upper body to the involved side, moving the center of gravity over the painful hip and decreasing the moment arm forces across the hip joint *(94)*. Evaluation of posture and limb position should look for pelvic obliquity, limb length inequality, muscle contractures, and scoliosis and includes both static and dynamic evaluations *(3)*.

Examination of the hip joint begins with palpation of specific regions of the hip to localize sites of tenderness, to delineate the integrity of the muscular structures about the hip, and to identify any areas of gross atrophy. If the source of the pain is truly intra-articular, palpation does not typically cause pain. Active and passive range of motion of both hips should be evaluated in the seated and supine positions. Any asymmetry in adduction, abduction, flexion, extension, external rotation, and internal rotation should be noted as well as any reproduction of symptoms in these positions.

Several diagnostic tests can be used to identify pathological conditions of the hip. The Thomas test will help to identify the presence of a hip flexion contracture by eliminating the effects of excessive lumbar lordosis on the perceived extension of the hip *(94)*. The patient is placed in the supine position, and both hips are flexed maximally toward the chest. The involved hip is then brought into extension. A hip flexion contracture is present if it is not possible to bring the hip to neutral. Typically, passive range of motion should match or exceed active range of motion; however, provocative maneuvers performed during passive range of motion evaluation may result in limited motion secondary to pain and are highly suggestive of intra-articular pathology. Painful hip flexion, adduction, and internal rotation can indicate acetabular rim problems or labral tears, especially if clicking or groin pain is elicited.

FABER (flexion, abduction, external rotation) is the classic examination for the distinction of hip pain with rotation in the abducted position, opposing the anterior superior rim of the femoral neck adjacent to the 12 o'clock position of the acetabulum. Pain may be referred to the spine or the sacroiliac joint, as well as the iliopsoas tendon, directing further evaluation to these areas.

The Ober test is used to evaluate tightness in the iliotibial band and may elicit symptoms in the presence of trochanteric bursitis. With the patient on his or her side, this test is positive when the affected leg remains in the abducted position after the hip is passively extended and abducted with the knee extended.

The piriformis test is performed by flexing the hip to 60°, stabilizing the hip, and exerting a downward pressure on the knee. If the piriformis is tight, then pain is elicited; if the sciatic nerve is compressed (piriformis syndrome), then the patient experiences radicular-like symptoms *(3,94)*.

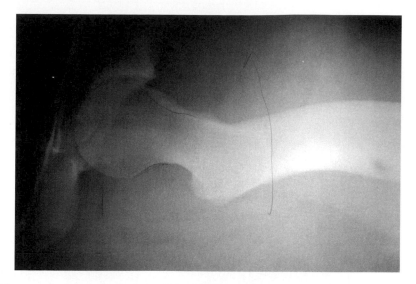

Fig. 10. Elongated neck lateral view of the hip demonstrating decreased offset at the head-neck junction.

Mechanical symptoms attributable to intra-articular pathology can also be elicited by loading the hip joint with both a resisted leg raise in the supine position as well as forced internal rotation while applying an axial load.

The complete physical examination should include motor strength testing of both hips to detect side-to-side differences. Finally, a neurovascular examination should be performed to rule out referred pain secondary to nerve problems or vascular abnormalities. If a patient presents with persistent hip pain that is reproducible on physical examination and does not respond to conservative measures, then hip arthroscopy may be of substantial value *(95,96)*.

DIAGNOSTIC IMAGING OF HIP PROBLEMS

All patients suspected of hip injury should undergo a series of radiographs, including a standing anteroposterior view of the pelvis, a cross-table lateral view, and false profile views of both hips. The main purpose of radiographs is to rule out joint space narrowing, the presence of acetabular dysplasia, and the presence of FAI. Radiographs facilitate the calculation of such indices as center-edge angle, anterior center edge angle, Tonnis angle, and neck-shaft angle and anterior offset *(84,97)*. Radiographic evidence of FAI is best seen on the cross-table lateral view, which will demonstrate decreased offset at the head-neck junction at the anterior-lateral portion of the neck (Fig. 10) *(84,98)*.

Magnetic resonance imaging has become the examination of choice for the evaluation of unexplained hip pain. The unique ability of MRI to provide detailed images of soft tissue and internal derangements of bone, in multiple planes of view, makes it superior to other imaging modalities that have been used in diagnostic hip imaging. Three-dimensional T_1-weighted gradient echo sequences with fat suppression have been reported to provide high accuracy in the detection of articular cartilage surface defects *(99)*. Some authors have suggested that contrast medium be used for the staging of chondral lesions within the hip joint *(100)*. Although gadolinium-enhanced MR arthrography is currently the most promising imaging

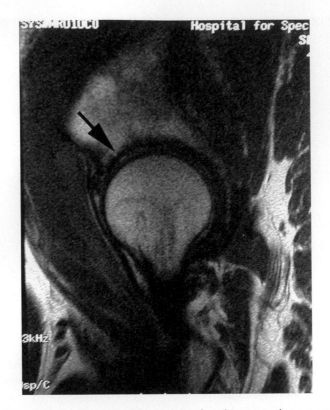

Fig. 11. Sagittal MRI with cartilage-sensitive sequencing demonstrating an anterior-superior labral tear with cartilage wear at the anterior-superior dome of the acetabulum, typical of CAM impingement.

modality, it still has some limitations in reliably demonstrating chondral injuries, perhaps because of the static nature of the imaging study and the lack of hip joint distraction during the test *(101,102)*. Potter et al. demonstrated the utility of cartilage-sensitive MRI for the detection of these lesions; it can be performed successfully without the use of gadolinium *(103,104)*. Specialized cartilage sequencing utilizing T_2 relaxation time mapping will likely improve our ability to detect early cartilage injury currently not detectable with standard imaging techniques (Fig. 11) *(105–107)*.

DIAGNOSTIC INTRA-ARTICULAR INJECTIONS

Intra-articular injections have been shown to be one of the most reliable indicators of intra-articular problems in the hip joint and should be used as an adjunct to the diagnostic workup *(101)*. Significant pain relief from an intra-articular injection provides good evidence that the affected patient will respond favorably to surgical management of a focal chondral lesions.

POSTOPERATIVE CARE

For arthroscopic procedures of the hip, patients are allowed to leave the hospital the same day of surgery. Weight-bearing status is predicated on the extent of the procedure. Simple debridements or lavage procedures generally require only 7–10 d of restricted weight bearing

(20 lb foot flat). If an extensive bony resection (osteoplasties) or microfracture procedure is performed, then 4–6 wk of restricted weight bearing is recommended.

Continuous passive motion is used for 4 h/d for 4–6 wk. This modality is used to maintain motion and to decrease the likelihood of postoperative stiffness. In addition, CPM has been shown to improve fibrocartilage ingrowth after microfracture procedures *(43)*. Early range of motion on a stationary bike is initiated on the first postoperative day, if possible.

The patient is placed in a hip brace to avoid hyperextension during the first 10 d after surgery. Postoperative medications include a narcotic, an anti-inflammatory agent, and an antiplatelet medication (enteric-coated aspirin, 325 mg per day). Sutures are removed on postoperative day 10, and follow-up visits are scheduled for 6 wk, 12 wk, 6 mo, and 1 yr. *(108)*.

REHABILITATION AND RETURN-TO-PLAY RECOMMENDATIONS

As a general guideline, we recommend 3 mo of supervised therapy after arthroscopic hip procedures. Month 1 is the tissue healing phase and focuses on decreasing inflammation, allowing the tissue to heal properly, and regaining full range of passive motion. During the first month, we prescribe 1 d of therapy each week. Month 2 is the early strengthening phase, during which patients receive therapy 2 d/wk. During the final month, when return of strength, coordination, and endurance are emphasized, patients should attend a physical therapy session three times per week.

The rehabilitation of patients undergoing debridement of chondral flaps with microfracture arthroplasty is particularly important in achieving a successful clinical outcome. The primary concern is to allow healing of the affected articular surfaces. The rehabilitation of such patients is designed to minimize the application of compressive and shear forces across the hip joint. Articular damage is often on the weight-bearing surface of the femur or acetabulum. Limited weight bearing of the operative limb is typically recommended for 6–8 wk. This time-period may vary depending on the extent and location of the chondral lesion. When transitioning from limited weight-bearing status to full weight bearing, the patient should be monitored for symptoms indicative of joint inflammation. If allowed to persist without a period of relative rest, such a synovitis can become extremely difficult to control. When such symptoms do occur, it is recommended that the patient resume a partial weight-bearing status (crutch use), utilize anti-inflammatories, and apply modalities locally to the hip joint (i.e., cryotherapy).

Rehabilitation after arthroscopic osteoplasty for FAI also requires a period of protective weight bearing if there is extensive bone resection along the femoral head-neck junction. Mardones et al. *(109)* demonstrated that resection of greater than 30% of the anterolateral quadrant of the head-neck junction significantly alters the load-bearing capacity of the proximal part of the femur and may decrease the amount of energy required to produce a fracture in the subcapital or femoral neck region. Although typical osteoplasties remove less than 30% of the anterolateral quadrant, we prescribe a period of protected weight bearing as a precautionary measure and obtain plain x-rays prior to advancing the weight-bearing status. In these patients, more aggressive early passive range of motion can be performed with particular attention to flexion and internal rotation.

Postoperative rehabilitation after surgical dislocation of the hip for chondral transplant or partial resurfacing procedures is much lengthier compared to arthroscopic hip procedures. Patients usually are hospitalized for 5–7 d. Because of the trochanteric flip osteotomy, these patients remain nonweight bearing for 12 wk to avoid nonunion across the osteotomy site.

Early hip motion is encouraged, as are isometric quadriceps contractions. Return to full activity occurs between 6 and 12 mo.

OUTCOMES AND FUTURE DIRECTIONS

There is no uniform classification system for osteochondral lesions in the hip. Most currently available classification systems are based on lesions in the knee. The widely used Outerbridge classification system, initially designed for chondromalacia patellae, is now widely used to describe cartilage lesions in joints throughout the body. Traditionally, assessment of chondral lesions within the hip joint has been difficult because of restricted access and visualization. Diagnostic imaging has also been challenging, and further improvements are needed to improve the sensitivity and specificity of radiographic and MRI evaluation of chondral lesions in the hip joint *(100,110)*. Noncontrast imaging techniques have demonstrated increased sensitivity for the evaluation of labral and chondral pathology through the use of optimized protocols. Such information may facilitate deciding which patients warrant surgical intervention, thus preserving hip arthroscopy as a therapeutic tool *(103)*.

To date, there is no universally accepted standardized outcome assessment tool for management of chondral injuries in the hip. Given this lack of a standard for both preoperative quantification of the injury and postoperative assessment of patient outcome, evaluation of surgical success is challenging. It is clear that improvements in outcome scoring criteria and prospective evaluation of clinical outcome are necessary to further advance this field. A new nonarthritic hip outcome score, the Hip Outcome Score (HOS), has been validated (Appendix) *(111)*. The HOS is comprised of two scales: the Activity of Daily Living and Sports scales. The primary purpose of the HOS is to function as an instrument that assesses the change in the patient's physical performance over time. It is an appropriate instrument for individuals with a wide range of musculoskeletal hip-related pathologies, both arthritic and nonarthritic. With respect to individuals with focal chondral pathology, these patients generally function at a high level and have few limitations except for sport-related activities. Therefore, a sports-specific scale was developed in an effort to be more responsive to changes in the physical performance of these individuals. The reliability, validity, and responsiveness of the HOS have been validated in 550 patients *(111)*.

CONCLUSIONS

Chondral injuries in the hip are becoming increasingly recognized as occult sources of hip pain that may be amenable to a variety of different surgical interventions. These cartilage injuries can be divided into focal chondral lesions on the femoral head (usually caused by direct trauma) and cartilage delamination lesions on the acetabular rim (usually caused by FAI). Appropriate management depends on the size and location of the lesion as well as a number of patient factors, including age, symptoms, activity level, and the patient's ability to comply with postoperative rehabilitation.

The majority of the procedures that are discussed in this chapter are relatively new and continue to evolve. Moreover, our ability to access and maneuver within the hip joint continues to develop as well. A uniform classification system that accurately characterizes these lesions and validated outcome tools are sorely needed in this area. As this field progresses and we develop a better understanding of the relevant disease processes, not only will we improve patients' symptoms, but also we will alter the natural progression of cartilage degeneration in the hip through the implementation of biological solutions to cartilage injury.

REFERENCES

1. Berend KR, Vail TP. Hip arthroscopy in the adolescent and pediatric athlete. Clin Sports Med 2001;20:763–778.
2. Byrd JW. Hip arthroscopy. The supine position. Clin Sports Med 2001;20:703–731.
3. Scopp JM, Moorman CT 3rd. The assessment of athletic hip injury. Clin Sports Med 2001;20:647–659.
4. Byrd JWT. Investigation of the symptomatic hip: physical examination. In: Byrd JWT, ed., Operative Hip Arthroscopy. New York: Thieme; 1998. p1–15.
5. Kelly BT, Williams RJ 3rd, Philippon MJ. Hip arthroscopy: current indications, treatment options, management issues. Am J Sports Med 2003;31:1020–1037.
6. Byrd JW. Lateral impact injury: A source of occult hip pathology. Clin Sports Med 2001;20: 801–815.
7. Cooper DE, Warren RF, Barnes R. Traumatic subluxation of the hip resulting in aseptic necrosis and chondrolysis in a professional football player. Am J Sports Med 1991;19:322–324.
8. Moorman CT 3rd, Warren RF, Hershman EB, et al. Traumatic posterior hip subluxation in American football. J Bone Joint Surg Am 2003;85-A:1190–1196.
9. Beck M, Leunig M, Parvizi J, Boutier V, Wyss D, Ganz R. Anterior femoroacetabular impingement: part II. Midterm results of surgical treatment. Clin Orthop 2004;418:67–73.
10. Ganz R, Parvizi J, Beck M, Leunig M, Notzli H, Siebenrock KA. Femoroacetabular impingement: a cause for osteoarthritis of the hip. Clin Orthop 2003;417:112–120.
11. Lavigne M, Parvizi J, Beck M, Siebenrock KA, Ganz R, Leunig M. Anterior femoroacetabular impingement: part I. Techniques of joint preserving surgery. Clin Orthop 2004;418:61–66.
12. Parvizi J, Ganz R, Beck M, Leunig M, Sibenrock K. Femoroacetbular impingement: mid-term clinical results. J Arthroplasty 2004;19:261–262.
13. Olson SA, Bay BK, Hamel A. Biomechanics of the hip joint and the effects of fracture of the acetabulum. Clin Orthop Relat Res 1997;339:92–104.
14. Greenwald AS, Haynes DW. Weight-bearing areas in the human hip joint. J Bone Joint Surg Br 1972;54:157–163.
15. Dussault RG, Beauregard G, Fauteaux P, Laurin C, Boisjoly A. Femoral head defect following anterior hip dislocation. Radiology 1980;135:627–629.
16. Repo RU, Finlay JB. Survival of articular cartilage after controlled impact. J Bone Joint Surg Am 1977;59:1068–1076.
17. Epstein HC. Traumatic dislocations of the hip. Clin Orthop Relat Res 1973;92:116–142.
18. Epstein HC, Wiss DA, Cozen L. Posterior fracture dislocation of the hip with fractures of the femoral head. Clin Orthop 1985;201:9–17.
19. Brumback RJ, Kenzora JE, Levitt LE, Burgess AR, Poka A. Fractures of the femoral head. Hip 1987:181–206.
20. Epstein HC, Wiss DA. Traumatic anterior dislocation of the hip. Orthopedics 1985;8:130,132–134.
21. DeLee JC, Evans JA, Thomas J. Anterior dislocation of the hip and associated femoral-head fractures. J Bone Joint Surg Am 1980;62:960–964.
22. Cruess RL. The current status of avascular necrosis of the femoral head. Clin Orthop Relat Res 1978;131:309–311.
23. Herndon JH, Aufranc OE. Avascular necrosis of the femoral head in the adult. A review of its incidence in a variety of conditions. Clin Orthop Relat Res 1972;86:43–62.
24. Glick JM. Hip arthroscopy using the lateral approach. Instr Course Lect 1988;37:223–231.
25. Glick JM. Hip arthroscopy. The lateral approach. Clin Sports Med 2001;20:733–747.
26. Sekiya JK, Ruch DS, Hunter DM, et al. Hip arthroscopy in staging avascular necrosis of the femoral head. J South Orthop Assoc 2000;9:254–261.
27. Lance D, Carlioz A, Seringe R, Postel M, Lacombe MJ, Abelanet R. Acute chondrolysis following slipped capital femoral epiphysis. A study of 41 cases [author's transl]. Rev Chir Orthop Reparatrice Appar Mot 1981;67:437–450.

28. Brandt KD. Animal models of osteoarthritis. Biorheology 2002;39:221–235.
29. Hartofilakidis G, Karachalios T. Idiopathic osteoarthritis of the hip: incidence, classification, natural history of 272 cases. Orthopedics 2003;26:161–166.
30. Lievense AM, Bierma-Zeinstra SM, Verhagen AP, Verhaar JA, Koes BW. Prognostic factors of progress of hip osteoarthritis: a systematic review. Arthritis Rheum 2002;47:556–562.
31. Maillefert JF, Nguyen M, Gueguen A, et al. Relevant change in radiological progression in patients with hip osteoarthritis. II. Determination using an expert opinion approach. Rheumatology (Oxford) 2002;41:148–152.
32. Tindall EA, Sharp JT, Burr A, et al. A 12-mo, multicenter, prospective, open-label trial of radiographic analysis of disease progression in osteoarthritis of the knee or hip in patients receiving celecoxib. Clin Ther 2002;24:2051–2063.
33. Jackson DW, Lalor PA, Aberman HM, Simon TM. Spontaneous repair of full-thickness defects of articular cartilage in a goat model. A preliminary study. J Bone Joint Surg Am 2001;83-A:53–A64.
34. Rosenberg TD, Weiss JA, Moulis PM, Deffner KT, Cooley VJ. Finite element simulation of stresses in chondral defects. Int Cart Repair Soc Newsl 1999;2:14.
35. Gilbert JE. Current treatment options for the restoration of articular cartilage. Am J Knee Surg 1998;11:42–46.
36. De Smet AA, Ilahi OA, Graf BK. Reassessment of the MR criteria for stability of osteochondritis dissecans in the knee and ankle. Skeletal Radiol 1996;25:159–163.
37. De Smet AA, Ilahi OA, Graf BK. Untreated osteochondritis dissecans of the femoral condyles: prediction of patient outcome using radiographic and MR findings. Skeletal Radiol 1997;26:463–467.
38. Shelbourne KD, Jari S, Gray T. Outcome of untreated traumatic articular cartilage defects of the knee: a natural history study. J Bone Joint Surg Am 2003;85-A(suppl 2):8–16.
39. Brittberg M, Peterson L, Sjogren-Jansson E, Tallheden T, Lindahl A. Articular cartilage engineering with autologous chondrocyte transplantation. A review of recent developments. J Bone Joint Surg Am 2003;85-A(suppl 3):109–115.
40. Cohen NP, Foster RJ, Mow VC. Composition and dynamics of articular cartilage: structure, function, maintaining healthy state. J Orthop Sports Phys Ther 1998;28:203–215.
41. Gill T. The role of microfracture technique in the treatment of full-thickness chondral injuries. Oper Tech Sports Med 2000;8:138–140.
42. Rodrigo JJ, Steadman JR, Silliman J. Improvement of full-thickness chondral defect healing in the human knee after debridement and microfracture using continuous passive motion. Am J Knee Surg 1994;7:109–116.
43. Steadman JR, Rodkey WG, Rodrigo JJ. Microfracture: surgical technique and rehabilitation to treat chondral defects. Clin Orthop 2001;(391 suppl):S362–S369.
44. Steadman JR, Rodkey WG, Singleton SB. Microfracture technique for full-thickness chondral defects: technique and clinical results. Oper Tech Orthop 1997;7:300–304.
45. Blevins FT, Steadman JR, Rodrigo JJ, Silliman J. Treatment of articular cartilage defects in athletes: an analysis of functional outcome and lesion appearance. Orthopedics 1998;21:761–767; discussion 767–768.
46. Lieberman JR, Berry DJ, Mont MA, et al. Osteonecrosis of the hip: management in the 21st century. Instr Course Lect 2003;52:337–355.
47. Linden B, Jonsson K, Redlund-Johnell I. Osteochondritis dissecans of the hip. Acta Radiol 2003;44:67–71.
48. Mont MA, Jones LC, Sotereanos DG, Amstutz HC, Hungerford DS. Understanding and treating osteonecrosis of the femoral head. Instr Course Lect 2000;49:169–185.
49. Zhang B, Zhu S, Guo Y. Treatment of ischemic necrosis of femoral head by focal cleaning and bone graft. Zhongguo Xiu Fu Chong Jian Wai Ke Za Zhi 2000;14:93–95.
50. Sledge SL. Microfracture techniques in the treatment of osteochondral injuries. Clin Sports Med 2001;20:365–377.
51. du Toit GT, Sweet MB. Arthroplasty by osteocartilaginous graft in primates. Clin Orthop 1982; 165:49–63.

52. Meyers MH, Jones RE, Bucholz RW, Wenger DR. Fresh autogenous grafts and osteochondral allografts for the treatment of segmental collapse in osteonecrosis of the hip. Clin Orthop 1983;174:107–112.
53. Roffman M, du Toit GT. Osteochondral hemiarthroplasty. An experimental investigation in baboons. Int Orthop 1985;9:69–75.
54. Buckwalter JA, Mankin HJ. Articular cartilage repair and transplantation. Arthritis Rheum 1998;41:1331–1342.
55. Fitzpatrick PL, Morgan DA. Fresh osteochondral allografts: a 6–10-yr review. Aust N Z J Surg 1998;68:573–579.
56. Brittberg M, Lindahl A, Nilsson A, Ohlsson C, Isaksson O, Peterson L. Treatment of deep cartilage defects in the knee with autologous chondrocyte transplantation. N Engl J Med 1994;331:889–895.
57. Easley ME, Scranton PE Jr. Osteochondral autologous transfer system. Foot Ankle Clin 2003;8:275–290.
58. Minas T. Autologous chondrocyte implantation in the arthritic knee. Orthopedics 2003;26:945–947.
59. Minas T, Chiu R. Autologous chondrocyte implantation. Am J Knee Surg 2000;13:41–50.
60. Peterson L, Brittberg M, Kiviranta I, Akerlund EL, Lindahl A. Autologous chondrocyte transplantation. Biomechanics and long-term durability. Am J Sports Med 2002;30:2–12.
61. Peterson L, Minas T, Brittberg M, Nilsson A, Sjogren-Jansson E, Lindahl A. Two- to 9-yr outcome after autologous chondrocyte transplantation of the knee. Clin Orthop 2000;374:212–234.
62. Cornell CN, Salvati EA, Pellicci PM. Long-term follow-up of total hip replacement in patients with osteonecrosis. Orthop Clin North Am 1985;16:757–769.
63. Meyers MH. Osteonecrosis of the femoral head. Pathogenesis and long-term results of treatment. Clin Orthop 1988;231:51–61.
64. Salvati EA, Cornell CN. Long-term follow-up of total hip replacement in patients with avascular necrosis. Instr Course Lect 1988;37:67–73.
65. Shinoda S, Hasegawa Y, Kawabe K, et al. Total hip arthroplasty for failed rotational acetabular osteotomy: a report of three cases. Nagoya J Med Sci 1998;61:53–58.
66. Barnes CL, Collins DN, Nelson CL. Cup arthroplasty, surface replacement arthroplasty, and femoral head resurfacing for osteonecrosis. Semin Arthroplasty 1991;2:222–227.
67. Campbell P, Mirra J, Amstutz HC. Viability of femoral heads treated with resurfacing arthroplasty. J Arthroplasty 2000;15:120–122.
68. Howie DW, Cornish BL, Vernon-Roberts B. Resurfacing hip arthroplasty. Classification of loosening and the role of prosthesis wear particles. Clin Orthop 1990;255:144–159.
69. Hungerford MW, Mont MA, Scott R, Fiore C, Hungerford DS, Krackow KA. Surface replacement hemiarthroplasty for the treatment of osteonecrosis of the femoral head. J Bone Joint Surg Am 1998;80:1656–1664.
70. Mont MA, Rajadhyaksha AD, Hungerford DS. Outcomes of limited femoral resurfacing arthroplasty compared with total hip arthroplasty for osteonecrosis of the femoral head. J Arthroplasty 2001;16(8 suppl 1):134–139.
71. Siguier T, Siguier M, Judet T, Charnley G, Brumpt B. Partial resurfacing arthroplasty of the femoral head in avascular necrosis. Methods, indications, results. Clin Orthop 2001;386:85–92.
72. Ushio K, Oka M, Hyon SH, Yura S, Toguchida J, Nakamura T. Partial hemiarthroplasty for the treatment of osteonecrosis of the femoral head. An experimental study in the dog. J Bone Joint Surg Br 2003;85:922–930.
73. Brand RA. Hip osteotomies: a biomechanical consideration. J Am Acad Orthop Surg 1997;5:282–291.
74. Gillingham BL, Sanchez AA, Wenger DR. Pelvic osteotomies for the treatment of hip dysplasia in children and young adults. J Am Acad Orthop Surg 1999;7:325–337.
75. Ko JY, Meyers MH, Wenger DR. "Trapdoor" procedure for osteonecrosis with segmental collapse of the femoral head in teenagers. J Pediatr Orthop 1995;15:7–15.

76. Mont MA, Fairbank AC, Krackow KA, Hungerford DS. Corrective osteotomy for osteonecrosis of the femoral head. J Bone Joint Surg Am 1996;78:1032–1038.

77. Tonnis D, Behrens K, Tscharani F. A modified technique of the triple pelvic osteotomy: early results. J Pediatr Orthop 1981;1:241–249.

78. Ito K, Minka MA 2nd, Leunig M, Werlen S, Ganz R. Femoroacetabular impingement and the cam-effect. A MRI-based quantitative anatomical study of the femoral head-neck offset. J Bone Joint Surg Br 2001;83:171–176.

79. Schmid MR, Notzli HP, Zanetti M, Wyss TF, Hodler J. Cartilage lesions in the hip: diagnostic effectiveness of MR arthrography. Radiology 2003;226:382–386.

80. McCarthy JC, Noble PC, Schuck MR, Wright J, Lee J. The Otto E. Aufranc Award: the role of labral lesions to development of early degenerative hip disease. Clin Orthop 2001; 393:25–37.

81. McCarthy JC, Noble PC, Schuck MR, Wright J, Lee J. The watershed labral lesion: its relationship to early arthritis of the hip. J Arthroplasty 2001;16(8 suppl 1):81–87.

82. Leunig M, Casillas MM, Hamlet M, et al. Slipped capital femoral epiphysis: early mechanical damage to the acetabular cartilage by a prominent femoral metaphysis. Acta Orthop Scand 2000;71:370–375.

83. Eijer H, Myers SR, Ganz R. Anterior femoroacetabular impingement after femoral neck fractures. J Orthop Trauma 2001;15:475–481.

84. Notzli HP, Wyss TF, Stoecklin CH, Schmid MR, Treiber K, Hodler J. The contour of the femoral head-neck junction as a predictor for the risk of anterior impingement. J Bone Joint Surg Br 2002;84:556–560.

85. Siebenrock KA, Schoeniger R, Ganz R. Anterior femoro-acetabular impingement due to acetabular retroversion. Treatment with periacetabular osteotomy. J Bone Joint Surg Am 2003;85-A:278–286.

86. Myers SR, Eijer H, Ganz R. Anterior femoroacetabular impingement after periacetabular osteotomy. Clin Orthop 1999;363:93–99.

87. Siebenrock KA, Wahab KH, Werlen S, Kalhor M, Leunig M, Ganz R. Abnormal extension of the femoral head epiphysis as a cause of cam impingement. Clin Orthop 2004;418:54–60.

88. Wagner S, Hofstetter W, Chiquet M, et al. Early osteoarthritic changes of human femoral head cartilage subsequent to femoro-acetabular impingement. Osteoarthritis Cartilage 2003;11: 508–518.

89. Goodman DA, Feighan JE, Smith AD, Latimer B, Buly RL, Cooperman DR. Subclinical slipped capital femoral epiphysis. Relationship to osteoarthrosis of the hip. J Bone Joint Surg Am 1997;79:1489–1497.

90. Leunig M, Beck M, Woo A, Dora C, Kerboull M, Ganz R. Acetabular rim degeneration: a constant finding in the aged hip. Clin Orthop 2003;413:201–207.

91. Guanche CA, Bare AA, Arthroscopic treatment of femoroacetabular impingement. Arthroscopy 2006;22(1):95–106.

92. Byrd JW, Jones KS. Prospective analysis of hip arthroscopy with 2 year followup. Arthroscopy 2000;16(6)578–587.

93. Kallas KM, Guanche CA. Physical examination and imaging of hip injuries. Operative Tech Sports Med 2002;10:176–183.

94. Hoppenfeld S. Physical examination of the hip and pelvis. In: Hoppenfeld S, ed., Physical Examination of the Spine and Extremities. Norwalk, CT: Appleton and Lange; 1976:143–144.

95. Villar RN. Hip arthroscopy. Br J Hosp Med 1992;47:763–766.

96. Villar RN. Hip arthroscopy. J Bone Joint Surg 1995;77B:517–518.

97. Erb RE. Current concepts in imaging the adult hip. Clin Sports Med 2001;20:661–696.

98. Armfield DR, Towers JD, Robertson DD. Radiographic and MR imaging of the athletic hip. Clin Sports Med 2006;25(2):211–239, viii.

99. Trattnig S, Mlynarik V, Huber M, Ba-Ssalamah A, Puig S, Imhof H. Magnetic resonance imaging of articular cartilage and evaluation of cartilage disease. Invest Radiol 2000;35:595–601.

100. Czerny C, Kramer J, Neuhold A. Magnetic resonance imaging and magnetic resonance arthrography of the acetabular labrum: comparison with surgical findings. Rofo Fortschr Geb Rontgenstr Neuen Bildgeb Verfahr 2001;173:702–707.
101. Byrd JW, Jones KS. Diagnostic accuracy of clinical assessment, magnetic resonance imaging, magnetic resonance arthrography, intra-articular injection in hip arthroscopy patients. Am J Sports Med 2004;32:1668–1674.
102. Edwards DJ, Lomas D, Villar RN. Diagnosis of the painful hip by magnetic resonance imaging and arthroscopy. J Bone Joint Surg 1995;77B:374–376.
103. Mintz DN, Hooper T, Connell D, Buly R, Padgett DE, Potter HG. Magnetic resonance imaging of the hip: detection of labral and chondral abnormalities using noncontrast imaging. Arthroscopy 2005;21:385–393.
104. Potter HG, Linklater JM, Allen AA, Hannafin JA, Haas SB. Magnetic resonance imaging of articular cartilage in the knee. An evaluation with use of fast-spin-echo imaging. J Bone Joint Surg 1998;80A:1276–1284.
105. Dardzinski BJ, Mosher TJ, Li S, Van Slyke MA, Smith MB. Spatial variation of T_2 in human articular cartilage. Radiology 1997;205:546–550.
106. Maier CF, Tan SG, Hariharan H, Potter HG. T_2 quantitation of articular cartilage at 1.5 T. J Magn Reson Imaging 2003;17:358–364.
107. Mosher TJ, Dardzinski BJ, Smith MB. Human articular cartilage: influence of aging and early symptomatic degeneration on the spatial variation of T_2—preliminary findings at 3 T. Radiology 2000;214:259–266.
108. Enseki KR, Martin RC, Draovitch P, Kelly BT, Philippon MJ, Schenker ML. The hip joint, arthroscopic procedures and postoperative rehabilitation. J Orthop Sports Phys Ther 2006;36(7):516–525.
109. Mardones RM, Gonzalez C, Chen Q, Zobitz M, Kaufman KR, Trousdale RT. Surgical treatment of femoroacetabular impingement: evaluation of the effect of the size of the resection. J Bone Joint Surg Am 2005;87:273–279.
110. Byrd JW, Jones KS. Traumatic rupture of the ligamentum teres as a source of hip pain. Arthroscopy 2004;20(4):385–391.
111. Martin RR, Kelly BT, Philippon MJ. Evidence of validity for the Hip Outcome Score (HOS). In: American Physical Therapy Association Combined Sections Meeting. New Orleans; 2005.

APPENDIX: THE HIP OUTCOMES SCORE (HOS)

Activities of Daily Living Subscale

Please answer *every question* with *one response* that most closely describes your condition within the past week.

If the activity in question is limited by something other than your hip, mark *not applicable (N/A)*.

	No difficulty at all	Slight difficulty	Moderate difficulty	Extreme difficulty	Unable to do	N/A
Standing for 15 min	☐	☐	☐	☐	☐	☐
Getting into and out of an average car	☐	☐	☐	☐	☐	☐
Putting on socks and shoes	☐	☐	☐	☐	☐	☐
Walking up steep hills	☐	☐	☐	☐	☐	☐
Walking down steep hills	☐	☐	☐	☐	☐	☐
Going up 1 flight of stairs	☐	☐	☐	☐	☐	☐
Going down 1 flight of stairs	☐	☐	☐	☐	☐	☐
Stepping up and down curbs	☐	☐	☐	☐	☐	☐
Deep squatting	☐	☐	☐	☐	☐	☐
Getting into and out of a bath tub	☐	☐	☐	☐	☐	☐
Sitting for 15 min	☐	☐	☐	☐	☐	☐
Walking initially	☐	☐	☐	☐	☐	☐
Walking approx 10 min	☐	☐	☐	☐	☐	☐
Walking 15 minutes or longer	☐	☐	☐	☐	☐	☐

Because of your hip, how much difficulty do you have with:

	No difficulty at all	Slight difficulty	Moderate difficulty	Extreme difficulty	Unable to do	N/A
Twisting/pivoting on involved leg	☐	☐	☐	☐	☐	☐
Rolling over in bed	☐	☐	☐	☐	☐	☐
Light-to-moderate work (standing, walking)	☐	☐	☐	☐	☐	☐
Heavy work (push/pulling, climbing, carrying)	☐	☐	☐	☐	☐	☐
Recreational activities	☐	☐	☐	☐	☐	☐

How would you rate (from 0 to 100) your current level of function during your usual activities of daily living, with 100 your level of function prior to your hip problem and 0 the inability to perform any of your usual daily activities?

☐☐☐.0%

Sports Subscale

Because of your hip how much difficulty do you have with

	No difficulty at all	Slight difficulty	Moderate difficulty	Extreme difficulty	Unable to do	N/A
Running 1 mile	☐	☐	☐	☐	☐	☐
Jumping	☐	☐	☐	☐	☐	☐
Swinging objects like a golf club	☐	☐	☐	☐	☐	☐
Landing	☐	☐	☐	☐	☐	☐
Starting and stopping quickly	☐	☐	☐	☐	☐	☐
Cutting/lateral movements	☐	☐	☐	☐	☐	☐
Low-impact activities like fast walking	☐	☐	☐	☐	☐	☐
Ability to perform activity with your normal technique	☐	☐	☐	☐	☐	☐
Ability to participate in your desired sport as long as you would like	☐	☐	☐	☐	☐	☐

How would you rate (from 0 to 100) your current level of function during your sports-related activities, with 100 your level of function prior to your hip problem and 0 the inability to perform any of your usual daily activities?
☐☐☐.0%

How would you rate your current level of function?
☐ Normal   ☐ Nearly normal   ☐ Abnormal   ☐ Severely abnormal

Since initiation of treatment, how would you rate your overall physical ability? (If this is your first visit to the doctor, please do not answer the question.)

_____ Much improved
_____ Improved
_____ Slightly improved
_____ No change
_____ Slightly worse
_____ Worse
_____ Much worse

20

Rehabilitation Strategies Following Articular Cartilage Surgery in the Knee

John T. Cavanaugh, MEd, PT/ATC

Summary

Advances in the understanding of the basic science inherent to articular cartilage has led to an evolution in the design of rehabilitation guidelines following articular cartilage surgery. Clinicians responsible for the rehabilitation of patients following articular cartilage surgery must respect the healing process associated with each individual procedure. Rehabilitation principles should be adhered to in order to safely progress the patient through the rehabilitative course. Treatment interventions to improve range of motion, enhance weight-bearing capability, develop strength, restore balance and proprioception, and enhance flexibility need to follow. A key task is to guide the patient into an active role in the rehabilitation process. Complying with activity modifications and practicing home therapeutic exercises are an important part of achieving a successful outcome.

Key Words: Rehabilitation; articular cartilage; surgery; range of motion; strength development; balance; proprioception; flexibility.

Rehabilitation guidelines following articular cartilage surgery continue to evolve as greater knowledge of this unique structure is appreciated. Articular cartilage allows nearly friction-less motion to occur between the articular surfaces of synovial joints (1). During the course of a lifetime, articular cartilage endures high compressive and shear forces that are inherent in activities of daily living and sports participation. Mechanisms of injury at the knee can include direct trauma, indirect impact loading, or torsional loading. Abnormal unloading at the knee joint can be detrimental to articular cartilage, and if deprived of the mechanical stimulus of load, cartilage becomes less stiff and is more vulnerable to injury (2,3).

Articular cartilage is avascular and aneural and therefore has minimal potential to regenerate after injury (4). Articular cartilage injury results in pain, mechanical symptoms, and an effusion that can interfere in an individual's activities of daily living and sports activity. Management of these lesions continues to be a significant challenge for orthopedic surgeons and rehabilitation specialists alike. In the United States, the most commonly performed cartilage repair procedures include (1) arthroscopic debridement or chondroplasty, (2) marrow stimulation techniques such as abrasion arthroplasty or microfracture procedure, (3) osteochondral autograft transplantation, (4) autologous chondrocyte implantation (ACI), and (5) osteochondral allograft transplantation.

REHABILITATION PRINCIPLES

Rehabilitation programs following articular cartilage surgeries of the knee are long and challenging assignments for the rehabilitation specialist. Throughout the rehabilitation

From: *Cartilage Repair Strategies*
Edited by: Riley J. Williams © Humana Press Inc., Totowa, NJ

process, it is important that the clinician considers the articular cartilage healing process that is associated with a given procedure. A progressive program to restore knee D (ROM) and to develop adequate lower extremity strength, flexibility, and proprioception needed for activities of daily living is crucial to optimize outcome following these surgical procedures. Certain rehabilitation principles should be followed to achieve these objectives.

1. Communication with the surgeon. The rehabilitation specialist should discuss the surgery performed with the orthopedic surgeon. Knowledge of the lesion location, size, and type of repair strategy applied will aid the therapist in designing a treatment program for each patient. Specific exercises or activities that could hinder the healing process by producing a shear or compressive forces should be avoided. Femoral condyle lesions are frequently found in areas that contact the tibia between 30 and 70° of knee flexion *(5)*. A rehabilitation guideline following surgery to address a lesion in this area will vary from a program designed for lesions on a nonweight-bearing femoral surface or patellofemoral defect. Communication with the surgeon regarding patient progress and symptoms throughout the rehabilitation period will directly influence the progression of the program (i.e., weight bearing, ROM, return to functional sport activity).

2. Maintain a safe environment. The rehabilitation specialist needs to apply a working knowledge of the function, structure, and biomechanics of articular cartilage to the rehabilitation program. This understanding combined with an awareness of the forces applied to the articular surfaces of the knee joint during specific activities will permit the clinician to progress the patient toward an optimal outcome. An ideal environment for articular cartilage healing must be maintained, especially in the early weeks following surgical intervention. Examples of such an approach include early monitoring of the weight-bearing status and limiting knee motion to arcs during strengthening exercises that result in minimal shear force application on the articular surfaces.

3. Criteria-based progression. Rehabilitation programs should be individualized. Progression of these programs should be predicated on the patient achieving certain goals that indicate a readiness to move into a broader rehabilitation program. Subjective and objective findings demonstrated throughout the rehabilitative course set the criteria for safe and effective advancement. A "cookbook" approach to treatment (i.e., rigid protocols based on postsurgical interval) can accelerate a program too quickly for the patient whose progress is delayed and can unnecessarily delay the patient who is progressing ahead of schedule. Treatment guidelines should be followed with flexible time frames to optimize patient outcome.

4. Functional progression. Throughout the rehabilitation process, progression is based on the return of knee function. Functional progression has been defined by Kegerreis *(6)* as an ordered sequence of activities enabling the acquisition or reacquisition of skills required for the safe, effective performance of athletic endeavors. The patient needs to display the necessary prerequisites to meet the demands of a certain task, then demonstrate the ability to perform such a task without pain or deviation (e.g., demonstrate quadriceps control by performing a straight leg raise [SLR] without lag or pain, establish a knee motion arc of at least 0–90°, and finally demonstrate the ability to ambulate with a normal gait without deviation).

   With continued gains in ROM, lower extremity muscle strength, flexibility, and balance, the patient will meet the criteria to meet the demands of the following progression: ascend stairs, descend stairs, run, perform plyometric and agility exercises, and eventually be tested functionally (Table 1).

5. Patient compliance. For a successful outcome following articular cartilage surgery, the patient must be ready and able to comply with the entire rehabilitation strategy. Changes in insurance reimbursement often limit the amount of authorized rehabilitation visits. A week consists of 168 h. Should a patient attend therapy three times per week for an hour per visit, this supervised effort represents just 2% of the entire week; 165 h (98% of the remaining time) is left for the patient to be responsible for personal care *(7)*. The patient should therefore adhere to the recommendations given by the surgeon and rehabilitation specialist. Compliance with prescribed home therapeutic exercises and activity modifications in daily routines are essential for consistent progress and the return of joint function.

Table 1
Functional Activities and the Recommended Criteria Needed to Perform Them

Task	Criteria
Normal gait without deviation	Quadriceps control—SLR without lag ROM 0–90°
Ascend 8-in. step	Normal gait, ascend 6-in. step ROM 0–100°
Descend 8-in. step	Ascend 8-in. step, descend 6-in. step ROM 0–120°
Running	Descend 8-in. step—good LE alignment ROM 0–130°
Plyometric exercises	Running ROM WNL
Functional testing	Plyometrics—unilateral power Normal flexibility
Return to sport	Functional testing > 85% limb symmetry Lack of apprehension with sport-specific movement

WNL, within normal limits.

TREATMENT STRATEGIES

Restoring Range of Motion

Following injury and periods of immobility, articular cartilage is less stiff and less capable of tolerating high loads *(8)*. Mobilization of the postsurgical knee is encouraged immediately following articular cartilage procedures to restore motion, diminish adhesion formation, and reduce pain. Research has supported early controlled motion following articular cartilage injury *(9–13)*. Suh et al. *(13)* demonstrated that joint motion following articular cartilage injury may facilitate healing as long as shear forces are minimized. The use of continuous passive motion (CPM) and unloaded active-assistive range of motion (AAROM) exercises are utilized as treatment strategies. Rodrigo et al. *(11)* concluded that CPM for 6 h daily for 8 wk after microfracture for full-thickness cartilage defects in the knee appears to result in better gross healing of the lesion when evaluated by arthroscopic visualization compared with the same treatment without CPM. Petersen *(10)* advocated the immediate application of CPM (within 48 h following surgery) for patients undergoing ACI on isolated femoral condyle lesions and has reported over 90% good-to-excellent results with this approach.

CPM is applied immediately after surgery using a motion arc in the 0–45° range for most articular cartilage procedures, and the flexion angle progresses as tolerated (Fig. 1). AAROM exercises are performed several times per day to compliment CPM utilization (Fig. 2). Achieving of full passive knee extension is a critical early goal following all knee surgeries. The development of a flexion contracture will result in gait abnormalities and ultimately patellofemoral symptoms *(14–16)*. Towel extensions are performed as the patient sits or lies with a towel under the heel, allowing gravity to apply a low-load prolonged stretch into extension (Fig. 3). This activity can be discontinued on the achievement of full passive extension. Patella mobilization should be performed by the rehabilitation specialist to assist in reestablishing normal patella mobility (Fig. 4). Superior mobility of the patella is required for complete knee extension. Inferior glide mobility of the patella is necessary for full knee flexion *(17)*. The patient is educated to incorporate this activity into daily home exercise program.

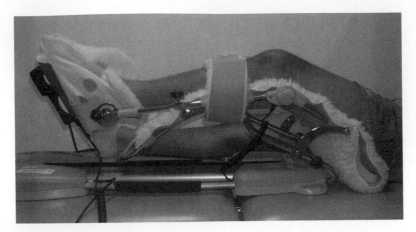

Fig. 1. Continuous passive motion (CPM) machine is applied immediately after surgery.

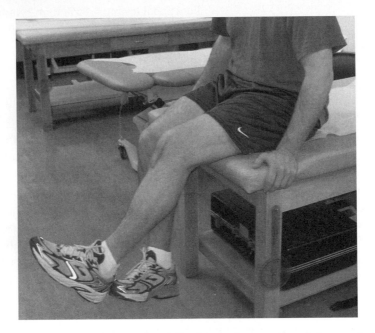

Fig. 2. The patient performs active-assisted flexion and extension of the surgical knee using the contralateral extremity for support.

Weight-Bearing Progression

Loading provides a mechanical stimulus to the articular cartilage of the knee; loading occurs with the simple act of ambulation. Under compression, interstitial fluid flows out of the permeable collagen-proteoglycan matrix inherent to articular cartilage. When the joint is unloaded, fluid flows back into the tissue. This reciprocal action (joint loading and unloading) facilitates the movement of nutrients from the synovial fluid into the matrix and the removal of catabolites *(18)*. Thus, load application to articular cartilage is vital for its long-term function.

However, articular cartilage repair procedures require that the clinician consider the type of repair tissue that is under development in a treated lesion following surgery. Weight-bearing status following articular cartilage surgery is dependent on the procedure performed, lesion

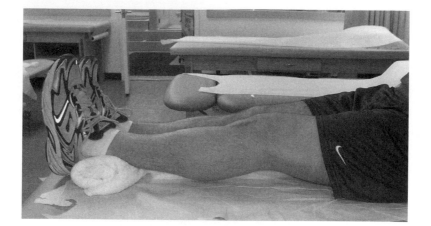

Fig. 3. Passive knee extension using a towel rolled up under heel to promote early full extension.

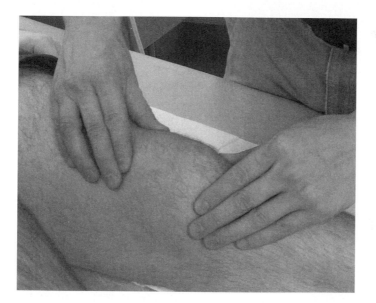

Fig. 4. Patella mobilization.

size, and lesion location. Following arthroscopic debridement or chondroplasty (Table 2), weight bearing is usually begun as tolerated with the support of crutches. As the patient demonstrates improved ROM and quadriceps control, the crutches are discontinued when a normal gait is demonstrated.

For procedures that include marrow stimulation (abrasion chondroplasty and microfracture) (Table 3), periosteal and perichondral grafting, osteochondral autograft transplantation, or fixation of an articular cartilage defect (i.e., osteochondritis dissecans pinning), weight bearing will be limited to toe-touch for the first 6 wk postoperatively. A double-upright knee brace is utilized, locked in extension during this protective phase. A progressive weight-bearing program is then initiated. For patients having undergone these procedures for a patellofemoral defect, weight bearing is initiated at 50%, with the postoperative brace opened between 0–20°. Weight bearing then gradually progresses as tolerated.

Table 2
Rehabilitation Guidelines Following Arthroscopic Debridement/Chondroplasty of the Knee

Weight-bearing status	Treatment strategies	Criteria for advancement	Precautions
Weeks 0–4			
Weight bearing as tolerated with appropriate assistive device D/C crutches when gait is nonantalgic	Active and AAROM exercises Quadriceps reeducation Multiple-angle quadriceps isometrics SLRs (all planes) Short crank → Standard ergometry Leg press 60° → 0° arc (avoid lesion) Hip progressive resisted exercises Proprioception/balance training Lower extremity flexibility exercises Cryotherapy Home therapeutic exercise program	ROM 0° → 130° Proximal muscle strength 5/5	Avoid ascending and descending reciprocally until adequate quadriceps control and lower extremity alignment is demonstrated Avoid pain with therapeutic exercise and functional
Weeks 4–8			
Full weight bearing with assistive device if needed	AAROM exercises Leg press (pain-free arc) Minisquats 60° → 0° arc (avoid lesion) Retrograde treadmill ambulation Proprioception/balance training: (bilateral → unilateral) Initiate forward step-up program Stairmaster SLRs (progressive resistance) Hamstring curls/progress proximal strengthening Lower extremity flexibility exercises Multiple-angle quadriceps isometrics (bilaterally, submaximal) (patellofemoral lesions: avoid lesion) OKC knee extension to 40°	ROM 0° → WNL Normal patella mobility Demonstrate ability to ascend 8-in. step Muscle strength 5/5 throughout involved lower extremity	Avoid descending stairs reciprocally until adequate quadriceps control and lower extremity alignment is demonstrated Avoid pain with therapeutic exercise and functional activities

	Weight bearing	Therapeutic exercises	Goals	Precautions
		(tibiofemoral lesions): CKC exercises preferred; Initiate forward step-down program; Home therapeutic exercise program		
Weeks 8–12	Full weight bearing with assistive device if needed	Progress squat program (PRE/pain-free arc); Leg press (emphasizing eccentrics); OKC knee extensions (pain-free arc); Isokinetic training (high velocities); Advanced proprioception training (perturbations); Elliptical trainer; Retrograde running; Lower extremity stretching; Forward step-down test (NeuroCom); Isokinetic test; Initiate forward running; Agility exercises (sport cord); Home therapeutic exercise program:	Ability to descend 8-in. stairs with good leg control without pain; 85% limb symmetry on isokinetic testing (tibiofemoral lesions) and forward step-down test	Avoid pain with therapeutic exercise and functional activities; Avoid running until adequate strength development and doctor's clearance
Weeks 12–16	Full weight bearing with assistive device if needed	Continue to advance lower extremity strengthening, flexibility, and agility programs; Advance forward running program; Plyometric program; Functional testing (hop test); Isokinetic testing; Monitor patient's activity level and volume of therapeutic exercise; Encourage compliance with home therapeutic exercise program; Home therapeutic exercise program	Hop test and isokinetic test (patellofemoral lesions) $\geq$ 85% limb symmetry; Lack of apprehension with sport-specific movements; Flexibility to accepted levels of sport performance; Independence with gym program for maintenance and progression of therapeutic exercise program at discharge	Avoid pain with therapeutic exercise and functional activities; Avoid sport activity until adequate strength development and doctor's clearance

WNL, within normal limits.

Table 3
Rehabilitation Guidelines Following Microfracture/Abrasion Chondroplasty Procedures of the Knee

Weight-bearing status/bracing	Treatment strategies	Criteria for advancement	Precautions
Weeks 0–6			
Toe-touch weight bearing with brace locked at 0° with crutches	CPM	Doctor's direction for progressive weight bearing (Wk 6)	Maintain weight-bearing restrictions
Partial weight bearing progressing to weight bearing as tolerated, brace 0° → 20° for patellofemoral lesions	AAROM	ROM 0° → 120°	Post-op brace locked at 0° 0° → 20° for patellofemoral lesion
	Towel extensions	Proximal muscle strength 5/5	Avoid neglect of CPM and ROM exercises
	Patella mobilization	SLR (supine) without extension lag	
	Quadriceps re-education (quad sets with EMS or EMG)		
	Multiple-angle quadriceps isometrics (tibiofemoral lesions; bilaterally, submaximal)		
	Short crank ergometry → standard ergometry		
	SLRs (all planes)		
	Hip progressive resisted exercises		
	Pool exercises		
	Lower extremity flexibility exercises		
	Upper extremity cardiovascular exercises		
	Cryotherapy		
	Home therapeutic exercise program:		
Weeks 6–12			
Progressive weight bearing with crutches	Computerized forceplate (NeuroCom) for weight-bearing progression/patient education	ROM 0° → WNL	Avoid descending stairs reciprocally until adequate quadriceps control and lower extremity alignment is demonstrated
Discontinue crutches when gait is nonantalgic	Underwater treadmill system (gait training)	Normal patella mobility	Avoid pain with therapeutic exercise and functional activities
Postoperative brace discontinued as good quadriceps control (ability to SLR without lag or pain) is demonstrated	Gait unloader device	Normal gait pattern	
Unloader brace/patella sleeve per doctor's preference	AAROM exercises	Demonstrate ability to ascend 8-in. step	
	Leg press (60° → 0° arc)		
	Minisquats/weight shifts		

Calf raises (bilateral)

Retrograde treadmill ambulation

Proprioception/balance training:

Initiate forward step-up program

Stairmaster

SLRs (progressive resistance)

Lower extremity flexibility exercises

OKC knee extension to 40° (tibiofemoral lesions)

CKC exercises preferred

Home therapeutic exercise program: evaluation based

Weeks 12–18

Full weight bearing with assistive device if needed

Unloader brace/patella sleeve per doctor's preference

Progressive squat program

Initiate step-down program

Leg press (emphasizing eccentrics)

OKC knee extensions 90° → 40° (CKC exercises preferred)

Advanced proprioception training (perturbations)

Agility exercises (sport cord)

Elliptical trainer

Retrograde treadmill ambulation/ running

Hamstring curls/proximal strengthening

Lower extremity stretching

Forward step-down test (NeuroCom) at 4 mo

Isokinetic test at 4 mo (tibiofemoral lesions)

Home therapeutic exercise program: evaluation based

Ability to descend 8-in. stairs with good leg control without pain

85% limb symmetry on isokinetic testing (tibiofemoral lesions) and forward step-down test

Avoid pain with therapeutic exercise and functional activities

Avoid running until adequate strength development and doctor's clearance

(Continued)

351

Table 3 (*Continued*)

Weight-bearing status/bracing	Treatment strategies	Criteria for advancement	Precautions
Weeks 18–?			
Full weight bearing with assistive device if needed	Continue to advance lower extremity strengthening, flexibility, and agility programs	Hop test ≥ 85% limb symmetry	Avoid pain with therapeutic exercise and functional activities
	Forward running	85% limb symmetry on isokinetic testing (including patellofemoral lesions)	Avoid sport activity until adequate strength development and doctor's clearance
	Plyometric program	Lack of apprehension with sport-specific movements	
	Brace for sport activity (doctor's preference)	Flexibility to accepted levels of sport performance	
	Monitor patient's activity level throughout course of rehabilitation	Independence with gym program for maintenance and progression of therapeutic exercise program at discharge	
	Reassess patient's complaints (i.e., pain/swelling daily, adjust program accordingly)		
	Encourage compliance to home therapeutic exercise program		
	Functional testing (hop test)		
	Isokinetic testing		
	Home therapeutic exercise program: evaluation based		

WNL, within normal limits; EMS, electrical muscle stimulation; EMG, electromyography.

352

Table 4
Rehabilitation Guidelines Following Autologous Chondrocyte Implantation Procedures of the Knee

Weight-bearing status/bracing	Treatment strategies	Criteria for advancement	Precautions
Weeks 0–6			
Non-weight bearing with brace locked at 0° with crutches (Wk 0–4)	CPM	Doctor's direction for progressive weight bearing (Wk 6)	Maintain weight-bearing restrictions
Toe-touch weight bearing with brace locked at 0° with crutches (Wk 4–6)	AAROM	ROM 0° → 120°	Postoperative brace locked at 0° 0° → 20° for patellofemoral lesion
Partial weight bearing with brace 0° → 20° for patellofemoral lesions	Towel extensions	Proximal muscle strength 5/5	Avoid neglect of CPM and ROM exercises
	Patella mobilization	SLR (supine) without extension lag	
	Quadriceps re-education (quad sets with EMS or EMG)		
	Multiple-angle quadriceps isometrics (tibiofemoral lesions)		
	Short crank ergometry → standard ergometry		
	SLRs (all planes)		
	Hip progressive resisted exercises		
	Pool exercises		
	Lower extremity flexibility exercises		
	Upper extremity cardiovascular exercises		
	Cryotherapy		
	Home therapeutic exercise program:		
Weeks 6–14			
Partial weight bearing with brace locked at 0° (Wk 6–8)	Computerized forceplate (NeuroCom) for weight-bearing progression/patient education	ROM 0° → 130°	Adhere to weight-bearing restrictions/progression
Progressive weight bearing as tolerated with brace opened 0° → 50° (Wk 8–10),	Underwater treadmill system (gait training)	Normal patella mobility	Postoperative brace locked at 0° until 8 wk postoperative, 0° → 20° for patellofemoral
Progressive weight bearing as tolerated with brace 0° → 20° for patellofemoral lesions with brace opened 0° → 50° at 8 wk	Unloader device (gait training)	Normal gait pattern	lesion until 8 wk postoperative
	AAROM exercises	Demonstrate ability to ascend 6-in. step	Avoid neglect of ROM exercises
	Bilateral leg press (60° → 0° arc)		
	Minisquats/weight shifts		
	Calf raises (bilateral)		

(Continued)

353

Table 4 (Continued)

Weight-bearing status/bracing	Treatment strategies	Criteria for advancement	Precautions
Discontinue crutches when gait is nonantalgic Unloader brace/patella sleeve per doctor's preference (Wk 8–10)	Proprioception/balance training: SLRs (progressive resistance) Lower extremity flexibility exercises OKC knee extension to 40° (tibiofemoral lesions) CKC exercises preferred Initiate forward step-up program Home therapeutic exercise program:		Avoid descending stairs reciprocally until adequate quadriceps control and lower extremity alignment is demonstrated Avoid pain with therapeutic exercise and functional activities
Weeks 14–26 Full weight bearing with assistive device if needed Unloader brace/patella sleeve per doctor's preference	Progress squat program Initiate step-down program Leg press (emphasizing eccentrics) OKC knee extensions 90° → 0° (pain/crepitus free) Advanced proprioception training (perturbations) Agility exercises (sport cord) Elliptical trainer Retrograde treadmill ambulation Hamstring curls/proximal strengthening Lower extremity stretching Forward step-down test (NeuroCom) at 6 mo Isokinetic test at 6 mo Home therapeutic exercise program:	ROM to WNL Ability to ascend an 8-in. stairs with good leg control without pain Ability to descend 8-in. stairs with good leg control without pain or deviations Isokinetic test >80% limb symmetry Forward step-down test > 85% limb symmetry	

354

Weeks 26–?

Full weight bearing with assistive device if needed	Continue to advance lower extremity strengthening, flexibility, and agility programs	Hop tests $\geq$ 85% limb symmetry	Monitor patient's activity level throughout course of rehabilitation
Unloader brace/patella sleeve per doctor's preference	Retro/forward running programs	85% limb symmetry on isokinetic testing (including patellofemoral lesions)	Reassess patient's complaint's (i.e., pain/swelling daily, adjust program accordingly)
Brace for sport activity (doctor's preference)	Plyometric program	Lack of apprehension with sport-specific movements	Encourage compliance to home and gym therapeutic exercise programs
flexibility, and agility programs	Functional testing (hop tests)	Flexibility to accepted levels of sport performance	
	Isokinetic testing	Independence with gym program for maintenance and progression of therapeutic exercise program at discharge	
	Home therapeutic exercise program: evaluation based		

WNL, within normal limits; EMS, electrical muscle stimulation; EMG, electromyography.

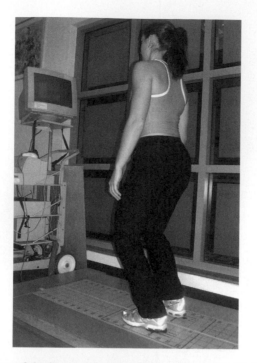

Fig. 5. Progressive loading of the involved extremity is performed utilizing the NeuroCom Balance Master (NeuroCom International, Clackamas, OR).

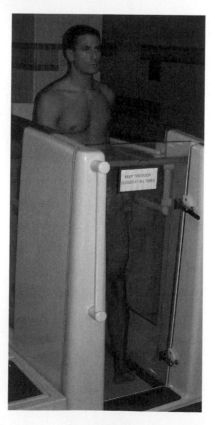

Fig. 6. Gait training using an underwater treadmill system.

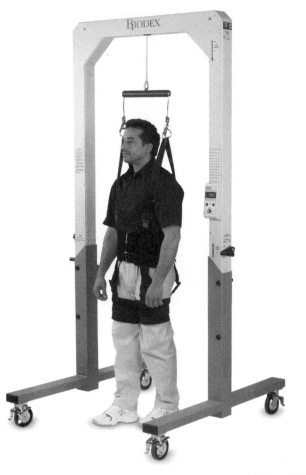

Fig. 7. Biodex Unweighing System (Biodex Inc., Shirley, NY).

For patients who have undergone an ACI procedure, weight bearing is deferred until 4 wk following surgery (Table 4). Patients will then progress from toe-touch weight bearing, to partial weight bearing at 6 wk, to progressive weight bearing as tolerated by 8 wk postoperatively. As weight-bearing restrictions are lifted, it is vital for the patient to adhere to a gradual progressive loading program. Excessive loads that are placed on the articular surfaces in the presence of a weakened muscular support system needed to disseminate compressive forces will result in increased knee effusion and pain. This will lead to quadriceps inhibition and further delay the rehabilitation process *(19)*.

A computerized forceplate system is utilized to assist the patient in the gradual loading of the involved extremity (Fig. 5). During this activity, the patient gradually loads the involved limb to the prescribed percentage of body weight, receiving visual feedback. This awareness is carried over into the progressive weight-bearing component of gait training during this phase.

Other treatment strategies utilized to gradually load a healing articular cartilage lesion include an underwater treadmill and a deweighting system (Figs. 6 and 7). Walking in chest deep water results in a 60–75% reduction in weight bearing; walking in waist deep water results in a 40–50% reduction in weight bearing *(20,21)*. Crutches are discontinued as a normal gait pattern without deviations is established. For patients with an excessive varus or valgus malalignment, an unloader brace is prescribed (Fig. 8).

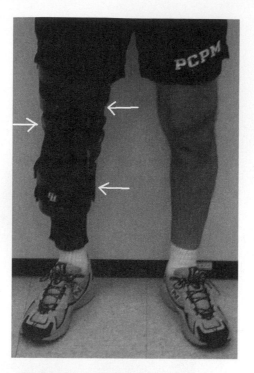

Fig. 8. Generation II Unloader brace.

Strength Development

The development of strength in the involved lower extremity is crucial following articular cartilage knee surgery to promote safe progression and optimal functional outcome. A strong muscle-tendon unit may dissipate compressive force and absorb shock from the articular surface. The rehabilitation specialist should consider the location and nature of the articular cartilage repair site before selecting strengthening interventions. The lubrication medium intrinsic with specific therapeutic exercises needs also to be considered. Exercises that provide a fluid film condition are preferred over those activities that employ a boundary condition. Healthy articular cartilage can withstand high loads, but exercises that result in shear stress application while under compression may adversely affect the healing response of articular cartilage *(13)*. Strengthening activities that induce shear in conjunction with compression forces on areas where the healing defect articulates with the opposing joint surface are therefore avoided. This is particularly crucial in the early postoperative period.

As most articular cartilage procedures entail a period of limited weight bearing, strengthening strategies employed during the early phases of rehabilitation concentrate on unloaded exercises. Muscle groups that are specifically targeted during this phase include the quadriceps and proximal muscle groups. Knee joint effusion from trauma or surgery are commonly associated with quadriceps inhibition *(19)*. Immediately following articular cartilage knee surgery, the patent is instructed to perform quadriceps setting in or as near to full extension as tolerated as most articular cartilage lesions are not engaged in this range. A small towel will promote co-contraction and allow for a more pain-free exercise (Fig. 9).

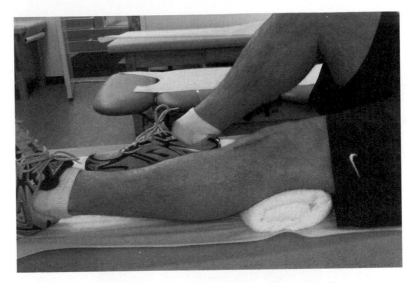

Fig. 9. Quadriceps setting. Towel is utilized for co-contraction and added comfort. Submaximal effort is encouraged.

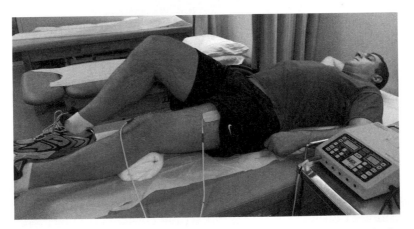

Fig. 10. Quadriceps reeducation utilizing an electrical stimulation device.

If a patient has difficulty eliciting a quadriceps contraction, a biofeedback unit or an electrical muscle stimulator can be used in conjunction with the quadriceps setting exercise to better facilitate quadriceps reeducation (Fig. 10). Straight leg raising is performed with the postoperative brace locked at 0° until sufficient quadriceps control is demonstrated (i.e., ability to SLR without pain or quadriceps lag).

Stationary bicycling can be used for strength development as soon as knee ROM approaches 85°. A short crank (90-mm) ergometer is initially utilized *(22)* (Fig. 11). Cycling is advanced to a standard ergometer when knee flexion improves to 110–115°.

Deep water exercises, including the use of a kick board or a flotation vest for deep water running, may be appropriate strengthening strategies during the limited weight-bearing period as quadriceps muscle control and ROM improvement are demonstrated (Fig. 12).

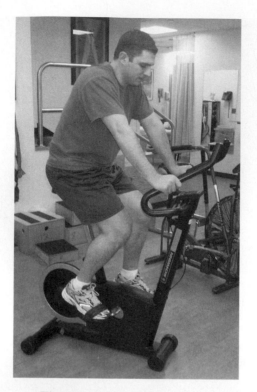

Fig. 11. Short crank ergometer.

Proximal (hip) musculature and core strengthening are initiated early in the postoperative program. SLRs in multiple planes, as well as stabilization activities, are introduced to establish a strong base for the functional demands placed on the knee joint in the weeks and months to follow. Progressive resistive exercises are used to further develop proximal strength by adding cuff weights to the SLRs and by utilizing progressive resistive exercise machines.

The understanding of specific compressive and shear forces induced on articular cartilage during strengthening exercises, although limited, needs to be considered with exercise selection. A combination of open kinetic chain (OKC) and closed kinetic chain (CKC) strengthening exercises in ranges that do not high load lesion sites are preferred. During OKC knee extension, an arc of motion from 60 to 90° appears to provide the greatest amount of compressive loading at the knee joint, whereas the greatest amount of shear appears in the 40–0° range *(23)*. Research has demonstrated that during CKC exercises the greatest amount of shear and compression occur in the 60–100° arc of motion *(23,24)*. Palmitier et al. *(25)*, in a biomechanical model of the lower extremity, demonstrated reduced tibiofemoral shear force when a compressive force is applied to the knee joint.

When increased weight bearing is permitted and tolerated, CKC strengthening interventions include a leg press inside a 60–0° arc of motion (Fig. 13) and minisquats inside a 45–0° range (Fig. 14). A high-repetition, low-load approach is utilized. Using a lateral or medial heel wedge under the involved extremity during the squatting exercise may protect the healing defect by creating a valgus or varus moment, respectfully, at the knee joint. This rehabilitation adjunct may aid in unloading the treated articular cartilage lesion from compressive forces while facilitating muscle strengthening. As the healing lesion matures,

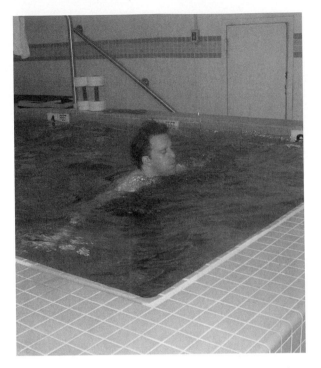

Fig. 12. Deep water exercises using flotation belt.

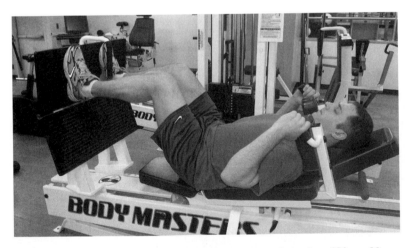

Fig. 13. Closed kinetic chain leg press. Arc of motion $60° \rightarrow 0°$.

ROM and progressive weights are added to these extremity-strengthening activities. As a normal gait is demonstrated, functional CKC exercises such as graduated forward step-ups and later step-downs are added for strength development. Retrograde treadmill ambulation on progressive percentage inclines is utilized to facilitate quadriceps strength development *(26)* (Fig. 15).

Multiple-angle OKC knee extension isometric exercises are utilized as long as the angle selected avoids any engagement with the healing articular cartilage defect. Isometric

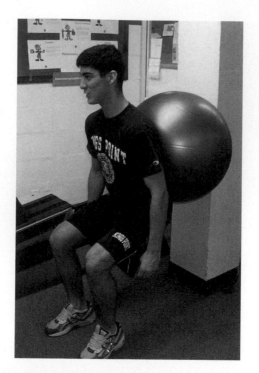

Fig. 14. Minisquats inside a 45° to 0° arc of motion using a physioball for support.

contractions should be short in nature as this condition supports a lubrication model of boundary friction *(2)*. These exercises, along with isotonic and isokinetic knee extension exercises, are to be used judiciously following articular cartilage procedures especially in procedures involving the patellofemoral joint. Signs of pain or crepitus are closely monitored. Wilk and colleagues demonstrated that OKC extension exercises produce significantly greater patellofemoral forces than CKC activities at knee angles less than 57° *(23)*.

Running as a treatment strategy for strength development is delayed until the patient demonstrates the ability to descend an 8-in. step without complaints of knee discomfort, normal extremity alignment without deviations, and good core pelvic strength. A functional forward step-down test *(27)* (Fig. 16) is employed to substantiate lower extremity strength. Retro running on a treadmill is progressed to forward running.

For an athlete wishing to return to sport participation, sport-specific agility activities and a plyometric program are introduced as strength, ROM, and flexibility demonstrate normal limits.

Balance and Proprioception

Research suggests that, following lower extremity joint trauma, de-afferentiation occurs *(28–31)*. Alterations in the afferent nerve pathway have been shown to disrupt proprioceptive function *(30,32)* Normal proprioception is necessary for good balance and joint function. *(33)* If proprioception is altered, then a direct negative effect on balance is expected. Proprioceptive and balance training following articular cartilage surgery are initiated as soon as the patient demonstrates the ability to bear 50% of his or her weight. An early treatment strategy utilizes a rocker board in the sagittal and coronal planes. The

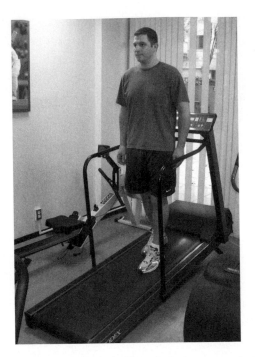

Fig. 15. Retrograde treadmill ambulation on an incline.

patient attempts to sustain a static position while even weight distribution is maintained. Uniplanar activities are advanced to multiplanar surfaces to enhance dynamic stabilization (Fig. 17).

As strength and balance demonstrate improvement, the patient is advanced to unilateral balance/strengthening by performing contralateral elastic band exercises (Fig. 18). Advanced treatment strategies include dynamic stabilization on unstable support surfaces (foam, cushions, balance boards), perturbation training, and sport-specific agility training.

Muscle Flexibility

Following extended periods of nonweight bearing, a loss of limb flexibility is expected. Hamstring and calf musculature stretching is encouraged early following all articular cartilage surgical procedures to the knee. As knee flexion approaches 120°, flexibility exercises for the quadriceps are initiated (Fig. 19). Flexibility exercises are further reinforced later in the rehabilitative course in preparation for higher-level and sport-specific activities.

Return to Sport

The decision to allow a return to sport activity for patients who have undergone an articular cartilage procedure is dependent on the patient meeting performance criteria, the type of surgical procedure, the sport in question, and the surgeon's final recommendation.

Performance criteria include full ROM and demonstration of sufficient flexibility to meet the demand of the desired sport. Muscle strength is assessed via isokinetic and functional testing. Isokinetic testing is performed at test speeds of 180° and 300° per second; these velocities have been shown to produce less compressive and shear forces than slower speeds *(34,35)*. Functional testing employs either the single-leg hop test or crossover hop test

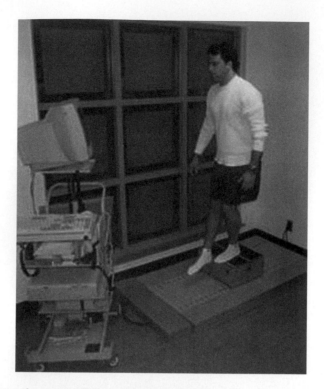

Fig. 16. Forward step-down test. The patient steps down an 8-in. step onto a forceplate (NeuroCom Balance Master System) as slowly and controlled as possible on each leg. Three trials are recorded. Mean impact and limb symmetry scores are calculated. Lower extremity control is observed for deviations. Normative data have established a mean impact of 10% body weight and limb symmetry of 85%.

(36,37). (Fig. 20). Tests are administered with the goal of achieving an 85% limb symmetry score. Apprehension during functional sport-specific movements and testing are closely monitored. These clinical findings are presented to the referring orthopedic surgeon for the final determination of a decision to return to sports.

Different surgical procedures entail a longer healing interval before the stress of athletic participation placed on the surgical lesion is allowed. Following arthroscopic debridement, return to sport is usually allowed on the patient meeting the aforementioned criteria. Following microfracture procedure, return to sport in activities such as basketball, soccer, football, or lacrosse are likely delayed for at least 6 mo. Following ACI, exclusion from these same sports may be encouraged for at least 1 yr or longer. Each individual case should be evaluated by the patient's surgeon.

SUMMARY

Basic science continues to evolve in understanding the properties and function of articular cartilage. The effects of loading and mechanical stress on articular cartilage when better understood will lead to improved evidence-based rehabilitation guidelines following articular cartilage surgical procedures. Successful outcome following articular cartilage surgery of the knee greatly depends on the rehabilitation specialist keeping current with the

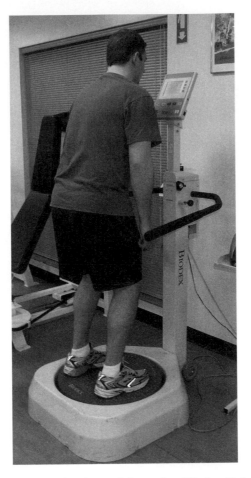

Fig. 17. Dynamic stabilization training using Biodex Balance System.

effects of forces at the knee joint during activities of daily living and with select rehabilitation exercises.

Following the surgical management of articular cartilage lesions, immobilization should be kept to a minimum. Proximal limb and core pelvic strengthening are important early interventions in the development of a stable, strong base in preparation for the joint reactive forces normally associated with weight bearing and the subsequent phases of the rehabilitation program. Weight bearing must be gradual so that the healing articular surface is progressively loaded. Care must be given to avoid those exercises and activities that may expose treated lesions to excessive shear stress while the knee joint is under compression. Criteria must be demonstrated throughout the rehabilitative course to ensure safe, effective progression toward a favorable outcome.

The rehabilitation specialist needs to communicate with the surgeon regarding patient progress in order to collaborate on the direction of the rehabilitation program. Throughout the rehabilitation course, the therapist should counsel the patient on monitoring the volume of activities, ensuring that ROM, muscle strength, and flexibility are appropriate for the desired length and type of activity performed. It is critical that the patient realize, at an early stage,

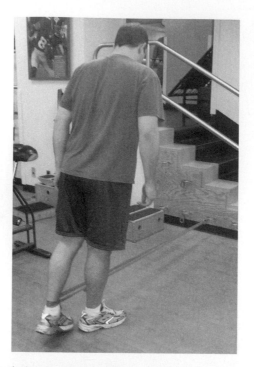

Fig. 18. Contralateral elastic band exercise. The patient stands and balances on involved extremity as noninvolved extremity performs movement in the frontal plane.

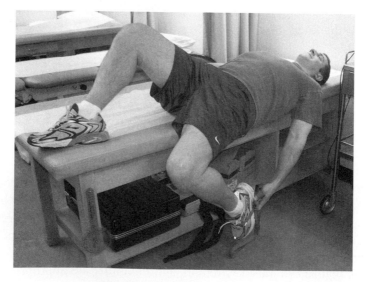

Fig. 19. Quadriceps stretching.

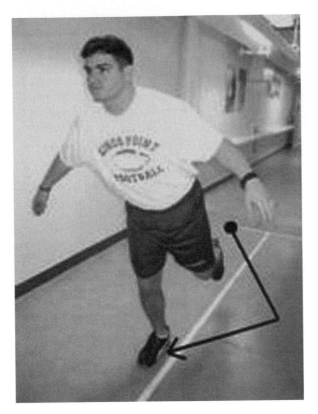

Fig. 20. Crossover hop for distance test. Patient performs three consecutive jumps on one leg, crossing over the drawn line with each jump. Total distance jumped is recorded. Three trials are performed on each leg and averaged. Limb symmetry is then calculated.

that compliance with the rehabilitation protocol is an integral part of ultimately achieving a successful outcome.

REFERENCES

1. Buckwalter JA, Mankin HJ. Articular cartilage I Tissue design and chondrocyte-matrix interactions. J Bone Joint Surg 1997;79A:600–611.
2. Walker JM. Pathomechanics and classification of cartilage lesions, facilitation of repair. J Orth Sports Phys Ther 1998;28:216–231.
3. Palmoski MJ, Colyer RA, Brandt KD. Joint motion in the absence of normal loading does not maintain normal articular cartilage. Arthritis Rheum 1980;23:325–334.
4. Mankin HJ. The response of articular cartilage to mechanical injury. J Bone Joint Surg 1982; 64A:460–466.
5. Rosenberg TD, Paulos LE, Parker RD, et al. The 45° posteroanterior flexion weightbearing radiograph of the knee. J Bone Joint Surg 1988;70A:1479–1483.
6. Kegerreis S. The construction and implementation of a functional progression as a component of athletic rehabilitation. J Orthop Sports Phys Ther July–August 1983:14.
7. Cavanaugh JT. Rehabilitation for Non Operative and Operative Management of Knee Injuries. In: Callaghan J, Simonian P, Wickiewicz T, eds., The Adult Knee. Philadelphia, PA: Lippincott Williams & Wilkins, 2003:380–430.

8. Walker JM. Pathomechanics and classification of cartilage lesions, facilitation of repair. J Orth Sports Phys Ther 1998;28:216–231.

9. Buckwalter JA. Effects of early motion on healing of musculoskeletal tissues. Hand Clin 1996; 12:13–24.

10. Petersen L. Autologous chondrocyte transplantation. Articular cartilage regeneration: chondro- cyte transplantation and other technologies. Paper presented at: Annual Meeting of the American Academy of Orthopedic Surgeons; February 1997; San Francisco.

11. Rodrigo JJ, Steadman JR, Silliman JF, et al. Improvement of full-thickness chondral defect heal- ing in the human knee after debridement and microfracture using continuous passive motion. Am J Knee Surg 1994;7:109–116.

12. Salter RB, Simmonds DF, Malcolm BW, Rumble EJ, MacMichael D, Clements ND. The biolog- ical effect of continuous passive motion on the healing of full- thickness defects in articular car- tilage. An experimental investigation in the rabbit. J Bone Joint Surg Am 1980;62:1232–1251.

13. Suh J, Aroen A, Mozzonigro T, et al. Injury and repair of articular cartilage: related scientific issues. Oper Tech Orthop 1997;7:270–278.

14. Benum P. Operative mobilization of stiff knees after surgical treatment of knee injuries and post- traumatic conditions. Acta Orthop Scand 1982;53:625–631.

15. Matsusue Y, Yamamuro T, Hama H. Arthroscopic multiple osteochondral transplantation to the chondral defect in the knee associated with anterior cruciate ligament disruption. Arthroscopy 1993;9:318–321.

16. Perry J, Antonelli D, Ford W. Analysis of knee-joint forces during flexed-knee stance. J Bone Joint Surg 1975;57A:961–967.

17. Fulkerson JP, Hungerford D. Disorders of the Patellofemoral Joint. 2nd ed. Baltimore, MD: Williams and Wilkins; 1990.

18. Mow VC, Rosenwasser M. Articular cartilage: biomechanics. In: Woo SL-Y, Buckwalter JA, eds., Injury and Repair of the Musculoskeletal Soft Tissues. Park Ridge, IL: AAOS; 1988:427–463.

19. Spencer JD, Hayes KC, Alexander LJ. Knee joint effusion and quadriceps inhibition in man. Arch Phys Med Rehabil 1984;65:171–177.

20. Bates A, Hanson N. The principles and properties of water. In Bates and Hanson, eds. : Aquatic Exercise Therapy. Philadelphia: Saunders; 1996:1–320.

21. Harrison RA, Hilman M, Bulstrode S. Loading of the lower limb when walking partially immersed: Implications for clinical practice. Physiotherapy 1992;78:164.

22. Schwartz RE, Asnis PD, Cavanaugh JT, et al. Short crank cycle ergometry J Orthop Sports Phys Ther 1991;13:95.

23. Wilk KE, Escamilla RF, Fleisig GS, et al. A comparison of tibiofemoral joint forces and elec- tromyographic activity during open and closed kinetic chain exercises. Am J Sports Med 1996;24:518–527.

24. Escamilla RF, Fleisig GS, Zheng N, et al. Biomechanics of the knee during closed kinetic chain and open kinetic chain exercises. Med Sci Sports Exerc 1998;30:556–569.

25. Palmitier RA, An KN, Scott SG, Chao EYS. Kinetic chain exercises in knee rehabilitation. Sports Med 1991;11:402–413.

26. Cipriani DJ, Armstrong CW, Gaul S. Backward walking at three levels of treadmill inclination: an electromyographic and kinematic analysis. J Orthop Sports Phys Ther 1995;22:95–102.

27. Cavanaugh JT, Stump TJ. Forward step down test. J Orth Sports Phys Ther 2000;30:A-46.

28. Borsa PA, Lephart SM, Irrgang JJ, et al. The effects of joint position sense on proprioceptive sen- sibility in anterior cruciate ligament deficient athletes. Am J Sports Med 1997;25:336–340.

29. Corrigan JP, Cashman WF, Brady MP. Proprioception in the cruciate deficient knee. J Bone Joint Surgery 1992;74B:247–250.

30. Freeman MA, Dean MR, Hanham IW. The etiology and prevention of functional instability of the foot. J Bone Joint Surg 1965;47B:669–677.

31. Skinner HB, Barrack RL, Cook SD, et al. Joint position sense in total knee arthroplasty. J Orthop Res 1984;1:276–283.
32. Beard DJ, Kyberd PJ, Ferfusson CM, et al. Proprioception after reconstruction of the anterior cruciate ligament. An objective indication of the need for surgery. J. Bone Joint Surgery Br 1993;73B:311–315.
33. Voight M, Blackburn T. Proprioception and balance training and testing following injury. In: Ellenbecker TS, ed., Knee Ligament Rehabilitation. Philadelphia: Churchill Livingston; 2000;361–385.
34. Nisell R, Ericson MO, Nemeth G, et al. Tibiofemoral joint forces during isokinetic knee extension. Am J Sports Med 1989;17:49–54.
35. Kaufman KR, An KN, Litchy WJ, et al. Dynamic joint forces during knee isokinetic exercise. Am J Sports Med 1991;19:305–316.
36. Daniel DM, Malcolm L, Stone ML, et al. Quantification of knee stability and function. Contemp Orthop 1982;5:83–91.
37. Barber SD, Noyes FR, Mangine RE, et al. Quantitative assessment of functional limitations in normal and anterior cruciate ligament deficient knees. Clin Orthop 1990;255:204–214.

Printed in the United States of America